Key Clinical Topics in

Obstetrics and Gynaecology

D0222627

Key Clinical Topics in

Obstetrics and Gynaecology

Emma J Crosbie PhD MRCOG
Senior Lecturer and Honorary Consultant in Gynaecological Oncology,
Institute of Cancer Sciences, University of Manchester;
St Mary's Hospital, Central Manchester University Hospitals
NHS Foundation Trust, Manchester, UK

Alexander Heazell MBChB (Hons) PhD MRCOG
Senior Clinical Lecturer and Honorary Consultant in Obstetrics,
Institute of Human Development, University of Manchester;
St Mary's Hospital, Central Manchester University Hospitals
NHS Foundation Trust, Manchester, UK

Andrew Pickersgill MB ChB MRCOG MD
Consultant Obstetrician and Gynaecologist,
Stockport NHS Foundation Trust, Stockport, UK

Richard J Slade MB ChB FRCS FRCOG
Consultant Gynaecological Surgeon,
The Christie Hospital NHS Foundation Trust,
Manchester, UK

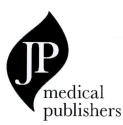

JP
medical
publishers

London • Philadelphia • Panama City • New Delhi

© 2014 JP Medical Ltd.
Published by JP Medical Ltd,
83 Victoria Street, London, SW1H 0HW, UK
Tel: +44 (0)20 3170 8910
Fax: +44 (0)20 3008 6180
Email: info@jpmedpub.com
Web: www.jpmedpub.com

ISBN: 978-1-907816-70-3

British Library Cataloguing in Publication Data
A catalogue record for this book is available from the British Library

Library of Congress Cataloging in Publication Data
A catalog record for this book is available from the Library of Congress

JP Medical Ltd is a subsidiary of Jaypee Brothers Medical Publishers (P) Ltd, New Delhi, India

Commissioning Editor:	Steffan Clements
Development Editor:	Thomas Fletcher
Design:	Designers Collective Ltd

Indexed, typeset, printed and bound in India.

Preface

The specialties of obstetrics and gynaecology have witnessed enormous changes in the last few years. This book has been written to reflect these changes and to provide a comprehensive overview of clinical practice, including topics such as HPV vaccination, female genital mutilation, recurrent miscarriage, vaginal birth after caesarean section, invasive fetal testing and HIV in pregnancy. It is not intended to be an exhaustive textbook, but a primer which provides up-to-date, relevant, evidence-based guidance for clinicians involved in the care of women during pregnancy and childbirth and the care of women with gynaecological disorders.

We have written this book primarily for specialty trainees in obstetrics and gynaecology. It is an exam revision tool and also facilitates clinical decision making at the point of care. It offers simple, concise explanations in an easily accessible format with extensive cross-referencing to NICE and RCOG guidelines. It is aimed specifically at prospective MRCOG Part 2 candidates, but it will also be useful for those studying for the DRCOG and for medical students preparing for their obstetrics and gynaecology finals. Each topic has been prepared by a specialty trainee in obstetrics and gynaecology or a consultant with expertise in a particular specialist area. Being based in England, the authors have referred to the English legislative and health service frameworks where these have relevance for clinical practice; in other countries there will be differences in detail, but the broad principles will apply.

We hope you find this book a useful resource for learning and clinical practice. We would like to thank all those who contributed to its authorship.

Emma J Crosbie
Alexander Heazell
Andrew Pickersgill
Richard J Slade
October 2013

Contents

Acknowledgements

The publishers wish to thank Series Advisors Dr Tim M. Craft and Dr Paul M. Upton for their assistance during the planning of the *Key Clinical Topics* series.

Contributors

Louise M Byrd MBBS MRCOG
Topics 59, 65 & 77
Consultant in High-Risk Obstetrics and
Maternal Medicine, St Mary's Hospital,
Central Manchester University Hospitals NHS
Foundation Trust Manchester, UK

Andrew Clamp BMBCh PhD MRCP
Topic 6
Senior Lecturer and Consultant in Medical
Oncology, University of Manchester;
The Christie Hospital NHS Foundation Trust,
Manchester, UK

Ruth O Cockerill MB BCh MRCOG
Topics 58, 69, 90, 105 & 106
Clinical Research Fellow, Maternal and Fetal
Health Research Centre St Mary's Hospital,
Central Manchester University Hospitals NHS
Foundation Trust, Manchester, UK

Emma J Crosbie PhD MRCOG
Topics 23, 31, 32, 35, 37 & 41
Clinical Senior Lecturer and Honorary
Consultant in Gynaecological Oncology,
Institute of Cancer Sciences, University of
Manchester; St Mary's Hospital, Central
Manchester University Hospitals NHS
Foundation Trust, Manchester, UK

Mark Davies BSc (Hons) MBChB MRCS (ed)
MRCOG
Topics 15, 20, 24 & 26
Speciality Registrar Obstetrics and Gynaecology,
North Western Deanery, Manchester, UK

Cheryl Fitzgerald MBChB MRCOG MD
Topics 3, 14, 43 & 44
Consultant in Reproductive Medicine,
St Mary's Hospital, Central Manchester
University Hospitals NHS Foundation Trust,
Manchester, UK

Joanna C Gillham BSc MBBS MD MRCOG
Topics 62, 78, 84, 100 & 102
Consultant Obstetrician and Sub specialist in
Fetal and Maternal Medicine, St Mary's Hospital,
Central Manchester University Hospitals NHS
Foundation Trust, Manchester, UK

Alexander Heazell MBChB (Hons) PhD MRCOG
Topics 56, 79, 82, 86, 93, 99 & 104
Senior Clinical Lecturer and Honorary
Consultant in Obstetrics, Institute of Human
Development, University of Manchester;
St Mary's Hospital, Central Manchester
University Hospitals NHS Foundation Trust,
Manchester, UK

Chibuike G Iruloh PhD MRCOG
Topics 64, 66, 74 & 85
Subspecialist Trainee, Maternal and Fetal
Medicine, Royal Hallamshire Hospital,
Sheffield, UK

Michelle L MacKintosh MBChB MRCOG
Topics 4, 5, 22, 51, 52, 53 & 70
Clinical Research Fellow in Gynaecological
Oncology, St Mary's Hospital, Central
Manchester University Hospitals NHS
Foundation Trust, Manchester, UK

Tessa BA Malone MBChB FFSRH MRCGP
DRCOG DipGUM
Topics 8 & 42
Consultant in Sexual & Reproductive Health,
Stockport NHS Foundation Trust, Stockport, UK

Nadine S Massiah MBBS MRCOG MA
Topics 31, 32, 35 & 37
Subspecialty Fellow in Gynaecological Oncology,
Department of Obstetrics and Gynaecology,
Princess Anne Hospital, Southampton
University Hospitals NHS Trust, Southampton,
UK

Anita J Merritt BSc PhD MBChB
Topics 2, 21, 28, 36 & 48
Specialty Trainee, Department of
Histopathology, Manchester Royal Infirmary,
Manchester, UK

Gadha Mohiyiddeen MBBS MRCOG
Topic 1
Specialty Trainee in Obstetrics and Gynaecology,
North-West Deanery, Manchester, UK

Lamiya Mohiyiddeen MBBS MRCOG MD
Topics 1, 27, 33 & 38
Subspecialty Trainee in Reproductive Medicine,
St Mary's Hospital, Central Manchester
University Hospitals NHS Foundation Trust,
Manchester, UK

Clare Mullan BSc, MBChB, MRCOG
Topics 71, 76, 81, 87 & 92
Specialty Registrar in Obstetrics & Gynaecology,
St Mary's Hospital, Central Manchester
University Hospitals NHS Foundation Trust,
Manchester, UK

Andrew Pickersgill MBChB MRCOG MD
Topics 7, 10, 11, 12, 29
Consultant Obstetrician and Gynaecologist,
Stockport NHS Foundation Trust, Stockport, UK

Fiona Reid MD MRCOG
Topics 13, 16, 18, 46 & 47
Consultant Urogynaecologist, The Warrell
Unit, St Mary's Hospital, Central Manchester
University Hospitals NHS Foundation Trust,
Manchester, UK

Sandra Sasson MB BCh (Hons) MRCOG
Topics 60, 68, 72, 88 & 103
Specialty Registrar in Obstetrics and
Gynaecology, St Mary's Hospital, Central
Manchester University Hospitals NHS
Foundation Trust, Manchester, UK

Vanitha N Sivalingam BSc MBChB
Topics 9, 30, 34, 40, 45 & 50
Clinical Research Fellow, Institute of Cancer
Sciences, University of Manchester, Manchester,
UK

Fatimah D Soydemir MBChB MRCOG MD
Topics 54, 83, 96, 98, 101 & 107
Consultant Obstetrician, Royal Preston Hospital,
Lancashire Teaching Hospitals NHS Foundation
Trust, Preston, UK

Gillian Stephen BSc MBChB MRCOG
Topics 73, 75, 80, 89 & 97
Subspecialty Trainee in Maternal/Fetal Medicine,
St Mary's Hospital, Central Manchester
University Hospitals NHS Foundation Trust,
Manchester, UK

Clare L Tower MBChB PhD MRCOG
Topics 55, 57, 61, 63, 67 & 108
Consultant in Obstetrics and Maternal and
Fetal Medicine, St Mary's Hospital, Central
Manchester University Hospitals NHS
Foundation Trust, Manchester, UK

Y Louise Wan MBBS MSc MRCS MRCOG
Topics 6, 19, 25, 39 & 49
Honorary Clinical Research Fellow, Women's
Cancer Group, Institute of Cancer Sciences,
University of Manchester; Specialty Registrar
in Obstetrics and Gynaecology, North-West
Deanery, Manchester, UK

Catherine White MBChB FFFLM FRCOG MRCGP
DCH DFFP DMJ
Topic 17
Clinical Director, St Mary's Sexual Assault
Referral Centre, Manchester, UK

Melissa K Whitworth MBChB (Hons) MRCOG MD
Topics 91, 94 & 95
Consultant Obstetrician, St Mary's Hospital,
Central Manchester University Hospitals NHS
Foundation Trust; Honorary Senior Lecturer,
Maternal & Fetal Health Research Centre,
Institute of Human Development, University of
Manchester, Manchester, UK

Abnormality of the genital tract

Overview

Congenital abnormalities of the genitourinary tract are seen in 3–4% of the population and they commonly coexist. Any abnormality in the reproductive tract should be an indication to establish the anatomy of the renal tract.

Vaginal

Vaginal agenesis   Congenital absence of the vagina occurs in 1:10,000 with 40–50% having associated genitourinary anomalies. The diagnosis is indicated by primary amenorrhoea and normal secondary sexual characteristics. Testicular feminisation needs to be excluded and upper tract ultrasound scan and/or intravenous urogram is indicated. If a uterus is present, an abdominal mass (haematometra) and pain will be present at puberty. Formation of a neovagina by repetitive dilatation to the Müllerian pit, fashioning of a perineal pouch, tissue expansion vaginoplasty, full-thickness skin flaps or intestinal grafts have all been described. Such management should be delayed until menstruation demands it.

Vaginal atresia   (**Figure 1**) Primary amenorrhoea is the most common presentation. Haematocolpos should be drained in theatre. Ultrasound scan and/or laparoscopy are indicated if there is associated haematosalpinx. Upper vaginal atresia may require an abdominoperineal approach.

Vaginal duplication or septae   (**Figure 1**) This occurs as a result of failure of full Müllerian duct fusion. The condition is harmless and such women have normal sexual function.

Cervical

Cervical atresia   (**Figure 1**) Congenital absence of the cervix is rare in the presence of a functional uterus and vagina. Formation of a uterovaginal anastomosis is necessary to prevent haematometra, haematosalpinx, adenomyosis and endometriosis. This is achieved via a laparoscopy or laparotomy. Hysterectomy is an alternative.

Cervical duplication   This is associated with uterine didelphis (**Figure 1**). Ensure that two intrauterine contraceptive devices (IUCDs) are used if this is the chosen method of contraception and that two cervical smears are performed.

Uterine

Uterine agenesis   Congenital absence of the uterus presents as primary amenorrhoea and will occur in conjunction with an absent cervix and upper vagina. It is caused by failure of development of the Müllerian ducts. A vestigial uterus and cervix may be present without evidence of a cavity or canal. The vagina in such women is usually shorter than normal, but is adequate for intercourse.

Uterine fusion variants   True Mullerian duct duplication on both sides is rare. Variants are common and include uterus didelphis, bicornuate uterus, rudimentary horn (communicating and non- communicating) and subseptate uterus (**Figure 1**). Most variants are innocuous if menstrual flow can occur. They are associated with an increase in spontaneous abortion, fetal malpresentation, intrauterine growth restriction (IUGR) and abnormalities of placentation.

Fallopian tubes

Hydatid cysts of Morgagni (paramesonephric remnants) are not uncommon. Torsion is rare. Atresia and undeveloped ostia are very rare.

Ovarian

Lack of ovarian function is due to aplasia or dysgenesis and requires hormone replacement therapy (HRT). Dysgenetic ovaries will require excision as up to 30% have malignant potential. Assisted reproduction with donor oocytes means that such women can bear children, so hysterectomy is not always required at oophorectomy.

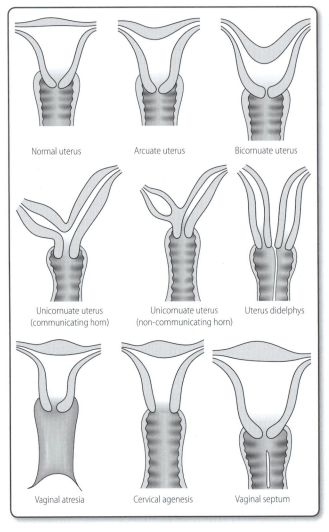

Figure 1 Congenital abnormalities of the female genital tract.

Normal uterus

Arcuate uterus

Bicornuate uterus

Unicornuate uterus (communicating horn)

Unicornuate uterus (non-communicating horn)

Uterus didelphys

Vaginal atresia

Cervical agenesis

Vaginal septum

Renal

Bilateral renal agenesis is known as Potter syndrome and is incompatible with life. Unilateral renal agenesis is relatively common. An ultrasound scan will establish the diagnosis. Simple remnants of the pronephros and mesonephros, the epoophoron, paroophoron and Gartner's duct cysts are benign. Other renal anomalies include multiple renal vessels, duplications of the upper tract, ectopic ureters, horseshoe kidneys, congenital bilateral polycystic kidneys (fatal), and urachal malformations including fistulae, ectopia vesicae, cloacal exstrophy and rectourinary fistulae.

Ambiguous genitalia/ disorders of sex development

Ambiguous genitalia are a birth defect where the external genitals do not have the typical appearance of either a male or a female.

The evaluation and management of neonates with ambiguous genitalia requires sensitivity, efficiency and accuracy. The approach to these neonates is facilitated by a multidisciplinary team including urology, endocrinology, genetics, and psychiatry or psychology.

Disorders of sex development (DSD) encompass chromosomal DSD, 46XX DSD, and 46XY DSD. The 46XX DSD is the most common DSD and in the majority of these children congenital adrenal hyperplasia (CAH) is the underlying aetiology. CAH results from a defect in the adrenal enzyme 21-hydroxylase resulting in excessive production of androgens and reduced production of cortisol and aldosterone. The effects of CAH vary from person to person. About 75% of babies born with CAH have the serious salt-wasting form. These babies do not produce enough aldosterone and as a result lose too much salt and water in their urine, causing dehydration and very low blood pressure. This can be life-threatening if not treated. About 25% have the simple virilising form where the adrenals produce enough aldosterone but excessive androgens. This causes virilisation of female genitalia. Babies born with non-classic CAH or late onset CAH are healthy and have normal genitals at birth. They have excess facial and body hair growth and male pattern baldness with mild virilising features in later life.

The 46XY DSD is a heterogeneous disorder that often results from a disruption in the production or response to testosterone, dihydrotestosterone, or Müllerian inhibitory substance. Chromosomal DSD includes conditions resulting from abnormal meiosis, including Klinefelter syndrome (47XXY) and Turner syndrome. The evaluation of children with DSD demands a thorough physical examination, medical history, karyotype, metabolic panel, 17-OH progesterone, testosterone, luteinising hormone, follicle stimulation hormone and urinalysis. A radiographic evaluation should begin with an abdominal and pelvic ultrasound but may include magnetic resonance imaging, endoscopy or laparoscopy.

Patients with salt-wasting CAH disorders need to be treated to avoid a crisis. This treatment includes glucocorticoid replacement with hydrocortisone. Apart from acute life-threatening issues, medical and surgical treatment will vary from case to case based on the diagnosis, the advice offered by the team of experts, and the wishes of the parents. For many patients whose gonads will never function at puberty, hormone replacement will eventually be needed in order to achieve puberty, regardless of the ultimate gender identity and assignment. Hormone replacement using oestradiol is carried out under the guidance of a paediatric subspecialist such as a paediatric endocrinologist, paediatric gynaecologist, or a paediatric urologist.

Although there has been a wide acceptance for surgical interventions in infancy, it is suggested that most surgeries be postponed until puberty. This recommendation is due to reports that many genitoplasties and vaginoplasties performed in infancy will need to be re done at puberty to achieve satisfactory outcomes and correct complications from previous surgeries such as vaginal stenosis.

Further reading

Murphy C, Allen L, Jamieson MA. Ambiguous genitalia in the newborn: An overview and teaching tool. Journal of Pediatric and Adolescent Gynecology 2011; 24:236–250.
Auchus RJ. Congenital adrenal hyperplasia in adults. Curr Opin Endocrinol Diabetes Obes 2010; 17:210–216.

Karnis MF. Fertility, pregnancy and medical management of Turner syndrome in the reproductive years. Fertil Steril 2012; 98:787–791.

Related topics of interest

Amenorrhoea

Primary amenorrhoea

Overview

This is defined as absence of menarche at age 16 years. It is categorised according to whether other secondary sexual characteristics are present using Tanner staging. The most common reason for primary amenorrhoea is constitutional delayed puberty; the natural anxiety of the patient and her parents may warrant basic investigations but reassurance may be all that is required, particularly if other secondary sexual characteristics are present.

Normal menstruation depends on normal female pelvic anatomy with appropriate stimulation of the pelvic target organs by the relevant hormones. Primary amenorrhoea can also be caused by genetic or structural factors. Two X chromosomes are necessary for ovarian development and maintenance of the menstrual cycle. Most causes of secondary amenorrhea can also cause primary amenorrhoea.

Clinical diagnosis

History   Cyclical abdominal pain may suggest either an anatomical obstruction to menstrual flow or menarche is about to start. A history of chronic severe illness or weight loss and heavy exercise would suggest the cause for delay.

Examination   A general clinical examination should be performed noting weight, height, body mass index, blood pressure, thyroid examination, evidence of dysmorphic signs, development of secondary sexual characteristics such as breasts, pubic and axillary hair, and performing an abdominal examination. An inspection of the external genitalia should give information about any structural abnormalities such as imperforate hymen.

Investigations   Primary amenorrhoea should be investigated in the following patients:

- Failure to menstruate by age 15 years in the presence of normal secondary sexual development or failure to menstruate within 5 years after breast development (if that occurs before age 10 years)
- Pregnancy should always be excluded with a urine human chorionic gonadotropin (hCG) test
- Pelvic ultrasound scan will confirm the presence/absence of a uterus and size of ovaries
- Serum follicle-stimulating hormone (FSH), prolactin and thyroid-stimulating hormone (TSH) will exclude ovarian or hypothalamic failure, pituitary adenomas and thyroid disease
- If serum FSH is raised (>20 IU/L) or the uterus absent, then a serum karyotype is indicated

Aetiology

1. Patients with absent breast development and high FSH levels
   - Premature ovarian failure (46XX)
   - Turner syndrome (46XO)
2. Patients with absent breast development and low FSH levels
   - Constitutional delay
   - Prolactinomas
   - Kallmann syndrome: hypogonadotropic hypogonadism caused by failure of fetal gonadotropin-releasing hormone (GnRH) neurons migrating to the thalamus, usually associated with anosmia or hyposmia. It is usually autosomal recessive but some cases are X-linked
   - Stress, exercise, weight loss and anorexia
   - Congenital adrenal hyperplasia
3. Patients with breast development
   - Uterus absent – androgen insensitivity syndrome (46XY) or Müllerian agenesis (46XX)
   - Uterus present – vaginal septum, imperforate hymen, polycystic ovarian syndrome (PCOS), constitutional delay

Management

The aim is to restore normal sexual function and fertility where possible.

- Ovarian failure is treated with exogenous sex hormones; pituitary failure with gonadotrophins
- Simple surgery will correct an imperforate hymen
- Successful treatment of absence of the lower genital tract has been achieved with the use of graduated glass dilators with full coital function resulting. Where these measures fail then complex plastic surgery procedures may be necessary in an attempt to achieve satisfactory coitus
- Phenotypic females, but with non-functioning gonads, either ovaries or testes, should have these gonads excised because of the high risk of malignant change
- Prolactinomas need a full endocrine review for subsequent management, usually involving dopamine-agonist treatment, e.g. bromocriptine; iatrogenic causes of hyperprolactinaemia may respond to domperidone and metoclopramide
- Kallmann syndrome (GnRH deficiency) can be treated with gonadotrophins
- Intracranial tumours require neurosurgical attention
- Weight loss and anorexia requires psychological and psychiatric input into management of weight

Secondary amenorrhoea

Overview

Secondary is defined as an absence of menstruation for 6 months or more in a female of reproductive years with previously established menstruation that is not the result of pregnancy, lactation or hysterectomy. Causes include long term treatment with hormones such as Depo-Provera, danazol or GnRH analogues.

Any severe illness may result in amenorrhoea and this should be excluded before definitive investigation is undertaken.

Clinical diagnosis

History   There may be a family history of premature menopause. Presentation may be preceded by a period of oral contraceptive usage or severe weight loss, associated with diet, anorexia nervosa or depression. Heavy exercise is associated with amenorrhoea and stress may be a factor. A hormonal cause may be suggested by galactorrhoea or virilising symptoms. An obstructive cause is suggested by cyclical pelvic pain and a history of gynaecological or obstetric surgery.

Examination   Signs of virilisation, nipple discharge, signs of a pituitary tumour (visual field disturbance and papilloedema), a pelvic mass (uterine or ovarian) or an abdominal mass (uterine, ovarian or adrenal) may lead to the diagnosis.

Investigation   This is decided by preceding history and examination. The most common causes are PCOS and premature menopause, which is confirmed by gonadotrophin estimation. A full hormone profile will determine a pituitary or adrenal aetiology and may suggest polycystic ovaries.

Ultrasound or examination under anaesthesia may reveal an ovarian or adrenal cause as well as identifying any site of obstruction to menstrual flow.

Aetiology

- Weight loss, anorexia and excessive exercise
- Non-specific hypothalamic causes
- PCOS and other causes of chronic anovulation
- Hypothyroidism
- Cushing syndrome – a relatively rare endocrine disorder resulting from excessive exposure to cortisol, which leads to a variety of symptoms and physical abnormalities
- Pituitary tumour
- Sheehan syndrome – a condition that follows postpartum uterine haemorrhage severe enough to cause circulatory collapse, resulting in pituitary necrosis and hypopituitarism
- Gonadal failure

- Abnormal karyotype
- Prolactinoma and idiopathic hyperprolactinaemia
- Asherman syndrome – a condition characterised by intrauterine adhesions
- Ovarian tumour

Management

Treatment is directed to the cause: hormone replacement for premature menopause, gonadotrophin stimulation for hormone-induced amenorrhoea or hypopituitarism (if fertility is desired, otherwise oral contraceptive pill or hormone replacement therapy if oestrogen deficient), counselling and psychiatric treatment for stress-related causes and depression, surgical correction of outflow obstruction and definitive treatment by the relevant specialists for pituitary and adrenal tumours.

Further reading

Edmonds D. Primary amenorrhoea. In: Edmonds, DK (Ed.). Dewhurst's Textbook of Obstetrics and Gynaecology, 7th edn. Oxford: Blackwell Publishing, 2007:369–376.

Child T. Investigation and treatment of primary amenorrhoea. Obstetrics, Gynaecology & Reproductive Medicine 2011; 21(2):31–35.

The Practice Committee of the American Society for Reproductive Medicine. Current evaluation of amenorrhea. Fertility and Sterility 2008; 90(5):S219–S225.

Related topics of interest

- Abnormality of the genital tract (p. 1)
- Polycystic ovarian syndrome (p. 118)
- Subfertility: aetiology and diagnosis (p. 139)

Assisted conception

Overview

Assisted conception is the term given to fertility treatments which involve manipulation of oocytes, sperm or embryos outside the body 'in vitro'. In vitro fertilisation (IVF) was first used to bring oocytes and sperm together for women with tubal disease, but since the birth of the first IVF baby more than 30 years ago, it has developed to treat couples with many types of fertility problems – tubal disease, male factor, endometriosis, anovulation and unexplained subfertility. Factors associated with a positive outcome after IVF treatment include a short duration of subfertility, female body mass index (BMI) 19–29 and a history of previous pregnancies; reduced ovarian reserve and advancing female age are associated with poorer outcomes. Assisted conception techniques are also used to treat patients who need oocyte or sperm donation. Almost 2% of all children born in the UK are now as a result of assisted conception treatment. All assisted conception treatment in the UK is regulated by the Human Fertilisation and Embryology Authority (HFEA), in accordance with the Human Fertilisation and Embryology Act.

In vitro fertilisation

Many couples require IVF treatment to help them conceive, but unfortunately this is not always available within the National Health Service (NHS). The majority of IVF cycles within the UK are still carried out in the private sector. The provision of funding for IVF treatment also varies between different areas, the so-called 'post-code lottery'. The National Institute for Health and Clinical Excellence (NICE) drew up guidelines several years ago which recommended that three cycles of IVF treatment should be offered to childless couples to help them conceive and demonstrated cost-effectiveness of such treatment. NICE also gave guidance on which patients should be treated within the NHS – only women under the age of 40 years, both partners should be non-smokers, the female partner should have a BMI of between 19 and 29, in order to optimise the chance of a successful outcome. Recent revision of NICE guidelines has increased the female age to 42 years in cases where the couple cannot conceive by other means. Unfortunately, the original guidance was not adopted by all purchasers, and we must await the response to the new guidelines. Within the NHS, most areas restrict IVF treatment to couples who are childless, although the definition of childless (one/both partners) varies. IVF treatment involves several stages:

Ovarian hyperstimulation

Many different regimens may be used for ovarian hyperstimulation, but the two commonest are the long agonist protocol and the short antagonist protocol.

Long agonist protocol

The patient is seen in the mid-luteal phase and commenced on a gonadotrophin releasing hormone (GnRH) agonist. After next menses, serum luteinising hormone (LH) and oestradiol levels are measured to confirm pituitary downregulation. Pituitary suppression is essential to prevent a spontaneous LH surge which would lead to premature ovulation. If pituitary downregulation is confirmed, daily follicle-stimulating hormone (FSH) or human menopausal gonadotrophin (hMG) injections are added. The patient is seen on day 8 of stimulation for an ultrasound scan and every day or two days thereafter. When a lead follicle of 18 mm is seen with two further follicles of 16 mm or more, an injection of human chorionic gonadotrophin (hCG) is given to act as an artificial LH surge. Throughout the period of monitoring, oestradiol and LH levels may also be measured to assess ovarian response and to confirm continued pituitary suppression.

Short antagonist protocol

The patient is seen on day 2 or 3 after menses, an ultrasound scan is carried out to exclude the presence of an ovarian cyst and serum levels of oestradiol may be checked. If no cyst is present, the patient is started on daily injections of FSH or hMG. After 4–6 days of stimulation, daily injections of a GnRH antagonist are added to prevent a premature surge of LH which could lead to spontaneous ovulation. The patient is seen on day 8 and monitoring is then similar to that seen in the long agonist protocol.

The short antagonist protocol is the treatment of choice for women with polycystic ovarian syndrome (PCOS) or high ovarian reserve as it is associated with a lower incidence of ovarian hyperstimulation syndrome (OHSS).

Oocyte recovery – day 0

34–36 hours after the injection of hCG, follicles that have developed during ovarian stimulation are aspirated via the vaginal route, under ultrasound guidance. The patient is sedated for the procedure.

Insemination – day 0

On the day of oocyte recovery, the male partner produces a semen sample. The sample is prepared and the oocytes retrieved inseminated (conventional IVF) or a single sperm injected directly into oocytes by the procedure of intracytoplasmic sperm injection (see below).

Fertilisation check – day 1

The day after oocyte recovery, on average 60–70% of collected oocytes will have fertilised normally.

Embryo culture and transfer – days 2–5

All normally fertilised oocytes are cultured in an incubator until they are transferred into the patient, 2, 3 or 5 days after oocyte collection (**Figure 2**). During embryo culture, some embryos will start to slow down their development or start to fragment. Embryos are observed during their development and the embryologist selects one or two embryos that are developing most normally. Culturing embryos therefore allows selection of the embryos most likely to give rise to a pregnancy. Due to regulation in the United Kingdom, only one or two embryos can be transferred. All IVF units draw up their own guidelines to decide when to transfer one or two embryos, taking into consideration factors such as female age and the response to treatment. The aim of such protocols is to reduce the number of twin pregnancies without compromising the chance of pregnancy. Exceptionally and only in a woman more than 40 years of age three embryos may be replaced. There is strict regulation in the UK about the number of embryos transferred, but patients are now travelling abroad for treatment and may return with high order pregnancies after having three or more embryos replaced.

Embryo transfer is carried out by placing a thin catheter into the uterine cavity, often under abdominal ultrasound control. The procedure is painless and no anaesthetic is needed. After embryo transfer, the woman can return to normal activity.

Luteal support

Following transfer, additional luteal support by progesterone is given, because of the risk of premature collapse of the corpus luteum. HCG injections can also be used but these are associated with a higher risk of OHSS.

Pregnancy testing

A pregnancy test is performed 16–18 days after embryo transfer. If the test is positive, luteal support is continued and an ultrasound scan performed 2–3 weeks later.

Intracytoplasmic sperm injection

Intracytoplasmic sperm injection (ICSI) is the procedure use to enable fertilisation in cases where there is a significant reduction in semen quality (concentration, motility or morphology) or when there has been a previous failure of fertilisation. If this is not the case, ICSI does not increase pregnancy rates and should not be used. The treatment for the patient is the same as IVF, the only difference occurring within the laboratory at the time of insemination. Rather than sperm being added to oocytes, a single sperm is injected into each mature oocyte (**Figure 3**). ICSI does not guarantee fertilisation. Approximately 70% of injected oocytes fertilise normally.

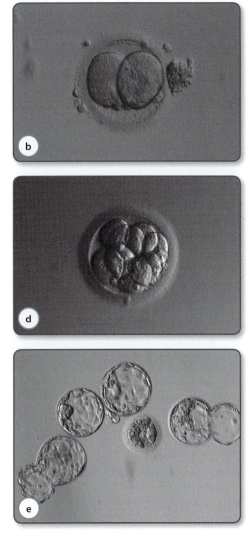

Figure 2 (a) Pronucleate embryos. Note two pronuclei in upper embryo confirming normal fertilisation; (b and c) Day 2 embryos with (b) 2 cells and (c) 4 cells. Note fragments within 4-cell embryo associated with reduced chance of implantation; (d) Day 3 embryo, usually 6-8 cells; (e) Day 5-6 embryos, four blastocysts. Note two blastocysts starting to hatch. Photos courtesy of Diane Critchlow.

Embryo cryopreservation

If there are additional good quality embryos available after embryo transfer, following IVF or ICSI, these embryos may be cryopreserved for the future. The process of creating embryos is difficult and costly, it is therefore important to ensure that all good quality embryos created may be used.

Oocyte, sperm and embryo donation

Some patients will require treatment using donated gametes as they may not be able to produce their own gametes, or they may choose to use donated gametes because of an underlying genetic condition. Donated oocytes can be used within IVF or ICSI

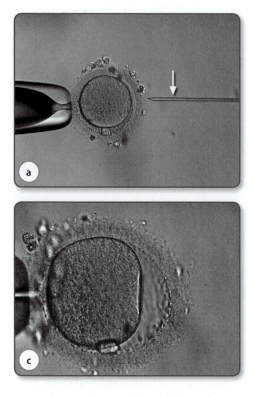

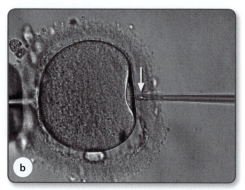

Figure 3 A single sperm is selected and injected into each mature oocyte – ICSI (a) A single sperm (arrow) inside the needle is lined up alongside the oocyte, which is held steady by the embryologist. (b) The sperm (arrow) is injected into the oocyte. (c) Oocyte following ICSI, with a clear indentation ('funnel') in the plasma membrane marking the site of sperm injection. Courtesy of Ruth Arneson.

treatment. If donor sperm is needed, this can be used either in insemination treatment or as part of IVF.

In the UK, all oocyte, sperm and embryo donation has to be undertaken without anonymity of the donor. This allows any child conceived from donation to approach the HFEA at the age of 18 years and gain access to identifying information about the donor. This is not the case in all other countries. There is a relative lack of both oocyte and sperm donors within the UK, although recent changes to the re-imbursement of donors has led to more donors coming forward. Some patients may undertake treatment with donated gametes from a known donor such as a family member or friend.

The woman receiving treatment with donated oocytes or sperm is the legal mother of any child conceived, and the donor has no legal rights over the child.

Patients receiving treatment with donated gametes must receive counselling prior to treatment.

Surrogacy

Surrogacy is a relatively rare treatment and is used in cases where the woman has had a hysterectomy, has an underlying medical condition which prohibits pregnancy or has a very poor obstetric history.

Surrogacy may be undertaken using oocytes from the couple requesting treatment (commissioning couple), oocytes from the surrogate herself or oocytes donated by a donor. Surrogacy treatment is complex as the surrogate host is the birth and hence legal mother. She cannot legally hand over parental rights until the child is 6 weeks old. It is therefore essential that all couples seek legal advice before embarking on such treatment.

Risks of IVF/ICSI treatment

Maternal

OHSS

This is the most significant risk after IVF treatment. Approximately 7% of patients will develop OHSS, 1% severe OHSS. The condition is frequently seen after excessive response to ovarian stimulation which usually presents early, within 2–3 days of oocyte recovery. Risk factors include low BMI, young age and a diagnosis of polycystic ovarian syndrome (POCS). Late onset OHSS occurs 7–10 days after oocyte recovery and is usually associated with an ongoing pregnancy. The syndrome is associated with capillary leak resulting in ascites, pleural and pericardial effusions with associated intravascular depletion. Early diagnosis with fluid replacement is critical. Dopamine agonists such as cabergoline have been shown to be of some benefit. Patients should be cared for in a specialist centre.

Long term risks

There is concern about the potential long term risks faced by women who have undergone IVF treatment, in particular the risk of breast and ovarian cancer. Although most of the data are relatively reassuring, there is a need for long term follow up.

Offspring

Multiple pregnancies

Multiple pregnancies carry higher risks for both mother and babies, in particular growth retardation and premature delivery. The HFEA has therefore stipulated that the multiple birth rates following IVF treatment should be no more than 10%.

Fetal abnormality

There is some evidence to suggest that there is an increased risk of fetal abnormality following ICSI treatment, although a significant increase after IVF treatment has not been shown. The need for ongoing follow-up of children conceived following assisted conception treatment is essential.

Adoption

Some couples may not achieve a pregnancy after treatment or may decide that they do not wish to undertake fertility treatment and instead look to adoption. This option must always be offered to couples and it is important that fertility units have access to counselling services to appropriately support and advise couples.

Further reading

RCOG Green Top Guideline No. 5. The management of ovarian hyperstimulation syndrome. London: RCOG, 2006.

van Rumste MME, Evers JLH, Farquhar C. Intra-cytoplasmic sperm injection versus conventional techniques for oocyte insemination during in vitro fertilisation in couples with non-male factor subfertility. Cochrane Database Syst Rev 2003; 2:CD001301.

Davies MJ, Moore VM, Willson KJ, et al. Reproductive technologies and the risk of birth defects. N Eng J Med 2012; 366:1803–1813.

Related topics of interest

Cervical cancer

Overview

Cervical cancer is the second leading cause of cancer-related death among women worldwide. In 2008, there were more than 500,000 new diagnoses and 275,000 deaths from cervical cancer. Nearly 90% of these were in developing countries. In the UK, cervical screening has been in existence since the 1960s and by the late 1980s, a highly organised call–recall system was in place. A reduction in the incidence of cervical cancer by 49%, and mortality rate by almost 70%, is testament to the success of this programme. Lifetime risk in the UK is now 1:134, with incidence peaking between the ages of 30–40 years, and again from 70 years onwards. Around 3000 new cases of cervical cancer are diagnosed in the UK each year, and almost 1000 women die from the disease annually. Across all stages, the 5-year survival rate from cervical cancer is 60%.

Clinical features

In the UK, cervical screening results in the detection of early invasive disease that is usually asymptomatic. In addition, women may be referred for urgent investigation if they are thought to have an abnormal-looking cervix on speculum examination. It is important to remember that a recent normal smear does not preclude the presence of cancer. Those with symptoms typically present with abnormal vaginal bleeding. Post-coital bleeding is characteristic but persistent heavy, irregular or post-menopausal bleeding is also common. Women may present with abnormal vaginal discharge. Late disease may present with more varied symptoms such as urinary or bowel symptoms, thrombosis, a mass protruding from the vagina, lower back or abdominal pain.

Aetiology

Cervical cancer is caused by persistent high risk human papillomavirus (HPV) infection. There are more than 100 subtypes of HPV, which is a small double stranded DNA virus, but not all are oncogenic. Low risk HPV types 6 and 11 cause anogenital warts, whilst high risk types, particularly HPV 16 and 18 cause cervical, anogenital and head and neck cancers. HPV infection is endemic within the adult population but the majority of women build immunity to it. Risk factors for cervical cancer therefore include early age at first coitus, multiple sexual partners, high parity and low socioeconomic status as well as smoking and immunosuppression. Squamous cell and adenosquamous tumours form 85% of cervical cancers, and adenocarcinomas the remaining 15%. Squamous tumours tend to be large cell keratinising, or large cell non-keratinising but occasionally may be small cell type. Small cell tumours have a poor prognosis as they do when they occur elsewhere in the body, i.e. the bronchus. Cervical cancer spreads by direct invasion (to parametrium, cervical stroma, uterus, bladder, rectum), and by lymphatic spread to pelvic and para-aortic lymph nodes. Haematogenous spread is uncommon. Prognosis is influenced by stage, grade, histological subtype and size of the tumour, and the presence of metastases.

Diagnosis

There may be a macroscopic lesion on the cervix or, alternatively, a microscopic focus of invasive disease may be detected during histopathological examination of a biopsy taken at colposcopy. A large loop excision of the transformation zone (LLETZ) or a knife cone biopsy is required to confirm the diagnosis, and to provide information regarding the histological type, grade and stage of disease to guide further management.

Management

Cervical cancer should be managed in a cancer centre with a specialised multidisciplinary team. Optimal management depends upon accurate staging of the disease (**Table 1**). Historically staging was purely clinical, and

Stage		Involvement	Positive pelvic lymph nodes (%)	5-year survival (%)
Table 1 International Federation of Gynaecology and Obstetrics (FIGO) staging of cervical cancer.				
I	I	Confined to cervix		
	Ia	Lesion identifiable microscopically		
	Ia1	≤3 mm depth, ≤7 mm diameter	0.6	
	Ia2	3–5 mm depth, ≤7 mm diameter	4.8	79
	Ib	Clinically detectable lesion, or bigger than Ia2	15.9	
	Ib1	≤4 cm lesion		
	Ib2	>4 cm lesion		
II	II	Extends beyond cervix, but not to pelvic wall or lower 1/3 of vagina		
	IIa	No obvious parametrial involvement, involves upper 2/3 vagina	24.5	47
	IIb	Obvious parametrial involvement	31.4	
III	III	Extends to pelvic sidewall or lower 1/3 of vagina, hydronephrosis or non-functioning kidney		
	IIIa	Involves lower 1/3 vagina	44.8	22
	IIIb	Extends to pelvic sidewall or hydronephrosis/non-functioning kidney		
IV	IV	Extended beyond pelvis or involves mucosa of bladder or rectum		
	IVa	Spread to adjacent pelvic organs	55	7
	IVb	Spread to distant organs		

Adapted from Sobin L, Wittekind CH. TNM Classification of Malignant Tumours (6th edn). Geneva: Union for International Cancer Control 2002:155–157.

based upon the findings of an examination under anaesthesia. However, increasingly cancer centres worldwide are moving to the use of imaging, particularly magnetic resonance imaging (MRI), to more accurately stage cervical cancer. Even when performed by an experienced clinician, clinical staging has been found to be inaccurate.

Stage Ia disease can be treated by cone biopsy with or without pelvic lymphadenectomy. Stage Ib-IIa disease is usually treated with radical hysterectomy and bilateral pelvic lymphadenectomy. Radical hysterectomy requires removal of the tumour with adequate disease free margins, and involves removal of the parametrial tissue, cardinal and uterosacral ligaments and upper vagina. Lymph node dissection aims to remove obturator, internal, external and common iliac nodes. Para-aortic nodes should be removed if there is suspicion that

pelvic nodes are involved or if at the time of surgery the para-aortic nodes are clinically suspicious. Intraoperative frozen section of suspicious para-aortic nodes may be performed as para-aortic node involvement is a contraindication to radical hysterectomy.

Serious complications include haemorrhage, damage to the bladder, ureter or bowel, venous thrombosis and pulmonary embolus. In the longer term, there is a risk of lymphoedema (3%), sexual dysfunction (2%) and bladder dysfunction (4%). Lymphoedema is more likely if adjuvant radiotherapy is given. Surgery is usually preferable in the medically fit younger patient, with the potential advantages of preservation of ovarian and sexual function. In addition, primary surgery has the advantage of allowing accurate surgical staging.

Adjuvant chemoradiotherapy is recommended in the case of positive lymph nodes, or close vaginal or parametrial resection margins, to reduce the risk of recurrence. Morbidity is increased when both surgery and radiotherapy are given.

With stage IIb disease or worse or sometimes bulky early disease, radical chemoradiotherapy is the treatment of choice. A course of radical chemoradiotherapy involves weekly cisplatin ($50\,mg/m^2$) chemotherapy with daily external beam radiotherapy (teletherapy) on an outpatient basis for 5 weeks (45 greys of radiotherapy/25 fractions). This is followed by an overnight stay for brachytherapy. Studies have shown up to a 30% survival benefit from this combined approach, and cure rates are 20–50%, but short and medium term complications are increased.

Cystitis, abdominal discomfort and diarrhoea are common adverse effects but are usually self-limiting. There are also the disadvantages of a radiation-induced menopause in younger patients. Vaginal stenosis is common but regular use of vaginal dilators can minimise the effects of this.

Fertility sparing treatment

As 43% of cervical cancers diagnosed are in women under the age of 45 years, fertility sparing treatment is increasingly being used.

1. Cone biopsy (knife or laser cone, depth at least 25 mm if adenocarcinoma):
- Stage Ia1 – < 1% risk of lymph node involvement
- Repeat if margins not clear (by at least 5 mm)
- Risks – cervical stenosis/incompetence, late miscarriage, preterm labour (2-fold increased risk)
- Avoid LLETZ as it limits pathological assessment of margins
2. Cone biopsy and laparoscopic pelvic lymph node dissection:
- Stage Ia2 squamous cell carcinoma (SCC) and adenocarcinoma – 5% risk of lymph node involvement
- Tumours < 1 cm in diameter have 0.6% risk of parametrial involvement
3. Radical trachelectomy (vaginal or laparoscopic) and pelvic lymph node dissection:

- Stage Ib1 SCC and adenocarcinoma – tumour < 2 cm in diameter, grade 1–2, no lymphovascular space invasion (LVSI)
- Radical excision of upper vagina, cervix, parametrium and placement of uterine suture
- Require caesarean sections in future pregnancies
4. Ovarian transposition and oocyte retrieval:
- Stage Ib2 +
- Reposition the ovaries outside the field of radiation, usually in the paracolic gutters level with ribs
- Still risk of ovarian failure from chemotherapy therefore pretreatment oocyte retrieval and freezing considered

Recurrent disease

Treatment of recurrence depends on the treatment which was given for the primary tumour. Women who were treated initially with surgery can have radiotherapy, women initially given radiotherapy can be considered for exenteration if there is no suggestion of distant disease. A positron emission tomography (PET)-CT scan is indicated prior to exenterative surgery to exclude lymph node or distant metastases. In carefully selected cases exenteration can have up to 50% 5-year survival, but thorough preoperative assessment and counselling is required to ensure patients understand the consequences of surgery to remove bowel and/or bladder. Operative mortality is in the region of 2–4%. Chemotherapy for recurrent disease is for palliation and should be considered if radiotherapy or exenteration is not feasible.

Palliation

Urinary tract symptoms are common in advanced cervical cancer, and ureteric obstruction can cause pain, infection and renal failure. Fistulae are also a feature of late disease, and can cause distressing symptoms. If survival may exceed 2 months, surgery to divert urine or faeces may be considered for symptom relief, but pain control and psychological support are essential.

Further reading

Ellis P, Mould T. Fertility-saving treatment in gynaecological oncology. The Obstetrician and Gynaecologist 2009; 11:239–244.

Martin-Hirsch PL. Cervical Cancer. In: Luesley DM, Baker PN (Ed.). Obstetrics and Gynaecology: An evidence-based text for MRCOG, 2nd edn. London: Hodder Arnold, 2010.

Keys HM, Bundy BN, Stehman FB, et al. Cisplatin, radiation and adjuvant hysterectomy compared with radiation and adjuvant hysterectomy for bulky stage Ib cervical cancer. N Engl J Med 1999; 340:1154–1161.

Related topics of interest

Cervical screening

Overview

Cervical cancer is the second most common cause of female cancer death worldwide and almost 3000 new cases per year are diagnosed in the UK alone. The introduction of an organised screening programme in the UK in 1988 saw a 49% reduction in incidence over the following 20 years. Over the last three decades, mortality rates from cervical cancer have fallen by almost 70%. It is estimated that the NHS cervical screening programme (NHSCSP) saves 4500 lives per year. Cervical precancer has a long natural history and exfoliative cytology is an acceptable test which detects a premalignant and treatable phase in the progression to cervical cancer.

Aim

The Papanicolaou (Pap) smear test is used worldwide to screen for precancerous changes in the cells of the cervix. Since October 2008 liquid based cytology has been used in the collection and processing of smear samples. This has reduced the number of inadequate smear results, increased the sensitivity of the smear test and also provided a medium in which to test for the presence of high risk human papillomavirus (hrHPV). The smear test aims to identify a subgroup of the population at increased risk of cervical cancer, for whom further tests should be carried out. It is believed that overall coverage of more than 80% will reduce deaths from cervical cancer by 95% in the long term. In 2010/2011 coverage in the UK averaged 78.6%.

Cervical cytology

Screening intervals

- 25 years   First invitation
- 25–49   3 yearly
- 50–64   5 yearly – can opt out if complete and normal smear history
- >65   Cease if screened since age 50 years and normal smears

Previously the first invitation for cervical screening was age of 20 years but in 2004, after assessing all evidence, it was concluded that cervical screening in under 25s was highly likely to detect and overtreat abnormalities which would spontaneously resolve, and furthermore that the overtreatment led to unjustifiable morbidity in young women in light of the link between loop excision and cervical incompetence/premature birth. There is no evidence that screening women under the age of 25 years improves survival.

Approximately 98% of all smears taken are adequate for diagnosis and more than 90% of smears taken are normal. The proportion of normal smears increases with age but the likelihood of abnormal smears representing invasive cancer also increases with age. Borderline and mildly dyskaryotic smears are very common in young women.

Referral to colposcopy

In the UK, further investigation of abnormal smears is by colposcopy (**Table 2**). In other countries colposcopy may be used as a primary tool, in the absence of organised screening programmes. The technique used for diagnostic colposcopy is described in **Table 3**. The aims of colposcopy are:

- Determine the size/position of the transformation zone
- Confirm or refute the cytological suspicion of cervical intraepithelial neoplasia (CIN)
- Recognise or exclude invasive cancer or glandular disease
- Facilitate treatment and monitoring of CIN

Colposcopic features suggestive of CIN are:
- Punctation
- Mosaicism
- Atypical vessels
- Density of acetowhite areas – high grade lesions are more dense
- Clarity of borders of acetowhite areas – high grade lesions are clearly demarcated

Colposcopic findings should record the type of transformation zone, whether colposcopy was satisfactory or not (i.e. whether the transformation zone was visualised in its entirety), and lesions should be recorded as low grade or high grade (suspected CIN 2 or 3).

In pregnancy the indications for referral for colposcopy are unchanged; however, due to

Table 2 The management of abnormal smears

Smear result	Interpretation	Management
Negative	No cellular abnormality	Routine recall
Inadequate	Unable to interpret	Repeat after 3 months
Borderline changes	Cellular appearance not normal	HPV triage
Mild dyskaryosis	Consistent with underlying CIN1	HPV triage
Moderate dyskaryosis	Consistent with underlying CIN2	Refer for colposcopy
Severe dyskaryosis	Consistent with underlying CIN3	Refer for colposcopy
Suspicious of invasive cancer	Possibility of invasive cancer	Refer for colposcopy
Glandular neoplasia	Possible abnormality in endocervix/endometrium	Refer for colposcopy/gynae assessment

Table 3 What does colposcopy entail?

Diagnostic colposcopy

1. Modified lithotomy position
2. Macroscopic examination of vulva
3. Wash cervix with normal saline
4. Examine cervix using colposcope, with and without a green filter to highlight blood vessels
5. Apply 3% or 5% acetic acid solution to cervix
6. Assess for acetowhite areas after at least 20 seconds. Premalignant disease is acetowhite
7. If transformation zone not visualised introduce endocervical speculum
8. Schiller's test, apply Lugol's iodine to demarcate abnormal areas. Premalignant cells don't take up iodine

changes in the cervix in terms of appearance and vascularity, colposcopy should be performed by an experienced colposcopist and biopsy should only be performed if malignancy is suspected. Otherwise the cervix should be assessed 3 monthly until biopsy can be safely performed.

Management of abnormal colposcopy

Normal practice is to biopsy lesions seen at colposcopy to determine further management. Some clinicians may 'See and Treat' in some cases. Although high grade lesions should all be treated, low grade lesions can be treated or kept under 6-monthly surveillance. A conservative approach is generally recommended for young women, with a biopsy and/or treatment being performed if there has not been regression of low grade disease after 24 months. Approximately, 50% of women with untreated low grade lesions will eventually regress. One factor to be considered in deciding how to manage low grade disease is the likelihood of the patient defaulting from follow-up. Another is her desire for future fertility.

Different approaches to treatment are seen. Techniques can be characterised as excisional or ablative (**Table 4**).

Excisional techniques have the advantage of allowing thorough histopathological assessment. Large loop excision of the transformation zone (LLETZ) is the technique most commonly employed in the UK, as it has less morbidity than other excisional options. With the exception of cryotherapy (where liquid nitrogen at –50°C is used to freeze and destroy superficial cervical tissue), all techniques consistently achieve cure rates of 90–98%. Cryotherapy has cure rates of around 84% in CIN3 and using a double freeze technique may be a reasonable mode of treatment in resource-poor countries as it is cheap and easy to use, with low morbidity. Although cold coagulation may sound similar

Table 4 Excisional and ablative methods for treating CIN			
Excisional		**Ablative**	
LLETZ	Local or GA	Electrodiathermy	GA
Laser cone	Local or GA	Cold coagulation	Local
Knife cone biopsy	GA	Cryocautery	No anaesthesia
Hysterectomy	GA, consider if other gynae problems	Laser	Local or GA
GA, general anaesthetic.			

to cryotherapy, it actually involves applying a probe heated to 120°C to the cervix, with better success rates.

Role of HPV testing

HPV 16 and 18 are thought to cause more than 70% of cervical cancers. Infection with high risk HPV can be detected using DNA amplification techniques such as the Hybrid Capture 2 assay, which detects 13 oncogenic HPV types. The Sentinel sites trials have seen the use of high risk HPV testing introduced to the UK national screening programme both as triage and as a test of cure (**Figure 4**).

In women with equivocal cervical cytology, determination of HPV status can help to separate those at high risk of disease from those at low risk of disease, and although initially increasing colposcopy referrals, it reduces the number of repeat smears and the time taken to return women to routine follow up (**Table 5**).

It also has a high sensitivity for detecting treatment failure in women who have been treated for CIN. By testing the first smear 6 months post-treatment for hrHPV, hrHPV negative smears with normal, borderline or mild dyskaryosis on cytology can be returned to routine recall.

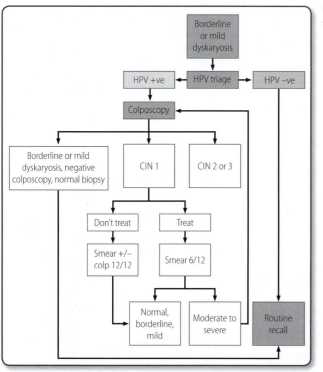

Figure 4 Human papillomavirus triage flowchart.

Table 5 Changes to national screening programme			
Cytology	Current management	HPV triage	
		Negative	Positive
Borderline	Repeat smear 6 months	Routine recall	Colposcopy
Mild dyskaryosis	Colposcopy	Routine recall	Colposcopy

In the future, hrHPV testing is likely to replace cytology as the initial screen for cervical precancer in the UK and across the world. Primary screening with hrHPV testing followed by reflex cytology for those who test positive has been shown in large randomised trials to offer several advantages, including high sensitivity for detection of high grade CIN, the potential for high-throughput automated testing, and extended screening intervals for those who are hrHPV negative. A negative hrHPV test provides a longer duration of negative prediction than cytology, allowing screening intervals to be safely extended to 6 years. The disadvantage of primary HPV screening is managing women who are hrHPV positive but cytology negative. Although the risk of underlying disease is low, such women are at a 2-fold higher risk of CIN during follow up than the general screening population. It may be appropriate to rescreen these women after 12–24 months, as most will have cleared their HPV infection by then. If they remain hrHPV positive, referral to colposcopy would then be indicated.

Follow-up

Previously women with treated low grade disease underwent 6, 12 and 24 months cytology before being discharged back to routine recall. Women with treated high grade disease required 6 and 12 months cytology and annual smears for a further 9 years. The implementation of HPV test of cure has changed this, with women being discharged back to routine recall sooner if HPV testing is negative post treatment (**Table 5**).

Women with low grade lesions that are not treated require 6-monthly follow-up until the lesions regress. If this has not occurred by 24 months a biopsy and/or treatment is indicated, particularly for women who have completed their family and those over 35 years of age.

Women treated for cervical glandular intraepithelial neoplasia (cGIN) are at higher risk of recurrent disease than those with high grade CIN, and it is harder to detect on smear tests. As a minimum they should be followed up as per high grade lesions, but ideally 6-monthly smears for 5 years followed by annual smears for 5 years is advisable.

Further reading

Kelly RS, Patnick J. Kitchener HC, et al. Human papillomavirus testing as a triage for borderline or mild dyskaryosis on cervical cytology: results from the Sentinel Sites study. Br J Cancer 2011; 105:983–988.

Sasieni P, Adams J. Effect of screening on cervical cancer mortality in England and Wales: analysis of trends within an age cohort model. BMJ 1999; 318:1244–1245.

Arbyn M, Kyrgiou M, Simoens C, et al. Perinatal mortality and other severe adverse pregnancy outcomes associated with treatment of cervical intraepithelial neoplasia: meta-analysis. BMJ 2008; 337:1284.

Kitchener HC, et al. Developing role of HPV in cervical cancer prevention. BMJ 2013; 347:4781.

Related topics of interest

Chemotherapy

Overview

Although the mainstay of curative management of gynaecological malignancies is surgery, chemotherapy has an increasingly important role in treatment. Chemotherapy may be employed with a number of intentions:

- Adjuvant therapy with the aim of increasing cure rates by eradicating micrometastatic disease
- Neoadjuvant therapy – administration before definitive surgery with the aim of disease control so reducing surgical morbidity and increasing rates of optimal surgical debulking
- Palliative therapy – in advanced/recurrent disease to increase survival and control disease-related symptoms

Chemotherapy may also be used to potentiate the effects of radiotherapy.

Indications

Ovarian cancer   Adjuvant chemotherapy with carboplatin should be offered to patients with optimally surgically managed high grade stage 1a and 1b cancer and all patients with stage 1c and stage II ovarian cancer (NICE, 2011). Adding in a second agent is of no survival benefit for these patients with early disease. In advanced disease patients are given combination therapy with carboplatin and paclitaxel. Neoadjuvant therapy is preferable in selected cases as it is associated with less surgical morbidity compared to primary surgery and adjuvant therapy. Bevacizumab, an antiangiogenic monoclonal antibody directed against vascular endothelial growth factor (VEGF) increases survival when given concurrently with carboplatin–paclitaxel chemotherapy and then as maintenance therapy in patients with disease at particularly high risk of recurrence (suboptimally debulked stage III and stage IV).

Endometrial cancer   Adjuvant platinum based chemotherapy is considered for patients with stage III/IV disease and might be beneficial in patients with lower stage disease with adverse prognostic factors (e.g. high grade, lymphovascular invasion). Trials exploring the most appropriate patients for adjuvant chemotherapy and how this is sequenced with radiotherapy are currently under way. In recurrent disease, carboplatin-paclitaxel is the standard of care. Hormonal therapies such as medroxyprogesterone acetate should be considered in patients with low grade or hormone receptor positive endometrioid cancers who are not suitable for surgery or radiotherapy.

Uterine sarcomas   Doxorubicin is the most commonly used first line therapy although it is of limited efficacy. There is no evidence to support its use in the adjuvant setting.

Cervical cancer   Chemotherapy (most commonly cisplatin) is given in conjunction with radiotherapy in stage Ib and above disease. Chemoradiation reduces the risk of relapse and death at the expense of serious haematological and gastrointestinal toxicity. For recurrent disease, platinum-paclitaxel or platinum-topotecan is often utilised.

Vulval or vaginal cancer   Chemotherapy is not commonly employed in the first line treatment of vulval or vaginal cancer.

Side effects and toxicity

Chemotherapy is cytotoxic and preferentially affects rapidly dividing cells. This includes normal tissues with high rates of cell turnover – in particular the bone marrow and gastrointestinal tract. Toxicity limits the dose of an individual cytotoxic drug which may be safely administered. However, as the side effect profile for each drug differs, multiple drug regimes are often utilised with the aim of increasing efficacy with manageable toxicities (see **Table 6**).

Haematological toxicity

Chemotherapy frequently causes myelosuppression which is usually transient but sometimes can cause significant morbidity and even mortality. Patients frequently become neutropenic thus susceptible to sepsis, thrombocytopenic increasing the risk of bleeding, or anaemic.

Table 6 Commonly used chemotherapeutic agents in gynaecological oncology: their actions and side effects				
Class and drug	Common uses	Administration	Action	Side effects
Platinum agents, e.g. Cisplatin, carboplatin	Epithelial ovarian, ovarian germ cell, cervical, endometrial, vulval	IV, Cisplatin is administered with IV hydration and forced diuresis. Requires adequate renal function	Bind to purine bases in DNA inhibiting DNA replication and repair leading to apoptosis	Carboplatin – less nephrotoxic than cisplatin, peripheral neuropathy, less emetogenic, more myelosuppression, Hypersensitivity reactions
				Cisplatin – nephrotoxic, ototoxic, peripheral neuropathy, highly emetogenic, less myelosuppression than carboplatin
Taxanes, e.g. paclitaxel	Epithelial ovarian, cervical, endometrial	IV with steroids, antihistamines and H2 antagonists	Bind to tubulin. Stabilise microtubules so inhibiting mitosis	Neurotoxicity, myelosuppression, alopecia
Topoisomerase inhibitors, e.g. Doxorubicin, Pegylated liposomal doxorubicin (Caelyx)	Epithelial ovarian, endometrial, uterine sarcoma	IV (IV/Oral with etoposide)	Inhibit DNA repair stimulating apoptosis	Doxorubicin – myelosuppression, alopecia, irreversible cardiac failure. Caelyx is associated with reduced risk of cardiac toxicity but increased mucositis/ skin toxicity (palmoplantar erythema)
Antimetabolites, e.g 5-fluorouracil, gemcitabine	5FU-vulval	IV/Topical	Interfere with metabolic pathways important in DNA synthesis	Myelosuppression, mucositis, hand-foot syndrome, coronary artery spasm
	Gemcitabine - Epithelial ovarian, cervical	IV		Myelosuppression, peripheral oedema, rash
Bevacizumab	Ovarian cancer	IV	Antiangiogenic. Monoclonal antibody against VEGF	Hypertension, proteinuria. Less commonly, arterial thromboembolic events, haemorrhage, gastrointestinal perforation/fistula. Delayed wound healing

Management of neutropenic sepsis

- Any patient receiving myelosuppressive chemotherapy who develops pyrexia or signs/symptoms of sepsis should be admitted urgently to a specialist oncology unit for assessment and managed according to local guidelines.
- Urgent blood tests and cultures should be taken and broad spectrum antibiotics should be administered immediately on admission. Antifungal and antiviral agents may be added if patients exhibit additional signs.

- Granulocyte colony stimulating factor (G-CSF) should be considered in severely neutropenic patients, those with evidence of pneumonia or septic shock.
- Blood and/or platelet transfusions may need to be considered in patients with concomitant anaemia or thrombocytopenia

Non-haematological toxicity

Common side effects include nausea and vomiting, fatigue, mucositis, alopecia and diarrhoea. Side effects can be reduced by the assessment of performance status and evaluation of renal and liver function following previous cycles. Dose reduction may sometimes be necessary to limit toxicity. Corticosteroids and antiemetics (e.g. ondansetron and metoclopramide) are given alongside emetogenic chemotherapy to ameliorate side effects. Hair loss may be reduced by the wearing of a cold cap during treatment. Long term side effects of some agents include nephrotoxicity, neuropathy, cardiac toxicity and infertility.

Bevacizumab has a distinct toxicity profile, most frequently hypertension and proteinuria. Less commonly it can cause arterial thromboembolic events and gastrointestinal perforation. Its use may also delay surgical wound healing and increase the risk of bleeding.

Follow-up

Assessment of response is monitored in three main ways: clinical examination, measurement of tumour markers (CA-125) and radiologically. Patients are monitored throughout their treatment and at regular but increasing intervals from their treatment if their disease is stable. Follow up protocols are individualised according to cancer type, stage, treatments employed and local guidelines. It is important to note that treating ovarian cancer patients with chemotherapy for low volume asymptomatic disease detected on the basis of rising CA-125 levels alone is not associated with improved survival but does reduce quality of life. This has lead to many centres not measuring CA-125 during routine follow-up after adjuvant therapy.

Treatment of recurrent disease

If patients with ovarian cancer relapse more that 6 months after completion of first line platinum based therapy, second line treatment with platinum-doublet chemotherapy is recommended (e.g. carboplatin–paclitaxel or gemcitabine–carboplatin). In patients with ovarian cancer that has become resistant or refractory to platinum agents (i.e. disease relapse within 6 months of platinum chemotherapy or disease progression during therapy), alternative treatment regimens such as weekly low dose paclitaxel, pegylated liposomal doxorubicin or topotecan can be considered. Bevacizumab has been shown to lengthen the duration of disease control when added to chemotherapy for both platinum-sensitive and resistant ovarian cancer.

Many patients will receive multiple lines of chemotherapy for recurrent ovarian cancer with significant prolongation of survival and control of disease-related symptoms. However, it is important that the patients are fully counselled about the likelihood of benefits from further treatment and potential toxicities associated with this.

Patients with relapsed or metastatic cervical cancer and endometrial cancer who have already received platinum-doublet chemotherapy should be considered for entry into clinical trials as no standard second line treatment regimens have been established.

Further reading

National Collaborating Centre for Cancer. Ovarian cancer: The recognition and initial management of ovarian cancer. NICE clinical guideline 122. London: NICE, 2011.

Winter-Roach BA, Kitchener HC, Dickinson HO. Adjuvant (post-surgery) chemotherapy for early stage epithelial ovarian cancer. Cochrane Database Syst Rev 2009; (1):CD004706.

Vergote I, Trope CG, Amant F, et al. Neoadjuvant chemotherapy or primary surgery in stage IIIc or IV ovarian cancer. N Engl J Med 2010; 363:943–953.

Related topics of interest

Chronic pelvic pain

Definition

What is pain? The International Association for the Study of Pain describe it as 'an unpleasant sensory and emotional experience associated with actual or potential tissue damage, or described in terms of such damage'.

It can be acute or chronic. Acute pain begins suddenly and is often severe, being associated with fresh tissue damage following acute injury. The pain resolves as the injury heals. Chronic pain is persistent and can become physically and emotionally exhausting. It may continue after the original injury heals or it can be associated with no obvious physical cause.

Chronic pelvic pain (CPP) is defined as intermittent or chronic pain in the lower abdomen or pelvis of at least 6 months' duration, not occurring exclusively with menstruation or intercourse and not associated with pregnancy.

Overview

CPP affects about 1 in 4–6 women. Over one-third of outpatient referrals to a gynaecologist are for pelvic pain. The majority do not have gross pelvic pathology.

CPP is a symptom and not a diagnosis. It can affect a woman's ability to function normally. 25% of women with CPP spend 2–3 days a month in bed and almost half feel sad or depressed some of the time.

Aetiology

CPP is often due to a combination of physical, psychological and social factors and should be treated holistically. There may be many underlying factors associated with the development of CPP. There is often poor correlation between the extent of these factors and the severity of the pain. Initial assessment of the patient must aim to identify these contributory factors rather than looking for a single pathology.

Clinical features

These factors include:

Gynaecological

- Chronic pelvic inflammatory disease
- Adenomyosis – difficult to diagnose. May have a tender uterus on palpation
- Endometriosis
- Adhesions – may be associated with pain if associated with organ entrapment or limited mobility. Particularly prevalent after fibroid and ovarian surgery and also hysterectomy. Commonly result from endometriosis and pelvic or intra-abdominal infections
- Residual ovary syndrome – symptoms from ovaries left at the time of hysterectomy. 75% present with pain
- Fibroids
- Pelvic organ prolapse
- Ovarian cysts
- Congenital anomalies – non-communicating rudimentary horn (frequently these are also associated with endometriosis)
- Pelvic venous congestion – the existence of this as a cause for CPP is widely disputed. There are no diagnostic tests for it but in women suspected of having it, gonadotropin-releasing hormone (GnRH) agonists may be the most useful therapeutic agent

Non-gynaecological

- Gastrointestinal disease – diverticulitis, inflammatory bowel disease, irritable bowel syndrome (IBS), hernia, anal fissures
- Urinary tract – kidney stones, infection, interstitial cystitis, urinary retention, malignancy
- Musculoskeletal – lumbosacral osteoarthritis, rheumatoid disease, prolapsed disc. This may be a primary cause or develop secondary to postural changes
- Nerve entrapment – in scar tissue, fascia or small foramen. Can be associated

with endometriosis. Can cause pain in the distribution of the nerve. Often develops after surgery, e.g. misplaced lateral tension-free vaginal tape (TVT), sacrospinous fixation, almost 4% after a Pfannenstiel incision
- Psychosocial problems – depression, sexual abuse, substance abuse, eating disorders. The association of CPP with abuse (either sexual or physical) is complex and needs careful assessment.

Diagnosis

The most important factors in the initial assessment of CPP include taking a detailed history (to include bowel, bladder and psychological symptoms) and performing a good clinical examination. A woman needs time in a clinical setting to feel that she has been able to tell her story and that she has been listened to and believed.

It is important to exclude organic causes of the pain. Basic investigations include:
- Screening for sexually transmitted infections (chlamydia, gonorrhoea) in all sexually active women
- Ca-125 especially if bloating, urinary urgency or frequency
- A transvaginal ultrasound scan and possible magnetic resonance imaging (MRI) to identify adnexal masses, fibroids and adenomyosis. MRI more sensitive and useful for evaluating rectovaginal endometriosis in the presence of nodules. MRI or 3D ultrasound in the assessment of uterine anomalies
- Laparoscopy to identify peritoneal endometriosis and adhesions. 33–50% may be negative and pathology identified may not be the cause of the pain
- X-rays are often indicated (e.g. plain X-rays of the lumbosacral spine and hips)
- Urinalysis, CT urogram or intravenous pyelogram (IVP) and cystoscopy may be necessary
- A barium enema, CT or colonoscopy may need to be considered

Management

Gynaecological pathology should be treated in the standard way. However, in many women with chronic pelvic pain, no clearly defined pathological cause will be found. In the absence of obvious pathology, reassurance is extremely important.

Patient symptoms are a very helpful guide to management:
- Treat underlying cause – offer medical or surgical treatment
- If a sexually transmitted infection (STI) is diagnosed ensure treatment is commenced and contact tracing arranged in conjunction with a genitourinary medicine physician
- Women with cyclical pain should be offered a therapeutic trial using hormonal treatment to suppress the ovaries, such as GnRH analogues or the oral contraceptive pill
- Adhesions – division of dense vascular adhesions may help, as will freeing of trapped organs but there is little evidence to suggest that fine adhesions cause CPP. There is very little scientific data to support use of antiadhesives at present, but these are not believed to be harmful
- Laparoscopic presacral neurectomy is the surgical removal of the presacral plexus that conducts pain signals from the uterus to the brain. It may be useful in central CPP. Can be effective – cure rates of up to 80% have been reported. Careful patient selection is essential. Complications include constipation, urinary disturbance and painless labour
- Laparoscopic uterosacral nerve ablation (LUNA) is not effective and should not be performed
- A negative laparoscopy may provide reassurance and symptoms may resolve
- Symptoms suggestive of IBS include: diarrhoea or constipation or both; episodes of pain more than once a month; relief of pain with defecation and abdominal distension, bloating, wind. There may also

be mucus passed per rectum, a feeling of faecal urgency and a feeling that symptoms are worse after eating. Women with IBS should be offered a trial of antispasmodics and advised to amend their diet and make lifestyle choices to eliminate precipitating factors. Regular meals and exercise help. Tea, coffee, alcohol and fizzy drinks should be restricted

- Psychotherapy is effective in this group of women along with careful explanation of the problem
- Referral to a pain team for optimum analgesia and medical treatment of neuropathic pain
- Support groups/cognitive behavioural therapy (CBT)

Further reading

RCOG Greentop Guideline No. 41. The initial management of chronic pelvic pain. London: Royal College of Obstetricians and Gynaecologists, 2012.

Lucas M, Pickersgill A, Smith RB. Chronic pelvic pain: Diagnosis and management. In: Christopher R Chapple et al., (Eds). Multidisciplinary Management of Female Pelvic Floor Disorders. Oxford: Churchill Livingstone, 2006.

NICE Clinical Guideline No. 61. Irritable bowel syndrome in adults. Diagnosis and management of irritable bowel syndrome in primary care. London: NICE, 2008.

Related topics of interest

Contraception: reversible methods

The ideal contraceptive (100% effective, completely reversible, totally acceptable and absolutely free of side effects) does not exist. Historically, contraceptive effectiveness has been expressed in the number of pregnancies per hundred women-years, also known as the Pearl Index. A more modern way of measuring contraceptive failure is life table failure probabilities which take into account women who leave a trial for a reason other than unintended pregnancy. Contraceptives can be divided into reversible methods, such as pills and condoms, and long-acting reversible contraception (LARC), such as implants and intrauterine methods. Reversible methods often have a significant difference in failure rates with typical and perfect use, whereas LARC methods do not. Contraceptive choice is dependent on lifestyle factors as well as medical contraindications. Factors affecting safety are detailed in the UK Medical Eligibility Criteria (UKMEC).

Fertility awareness methods

The time of maximum fertility is predicted from a combination of menstrual calendars, temperature charting, cervical secretion changes and fertility monitoring devices. To be effective, abstinence of intercourse must be practiced during the fertile days. The failure rate can be low with perfect use, but with typical use can be as high as 24%.

Barrier methods

These work on the principle of preventing the sperm gaining access to the upper genital tract. They are also used to reduce the spread of sexually transmitted infections. They include male and female condoms, diaphragms and cervical caps, and must be used before penetration occurs. Failure rates of barrier methods are very different with perfect and typical use, ranging from 2–15% with male condoms and 6–16% with the diaphragm. Diaphragms and caps should be used with additional spermicide.

Intrauterine contraception

This encompasses the intrauterine device (IUD) and intrauterine system (IUS). These are very effective methods as they do not rely on correct use by women, with failure rates of less than 1%. The main mode of action of copper IUDs is prevention of fertilisation with a backup mechanism of interfering with blastocyst implantation. Copper IUDs can be framed (banded or unbanded) or frameless (Gynefix), and have a surface area of copper of 300–380 mm^2. They can be left in situ for 5–10 years and in a woman of > 40 years may be left until the menopause. The IUD can be also used as emergency contraception – see below.

The IUS is a framed device with a slow release progestogen (levonorgestrel) sleeve around its stem. Its mode of action is hormonal, causing atrophy of the endometrium preventing implantation, and thickening of cervical mucus, making it impenetrable to sperm. The IUS is licensed for 5 years for contraceptive use and if fitted in a woman of > 45 years of age can be left until the menopause. The effect on the endometrium also leads to improvement in menstrual disorders, in contrast to the copper IUD which can increase menstrual blood loss and pain. Disadvantages of both IUD and IUS include uterine perforation (up to 2 in 1000), expulsion (one in 20), pelvic infection, and if pregnancy occurs, an increased risk of ectopic pregnancy, spontaneous abortion and preterm delivery. A sexual history should be taken at initial assessment and chlamydia/gonorrhoea tests performed in high risk women. Even if tests are negative, there is a 6-fold risk of pelvic inflammatory disease (PID) in the 20 days following insertion, after that infection rates fall to baseline levels. Emergency equipment including atropine should be available at time of fitting in case of cervical shock.

Combined hormonal contraception

Combined hormonal contraception (CHC) contains the hormones oestrogen and progestogen, and can be delivered orally, via a transdermal patch or a vaginal ring. Failure rates are 0.3% with perfect use but 9% with typical use. Non-contraceptive benefits include regulation of periods and reduced menstrual loss; reduction of androgenic effects such as acne; reduction of benign ovarian cysts; reduction in ovarian (20% for every 5 years of use), endometrial (50% reduction) and colorectal cancer and improvement of endometriosis. Risks include an increased risk of venous thromboembolism (VTE) and arterial disease, which escalate with age, obesity, cigarette smoking and other risk factors; and a small increased risk in cervical cancer, related to duration of use. Risk of breast cancer associated with CHC use is likely to be small, and will reduce with time after stopping.

Contraindications include conditions that increase risk of VTE, arterial disease (including some types of migraine) or liver disease, or where the condition is adversely affected by the hormones in CHC (refer to UKMEC). Before starting, CHC assessment should include a thorough medical history and measurement of blood pressure and body mass index. It can be continued until age 50 years in healthy women. Effectiveness is reduced by liver enzyme inducing drugs. A higher dose of combined oral contraceptive (50–70 µg oestrogen) can be given but it is usually more appropriate to change to an alternative method. Concomitant use of CHC and Lamotrigine is not recommended as CHC reduces the therapeutic effect of Lamotrigine. Side effects of CHC include breakthrough bleeding and mood changes. There is no evidence that it causes weight gain. CHC can be started up to day 5 of the cycle without the need for extra precautions or at any time (with extra precautions for 7 days) if there is no pregnancy risk.

Combined oral contraceptive (COC)
Commonly used pills contain 20–35 µg ethinylestradiol, and come in monophasic, phasic and every day regimes. They contain seven different progestogens, each with a slightly different profile. The risk of VTE amongst COC users is approximately twice that of non-users (9–10/10,000 woman-years), greatest in the first few months of starting. Pills with levonorgestrel (LNG) have been shown to have the lowest risk of VTE so should be used first line. Dianette contains an antiandrogen and is useful for treatment of severe acne and hirsutism, but is not licensed for use solely as a contraceptive. Effectiveness of COC is limited by vomiting and diarrhoea, and if pills are missed that extend the pill free interval to 9 days or more. Broad spectrum antibiotics do not reduce effectiveness of COC.
Transdermal patch   One patch containing ethinylestradiol and norelgestromin is applied weekly for 3 weeks, followed by a patch-free week.
Vaginal ring   This contains ethinylestradiol and etonogestrel and is inserted vaginally and retained for 3 weeks, followed by a ring-free week.

Progestogen methods

These methods work by enhancing cervical mucus hostility towards sperm, suppressing ovulation and affecting implantation. All progestogen methods can cause menstrual irregularity or amenorrhoea. Other side effects include mood changes and weight gain. Contraindications are few, with current breast cancer being the only absolute contraindication (refer to UKMEC). Effectiveness of progestogen-only pill (POP) and implants are reduced by liver enzyme inducing drugs, in contrast to injectable methods, which are unaffected.
POP   All POPs thicken cervical mucus and can inhibit ovulation. POP containing desogestrel (Cerazette) more reliably inhibits ovulation than traditional POPs. Efficacy is decreased if the time of taking is delayed by > 3 hours for traditional POPs and 12 hours for desogestrel pills. Failure rates vary from 0.3–9%.

Implants   Nexplanon is the only contraceptive implant currently available in the UK. It is a semi-rigid rod releasing etonorgestrel over 3 years, which is inserted subdermally over the triceps in the non-dominant arm. The main mode of action is prevention of ovulation. Failure rates are very low (< 1 in 1000 over 3 years). Levonorgestrel implants (Norplant and Jadelle) are available outside the UK.

Injectable contraception
Medroxyprogesterone acetate (DMPA, Depo-Provera) is a long-acting (12 weeks) progestogen given by intramuscular injection. It causes amenorrhoea in 70% of women at 1 year, and a delay in return to fertility after discontinuation. It is associated with a small reduction in bone density which is recovered on discontinuation. Norethisterone enantate is also available but rarely used. Failure rates for both are low (0.1–0.7%).

Emergency contraception   There are two types of oral methods. Levonorgestrel is licensed for use up to 72 hours, but has been shown to be effective up to 96 hours after risk. It was licensed for pharmacy sale in 2001. Ulipristal Acetate (UPA) (a selective progesterone receptor modulator) is licensed for use up to 120 hours after unprotected sexual intercourse (UPSI). Clinical trials comparing LNG with UPA have shown statistically significantly lower pregnancy rates in the UPA group. Effectiveness of both oral methods is reduced by liver enzyme inducing drugs, and UPA can reduce effectiveness of progesterone containing contraceptives. The IUD is the most effective method of emergency contraception, and should be inserted within 120 hours of UPSI, or up to 5 days after the earliest predicted time of ovulation.

Special groups

Contraceptives can be prescribed to girls under the age of 16 years without parental knowledge or consent, if they are assessed as competent to consent to treatment using the 'Fraser' guidelines, with specific reference to the risk of harm without treatment, the girl's ability to understand the implications of sexual activity/treatment and encouraging the girl to talk to parents/carers.

On reaching the menopause, contraception should be continued for 2 years after the last period if a woman is < 50 years and 1 year after the last period if a woman is > 50 years. If women are on hormonal contraceptives that mask their natural cycle, menopause can be diagnosed by raised follicle-stimulating hormone (FSH) levels (stop oestrogen containing contraceptives before testing).

Further reading

RCOG Faculty of Sexual and Reproductive Healthcare. UK Medical Eligibility Criteria for Contraceptive Use, 2009

Trussell, J. Contraceptive Failure in the United States. Contraception 2012; 83:397–404.

Related topics of interest

Contraception: sterilisation

Overview

Sterilisation provides a long term, permanent form of contraception and is the principal method used worldwide. In 2005, over 18,000 female sterilisations and over 28,000 vasectomies were performed in National Health Service (NHS) hospitals or clinics. The role of this form of contraception is changing as a greater choice of long term reversible methods of contraception has become available. More recent statistics have demonstrated that vasectomy rates have more than halved in 2011–2012, compared with 2001–2002. The declining numbers could be prompted by a number of factors, including awareness among men that a relationship may break down and that second families are becoming more common.

Both male and female sterilisations are surgical procedures and it is important that patients should be aware of the permanence of these fertility removing procedures. Alternative long-acting reversible methods of contraception and both male and female methods of sterilisation should be discussed at each consultation. Women in particular should be informed that vasectomy carries a lower failure rate in terms of post-procedure pregnancies and less surgical risks.

Male sterilisation

Procedure

Vasectomy can be performed under local anaesthetic and does not carry the risks associated with achieving a pneumoperitoneum necessary for female sterilisation. The vas deferens is exposed out of the scrotum through an incision and the vas is occluded or interrupted. A no-scalpel technique has been developed, where a fixation clamp is used to secure the vas without penetrating the skin, and a sharp dissecting forceps punctures the skin allowing the scrotum to be opened.

Effective contraception should be used until azoospermia (no sperm in the ejaculate) is confirmed. Postvasectomy semen analysis allows confirmation of clearance of stored spermatozoa downstream of the vasectomy site and allows detection of early recanalisation. In the UK, two postvasectomy samples are usually examined before clearance to stop contraception is given. The timing of the postvasectomy samples varies but the British Andrology Society guidelines for the assessment of postvasectomy semen samples recommend that initial assessment is undertaken 16 weeks postvasectomy and after the patient has produced at least 24 ejaculates.

Complications

Immediate complications following vasectomy include bruising and haematoma. Chronic testicular or scrotal pain may develop months or years after vasectomy. The incidence of chronic postvasectomy pain ranges from 12–52%. Previous concerns arising from epidemiological studies that suggested an increased risk of testicular cancer and cardiovascular disease following vasectomy were unfounded. There is no increase in testicular cancer or heart disease associated with vasectomy. Men should be reassured that the association of an increased risk of prostate cancer is non causative.

Failure rate

The failure rate of vasectomy is 1/2000 procedures after clearance has been given. Recanalisation or 'natural vasectomy reversal' is a rare event that develops in only 1 in 4000 vasectomies. This occurs when the cut ends of the vas deferens spontaneously connect.

Reversal

Vasectomy reversals or intracytoplasmic sperm injections (ICSI) are rarely provided within the NHS. The success rate of vasectomy reversal depends on the time since vasectomy, the type of vasectomy being reversed (open-ended, sealed with suture, sealed with heat), the type of reversal (vasovasostomy or vasoepididymostomy, unilateral or bilateral), the technique used (macrosurgical or microsurgical, one-layer or two-layer anastomosis), the surgical expertise, the presence of anti-sperm antibodies or other scrotal pathology. Success rates vary between 52% and 82%.

Female sterilisation

Procedure

Tubal occlusion can be performed either laparoscopically or by laparotomy under general anaesthesia. A mini-laparotomy can be performed if the laparoscopic approach has failed or been rejected because of previous abdominal surgery or obesity. Filshie clips are the most commonly used method of female sterilisation in the UK.

For mechanical occlusive methods (e.g. Filshie clip) to be successful, they must be applied to the right part of the tube, at right angles to the isthmic portion of tube, 1–2 cm from the cornu, making sure the whole width of the tube is encased. It is important that the ease of access to the tubes, clarity of identification of the tubes and accurate placement of the occlusive device is explicitly stated in the patient record. Multiple clips are not necessary for the procedure to be effective, unless there is doubt about the security of the first clip. The use of multiple clips may cause difficulties if a reversal is undertaken in the future. Tubal occlusion is associated with much more postoperative pain than a diagnostic laparoscopy. This may be due to tubal ischaemia and necrosis.

Hysteroscopic sterilisation by tubal cannulation and placement of intrafallopian implants can be performed under local anaesthetic or sedation. A flexible microinsert is passed through the hysteroscope and placed into each fallopian tube. This induces scar formation, which occludes the fallopian tubes and prevents conception. Additional contraception should be used until imaging by X-ray, ultrasound scanning and hysterosalpingogram demonstrates that the fallopian tubes have been occluded. This method is particularly suitable for women in whom general anaesthesia carries unacceptable risks or may require conversion to laparotomy.

Both laparoscopic tubal occlusion and hysteroscopic sterilisation can be performed as day case procedures.

Complications

Laparoscopic sterilisation carries risks of morbidity and mortality. Major complications include injuries to bowel, bladder and blood vessels that require laparotomy and in rare cases can lead to death. The risk of laparotomy in one large prospective study was 1.9/1000 procedures. Patients should be counselled of the risk of regret and the difficulties associated with reversal. Tubal occlusion in association with delivery or termination of pregnancy carries a higher regret rate. Women should be informed that if a tubal occlusion fails, there is an increased risk of an ectopic pregnancy.

Hysteroscopic sterilisation is associated with uterine perforation and the microinsert being placed into the peritoneal cavity. There is an increased risk of ectopic pregnancy if failure occurs.

Failure rate

The lifetime failure risk of tubal occlusion is 1/200. The longest period of follow up data available for the Filshie clip suggests a failure rate after 10 years of 2–3/1000 procedures. A lower failure rate is associated with a mini-laparotomy and a partial salpingectomy (usually a modified Pomeroy technique). The highest failure rates are amongst those performed at caesarean section or done in the immediate puerperium.

Studies on hysteroscopic sterilisation have reported a failure rate (pregnancy) of 1.1% after 1 year in 645 women. Women need to use an alternative form of contraception for up to 3 months after implant placement and the procedure may need to be repeated. In one study, approximately 15% of women did not have complete blockage of tubes after 3 months.

All women should be advised to continue effective contraception until the procedure and continue until the next menstrual period. If contraception was not being used, the operation should be deferred until the follicular phase of a subsequent menstrual cycle. A pregnancy test should be performed prior to tubal occlusion to exclude the possibility of a pre-existing pregnancy, but a negative test does not exclude the possibility of a luteal-phase pregnancy.

Further reading

RCOG. National Collaborating Centre for Women's and Children's Health, Male and Female Sterilisation. Evidence-based Clinical Guideline No. 4. London: RCOG, 2004.

National Institute for Health and Clinical Excellence. Female sterilisation using implants (inserted through the vagina) to block the fallopian tubes. Interventional Procedure Guidance. London: NICE, 2009;315.

Peterson HB. Sterilization. Obstet Gynecol 2008; 111:89–203.

Related topics of interest

- Contraception: reversible methods (p. 26)
- Ectopic pregnancy (p. 34)
- Subfertility: medical and surgical management (p. 142)

Dyspareunia

Overview

Dyspareunia (from the Greek meaning 'badly matted') is defined as pain during or after sexual intercourse. It can be associated with physical or psychological factors. It affects up to 20% of women at some point during their lives.

Definition

The Diagnostic and Statistical Manual of Mental Disorders (DSM-IV) defines it as being when a woman complains of recurrent or persistent genital pain before, during or after sexual intercourse that is not caused exclusively by lack of lubrication or by vaginismus.

It must be differentiated from vaginismus which is due to spasm of the pubococcygeus muscle leading to closure of the vaginal introitus, preventing penetration. However, it should be noted that vaginismus may occur secondary to dyspareunia or cause it.

It can be divided into two distinct groups. Superficial is defined as introital pain and deep is defined as pelvic pain. There can be an overlap and some women experience both.

Aetiology

The aetiology of dyspareunia is complex and may be multifactorial. It can be due to congenital conditions (e.g. vaginal septum or hypoplasia of the introitus) or acquired. There may be several factors involved and as well as physical elements, there is often a psychological overlay in either causing or prolonging the pain.

Causes

(Not in order of frequency and not exhaustive)

Superficial
1. Vulval causes
- Impersforate hymen, vaginal atresia
- Infective – herpes simplex virus (HSV), human papillomavirus (HPV), candidiasis
- Vulval dystrophy
- Localised vulval dysaesthesia (LVD) (common premenopausally)
- Traumatic
- Atrophic changes (common postmenopausally)
- Vulval carcinoma
- Female genital mutilation
- Postpartum, e.g. poor perineal repair or scarring, granulation tissue, dryness secondary to breastfeeding
- Iatrogenic – after a posterior repair
2. Vaginal causes
- Congenital – stenosis, bands
- Infective – HSV, HPV, *Candida, Chlamydia*
- Atrophic changes
- Behcets syndrome
- Bartholin's cysts/abscess
- Urethral caruncle
- Fistula
- Vaginal carcinoma
- Postradiotherapy
- Sjögren's syndrome – associated with vaginal dryness
- Mesh erosion (following prolapse or incontinence surgery)

Deep
1. Cervical
- Cervicitis secondary to infection
2. Uterine
- Endometritis: *E. coli, Chlamydia*, anaerobic streptococci, etc.
- Adenomyosis
- Retroversion – secondary to any cause [endometriosis, fibroids, pelvic inflammatory disease (PID)]
- Prolapse
3. Adnexae
- Ovaries – prolapsed into the Pouch of Douglas (POD) due to retroversion, adherent, retained after hysterectomy
- Endometriosis
- Ovarian cysts
- Pelvic inflammatory disease
- Ectopic pregnancy
- Hydrosalpinx
- Ruptured uterosacral ligament
- Adhesions

4. Extrapelvic
- Appendicitis
- Inflammatory bowel disease
- Diverticular disease
- Tuberculosis
- Constipation
- Irritable bowel syndrome
- Interstitial cystitis
- Urinary infections
5. Psychological associations
- Traumatic delivery
- Sexual abuse
- Depression and anxiety

The most important factors in the initial assessment of dyspareunia include taking a detailed history (to include bowel, bladder and psychological symptoms) and performing a good clinical examination. The aim of the clinical examination is to try and duplicate the site or source of pain.

Any findings of trauma and the suspicion of female genital mutilation will require careful management.

Simple diagnostic investigations include urinalysis and a transvaginal scan or magnetic resonance imaging (MRI), screening for sexual diseases.

Laparoscopy is the investigation of choice for deep dyspareunia.

If all these logical causes have been ruled out, or appropriately treated, then the more difficult diagnosis of dyspareunia secondary to a psychosexual cause may be made and expert counselling should be introduced.

Management

The management depends upon the diagnosis and the woman's reproductive status:
- Infections should be treated with antibiotics
- Vaginal atrophy responds to topical oestrogens
- Surgery may be useful in the treatment of hydrosalpinges, endometriosis, ovarian pathology, prolapse, adhesions and fibroids
- Advice regarding sexual positions and referral onwards to a specialist in psychosexual disorders

Further reading

RCOG Green-top Guideline No. 36. Female Genital Mutilation and its Management. London: RCOG, 2009.
Ryan L, Hawton K. Female dyspareunia. BMJ 2004; 328:1357

Kettle C, Ismail KMK, O'Mahony F. Dyspareunia following childbirth. The Obstetrician and Gynaecologist 2005; 7:245–249.

Related topics of interest

- Female genital mutilation (p. 41)
- Sexual function (p. 132)
- Vulval pain syndromes and pruritus vulvae (p. 171)

Ectopic pregnancy

Overview

Ectopic pregnancy is defined as the implantation of a pregnancy outside the uterine cavity. Some definitions define it as the embryo developing outside the uterus, others the fertilised egg. It is uncommon to find a fetus developing and most are purely trophoblastic tissue.

The incidence and mortality associated with ectopic pregnancies varies worldwide. The rate is estimated to be 11/1000 with a death rate of 0.2/1000. Two-thirds of the deaths are associated with substandard care. This may be due to the failure to recognise the signs and symptoms, a lack of continuity of care via contact with several health care professionals or lack of understanding by some women of the need to access the health care system (e.g. refugees/asylum seekers) with sometimes vague symptoms.

The most common site of ectopic pregnancy is the ampulla of the Fallopian tube (about 80%) followed by other sites within the tube, the isthmus (12%) the fimbrial end and the cornua; these constitute 98% of the total. Other sites include the ovary, cervix, caesarean section scar, broad ligament and the abdomen. Rarely abdominal pregnancies can progress to viability and live babies have been delivered at a laparotomy.

Heterotopic pregnancy describes a rare situation (1 in 40,000) with coexisting ectopic and intrauterine pregnancies. The intrauterine pregnancy often progresses uneventfully.

Clinical features

Presenting symptoms:
- 93% abdominal or pelvic pain
- 73% with amenorrhoea
- 64% with vaginal bleeding (with or without clots)
- 20–30% with vague abdominal symptoms, fainting, syncope and breast tenderness
- 10–20% with shoulder tip pain. This results from peritoneal irritation secondary to bleeding from the tube

- < 10% with urinary symptoms, rectal pain, pressure or the passage of tissue

On examination:
- 91% pelvic tenderness
- 82% adnexal tenderness
- 78% abdominal tenderness
- 40–75% cervical motion tenderness/ peritoneal signs, e.g. rebound tenderness
- < 40% abdominal distension, an enlarged uterus or adnexal mass and signs of hypotension or tachycardia
- < 20% palpable mass or are shocked

A pregnancy test must be performed on women of reproductive age who present with any of the above symptoms to any health care worker.

If an ectopic pregnancy is considered then they should be referred to the local Early Pregnancy Assessment Unit (EPU).

Aetiology

There is no high quality evidence with regard to risk factors due to the numbers in the studies analysed. The data below is only of moderate quality at best:
- 33% – no identifiable risk factors
- 48% – smoking (low-quality evidence)
- 23% – prior pelvic or abdominal surgery
- 10–20%
  - Pelvic inflammatory disease – chlamydia, gonorrhoea
  - Infertility
  - Miscarriage
  - Previous temination of pregnancy
  - Previous ectopic pregnancy
  - Intrauterine contraceptive device (IUCD)
- < 10%
  - Oral contraceptives
  - Endometriosis (low quality evidence)
  - Previous tubal surgery, e.g. sterilisation, re-anastomosis
- Other reported risk factors include:
  - Exposure to diethylstilboestrol in utero
  - Non-caucasian and > 35 years old

Diagnosis

The diagnosis is normally based on scans, serum human chorionic gonadotropin (hCG) measurement and clinical symptoms.

- The date of the last period may not be accurate and should be ignored
- Transvaginal scan
  - Look for fetal pole. Fetal non-viability is diagnosed if no fetal cardiac activity with a crown-rump length (CRL) > 7 mm or a mean gestational sac diameter of 25 mm (otherwise repeat one week)
  - A pregnancy of unknown location (PUL) – an empty uterus with free fluid +/- adnexal mass
- Quantitative serum hCG helps distinguish ectopic pregnancies from early intrauterine ones and complete miscarriage. Progesterone is of little help:
  - If hCG increases > 63% after 48 hours – likely it is intrauterine. Repeat scan in one week
  - If hCG decreases > 50% after 48 hours – pregnancy unlikely to continue. Repeat urinary test at 2 weeks and if positive review
- With collapse (in a woman of reproductive age and a positive pregnancy test), the diagnosis may only be made at laparoscopy or laparotomy

Management

In shocked patients, immediate resuscitation followed by laparotomy (laparoscopy in experienced hands) usually resulting in a salpingectomy.

Medical

- Systemic methotrexate (50 mg/m^2 intramuscular) – successful in up to 92%
- Potassium chloride, adrenaline, PGE$_2$ and PGF$_{2\alpha}$ have been successfully injected into gestation sacs but are not recommended
- No differences in long term follow-up or repeat ectopic or intrauterine pregnancy compared with surgical management

- Methotrexate is recommended if there is:
  - minimal pain
  - an unruptured, adnexal mass < 35 mm
  - hCG < 1500 IU/L
  - no evidence of fetal heart (FH)

βhCG may rise (1–4 days) initially but then fall. Check levels on days 4 and 7 and monitor until negative. About 15% may require a second dose.

Surgery

- Surgery is recommended if there is:
  - significant pain
  - an adnexal mass > 35 mm
  - a viable ectopic (rare)
  - serum hCG > 5000 IU/L

(A choice of treatment can be offered for women with hCG between 1500 and 5000 IU/L with minimal pain.)

- Laparoscopic surgery is the treatment of choice. It is safe, as effective as a laparotomy, with shorter hospital stay, lower costs and quicker return to work
- Salpingectomy is the treatment of choice if the other tube is healthy (Figure 5). It is associated with lower rates of repeat ectopic pregnancy and similar rates of intrauterine pregnancy
- Linear salpingostomy and removal of the pregnancy is the operation of choice if the other tube is damaged. Trophoblastic tissue may persist (3–20%), and this is higher than with open surgery. Weekly serum hCG estimations should fall, becoming undetectable within an average of 4 weeks. Methotrexate given prophylactically significantly lowers the rate of persistent trophoblastic disease

Cervical ectopic

- Often unrecognised until the pregnancy has been evacuated, with the patient presenting as an incomplete miscarriage. The first signs of a problem are continual heavy bleeding; examination may reveal a sac-like cavity in the cervix with the body of the uterus palpable above
- Insert a 14-gauge Foley catheter into the uterus and inflate the balloon (up to

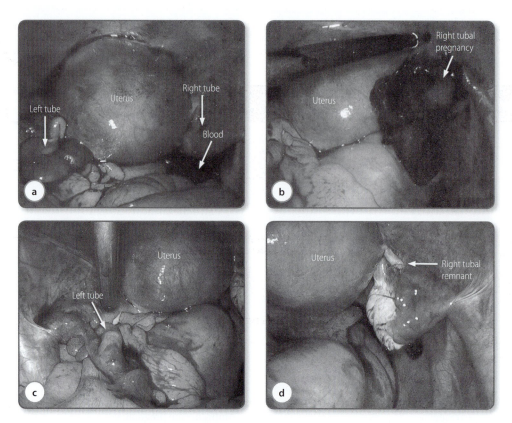

Figure 5 Laparoscopic right salpingectomy for tubal pregnancy. Laparoscopic view of pelvis showing (a) haemoperitoneum; (b) bleeding right tubal pregnancy; (c) normal left fallopian tube; and (d) right adnexa following salpingectomy. Photos courtesy of Dr Rick Clayton.

50 mL) until the locally applied pressure controls the bleeding. Release the pressure after 24 hours and remove the catheter. The catheter allows only blood from above the balloon to drain. The use of a circumcervical suture may be necessary to prevent the balloon slipping out
- Hysterectomy may be required

Cornual ectopic
- 2–4% of ectopics, with a relatively high mortality rate (2–2.5%)
- Difficult to diagnose – use magnetic resonance imaging (MRI) or 3D transvaginal scan

- Laparoscopic and hysteroscopic resection is required
- Systemic methotrexate may be needed as well
- Ultrasound or laparoscopic guided medical treatment is an option

Sequalae
Over 50% of women who have had an ectopic pregnancy wish to conceive again:
- 33% achieve a live infant
- 15% have another ectopic
- The risk of ectopic pregnancy after conservative surgery is:
  - 7% after laparoscopy
  - 14% after laparotomy

Further reading

NICE Clinical Guidance No. 154. Ectopic pregnancy and miscarriage: diagnosis and initial management in early pregnancy of ectopic pregnancy and miscarriage. London: NICE, 2012.
RCOG Green-top Guideline No. 21. The Management of Tubal Pregnancy. London: RCOG, 2010.

Hajenius PJ, Mol F, Mol BWJ, et al. Interventions for tubal ectopic pregnancy. Cochrane Database of Systematic Reviews 2009; 1:CD000324.

Related topics of interest

- Minimal access surgery (p. 91)
- Miscarriage (p. 94)
- Pelvic inflammatory disease (p. 112)

Endometriosis

Definition

Endometriosis is defined as the presence of endometrial glands and stroma outside the uterine cavity. It induces a chronic inflammatory reaction. It may affect as many as 2 million women in the UK. Its exact aetiology and pathogenesis is unknown. There is no known cure but it can be treated. Its associated symptoms can impact on every aspect of a woman's life and affect her partner too.

Aetiology

Endometriosis is a common disorder, especially in white British women, having a prevalence of 6–25% in most reported series. It is a disorder of the reproductive years, although postmenopausal endometriosis has been reported. There is no single theory that can account for endometriosis and it has been suggested that peritoneal disease and more infiltrative disease may actually be caused by different mechanisms.

- The most widely held theory is that of Sampson from 1921, who proposed the cause to be implantation of endometrial cells transported to the pelvic cavity by retrograde menstruation. Retrograde menstruation is an extremely common phenomenon as witnessed by laparoscopy. Most endometrium is probably cleared but perhaps in some women, in association with other unknown stimuli such as an autoimmune reaction, the presence of toxins (like dioxides) or a genetic predisposition, this tissue could establish as endometriotic deposits. However, endometriotic implants are not identical to eutopic endometrium, having structural and functional differences which may be relevant in explaining the pathogenic effects. It has also been identified in men

- **Müllerianosis** suggests that during embryological development, cells which have the potential to develop into endometrial cells are laid down outside the uterus. These migrating cells act like seeds. This theory is supported from fetal postmortem examinations

- **Coelomic metaplasia** (Meyer) suggests that the peritoneum can undergo metaplasia as the coelomic epithelium is the common ancestor of both the endometrium and peritoneum. Again there may be other stimuli associated with this

- **Vasculogenesis** is the process whereby ectopic endometrial tissue may originate from endothelial progenitor cells

- **Risk factors**
  - Genetics – changes in Chromosome 10 at 10q26
  - Environmental factors – dioxins (equivocal data)
  - Other – shorter menstrual cycle, early menarche

Clinical features

The main symptoms are cyclical pelvic pain, deep dyspareunia and infertility.

Other symptoms can include menorrhagia, ovulatory pain, dysmenorrhoea, fatigue, depression and symptoms suggestive of irritable bowel syndrome (IBS). Pains with voiding (dysuria) and defaecation (dyschezia) are frequently found. Thus, it is important to take a complete history to elucidate these symptoms. Cyclical bleeding from other organs may occur and rarely severe symptoms of intestinal obstruction or intraperitoneal bleeding are a feature.

Women with endometriosis often have fibroids, adenomyosis and non-gynaecological disease including hypothyroidism, rheumatoid arthritis, chronic fatigue syndrome, fibromyalgia, allergies and asthma. There is also a link with certain cancers including ovarian, brain and non-Hodgkin's lymphoma. Endometriosis increases the risk of preterm birth.

Endometriosis occurs more commonly on the left (except for the diaphragm). The main sites for endometriosis are:

- Ovaries
- Fallopian tubes

- Uterosacral ligaments
- Pouch of Douglas (cul-de-sac)
- Pelvic side wall
- Uterovesical pouch
- Large intestine – rectum and sigmoid more frequently than the caecum or appendix
- Bladder, ureters
- Distant sites – diaphragm, abdominal wall, umbilicus, skin, lungs, nose

It can be mild, affecting small areas, or be extensive and associated with severe adhesions and fibrosis.

Diagnosis

A good history and thorough clinical examination at the time of menstruation are helpful.

Biomarkers – a systematic review in 2010 concluded that none were of clear value at the present time.

Ca-125 has a low sensitivity and specificity in detecting endometriosis; it may indicate severe disease and cause confusion in the differential diagnosis of ovarian cysts.

Imaging techniques are poor at detecting superficial disease. Transvaginal scanning is useful in diagnosing adnexal masses and is almost as sensitive as magnetic resonance imaging (MRI). MRI is superior in looking at infiltrative disease either anterior or posterior to the uterus.

For a definitive diagnosis, laparoscopy remains the 'gold standard' to visualise the peritoneal cavity and assess the sites and severity of the disease, unless there are visible lesions infiltrating the posterior fornix of the vagina. Good practice includes examination of the Pouch of Douglas and the introduction of a secondary port to ensure adequate visualisation of the peritoneum. Laparoscopy is associated with about a 3% risk of minor complications and a 0.06–0.18% chance of major complications.

As there are many different types of endometriosis (powder burns, flame lesions, vesicular lesions, white glands, nodular disease) it is important that the surgeon thoroughly and closely inspects the peritoneum and familiarises themselves with the different appearances of the disease (**Figure 6**).

Positive histology is the only way that the disease can be confirmed.

Surgical staging uses the Revised Classification of the American Society of Reproductive Medicine and defines the disease as stage I (mild) to 4 (severe). This only identifies the physical disease and it does not correlate with symptoms and may not score highly for significant rectovaginal disease.

Management

A wide range of medical treatment options are currently available aimed at suppressing ovarian function and providing symptom relief. Supportive treatment with a range of simple analgesics may be helpful. Surgery is often relied upon and can be conservative or radical.

Medical

- Non-steroidal anti-inflammatory drugs may have a role in controlling the pain of endometriosis. However, there is

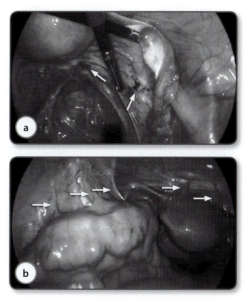

Figure 6 Laparoscopic view of endometriosis: (a) Typical small, flat dark patches or flecks of blue/black (powder burns) in right ovarian fossa and on the right uterosacral ligament (arrows). (b) Fine adhesions between the sigmoid colon and the left pelvic sidewall, and between the anterior surface of the uterus and the anterior abdominal wall (arrows). Photos courtesy of Dr Andrew Pickersgill.

no conclusive evidence about their effectiveness

- Suppressive therapy to mimic pregnancy – oral contraceptive pill, progestins
- Suppressive therapy to mimic menopause – gonadotropin-releasing hormone (GnRH) analogues with add-back hormone replacement therapy (HRT), aromatase inhibitors
- Danazol and gestrinone are suppressive steroids with androgenic activity and side effects limit their use

All medical options are equally effective and vary in their side effect profile. There is no role for medical treatment in women trying to conceive. Symptom recurrence is common on cessation of treatment. The levonorgestrel intrauterine system (LNG-IUS) reduces endometriosis-associated pain.

Surgical

- Conservative therapy consists of excising or destroying the ectopic endometrium (laser, diathermy, and Helium gas), removing the ovarian cysts and dividing the adhesions to restore normal anatomy

- The laparoscopic approach is recommended
- Surgery is recommended where fertility is required
- Recurrence rates of 20–40% within 5 years have been reported after conservative surgery. There is insufficient evidence to recommend hormonal treatment before or after surgery
- Laparoscopic ovarian cystectomy for endometriomas >4 cm improves fertility when compared to drainage and coagulation and is associated with a lower rate of recurrence
- A hysterectomy may be necessary if there is disease infiltrating it or adenomyosis is present. Other endometriosis should also be treated at the same time

Assisted conception

- Intrauterine insemination improves fertility if endometriosis is mild
- In vitro fertilisation (IVF) may be necessary especially if there are tubal or other factors
- GnRH for 3–6 months before IVF/intracytoplasmic sperm injection (ICSI) improves pregnancy rates

Further reading

Sampson JA. Perforating haemorrhagic (chocolate) cysts of the ovary. Their importance and especially their relation to pelvic adenomas of the endometrial type. Arch Surg 1921; 3:245–323.

RCOG Green-top Guideline No. 24. Endometriosis, Investigation and Management. London: RCOG, 2006.

ESHRE Guideline for the diagnosis and treatment of endometriosis. Grimbergen: ESHRE, 2007.

NICE Clinical Guidance No. 156. Assessment and treatment for people with fertility problems. London: NICE, 2013.

Related topics of interest

Female genital mutilation

Overview

Female genital mutilation (FGM) is defined as all procedures involving partial or total removal of the external female genitalia or other injury to the female genital organs, whether for cultural or other non-therapeutic reasons. It is estimated by the World Health Organization (WHO) that 130 million women worldwide have undergone genital mutilation and that in Africa, 3 million girls are at risk of undergoing some form of genital mutilation annually.

Traditionally FGM is carried out by an older woman with no medical training. Anaesthetics and antiseptics are not generally used. It is usually carried out using basic tools such as knives, scissors, scalpels, pieces of glass and razor blades. Often iodine or a mixture of herbs is placed on the wound to tighten the vagina and stop the bleeding. Girls are often between 4 and 10 years of age.

There are controversies over the use of the term 'mutilation': however, the use of the word reinforces the idea that this practice is a violation of human rights and thereby helps to promote international advocacy towards its abandonment. However, at the individual level, the term can be problematic and stigmatising and both the United Nations (UN) and WHO call for tact when dealing with individual patients. They suggest that the term 'cutting' or circumcision may be more acceptable.

FGM is an abuse of human rights and is also a child protection issue.

UK law

FGM is prohibited by law in England, Scotland and Wales, whether it is committed against a UK national or permanent UK resident in the UK or abroad. The 1985 Female Genital Mutilation Act states that it is an offence for any person: (a) to excise infibulate or otherwise mutilate the whole or any part of the labia majora or clitoris of another person; or (b) to aid, abet, counsel or procure the performance by another person of any of those acts on that other person's own body. In 2003, the penalty for a person found guilty of an offence under the Female Genital Mutilation Act was stipulated as a prison sentence of up to 14 years. No offence is committed if the cutting takes place while a woman is giving birth, provided that the purpose is connected with the labour or birth.

Classification

Female genital mutilation is classified by the WHO into four categories (**Table 7**).

Clinical features

FGM can cause many physical and emotional sequelae. Haemorrhage and infection are common and can be life-threatening.

It is estimated that 15% of fistulae are caused by FGM. One particular type, 'Gishiri cutting', commonly practised in Nigeria amongst the Hausa people, is more commonly associated with fistulae. A cut is made in the anterior wall of the vagina with an unsterilised sharp instrument. If the cut is made too deep, a hole is created between the bladder and the vagina resulting in a vesicovaginal fistula (VVF).

Later, women can experience post-traumatic stress syndrome and flashbacks,

Type	Description
Table 7 WHO classification of female genital mutilation	
I	Partial or total removal of the clitoris and/or the prepuce (clitoridectomy)
II	Partial or total removal of the clitoris and the labia minora, with or without excision of the labia majora (excision)
III	Narrowing of the vaginal orifice with creation of a covering seal by cutting and appositioning the labia minora and/or the labia majora, with or without excision of the clitoris (infibulation)
IV	All other harmful procedures to the female genitalia for non-medical purposes, e.g. pricking, piercing, incising, scraping and cauterising

inclusion cysts, neuroma, anorgasmia, apareunia, dyspareunia, dysmenorrhoea and recurrent urinary tract infection (UTI).

Management

To date there have been no cases brought to court of FGM being performed on a UK national; however, it is thought to be occurring covertly. Any female child born to a woman who has had FGM herself should be considered at risk. The mother should be informed of the UK law.

In the UK, rather than acute complications, it is the later sequelae of FGM that clinicians may need to manage. These are encountered in migrants to the UK.

Women may experience a range of sexual dysfunction including anorgasmia, dyspareunia or apareunia. Penetrative sexual intercourse is not possible following type III FGM. Some women will require deinfibulation to open the vagina. This procedure is normally performed under local anaesthetic.

Clinicians may also encounter women who have undergone FGM when they are in labour. An anterior episiotomy may be required to enable examination in labour, catheterisation and delivery of the baby. If an anterior episiotomy is performed it is illegal to resuture the labia in apposition effectively closing the vagina again. The edges of the open labia should be over sewn to prevent bleeding.

Prevention

In several countries many women believe that FGM is necessary to ensure acceptance by their community; they are unaware that FGM is not practiced in most parts of the world. There are many organisations working to educate women and thereby prevent FGM.

Further reading

RCOG Green-top Guideline No. 53. Female Genital Mutilation and its Management. London: RCOG, 2009.
Hussein E. Women's experiences, perceptions and attitudes of female genital mutilation: the Bristol PEER Study. Foundation for Women's Health Research and Development (FORWARD), 2010.
Anderson SHA, Rymer J, Joyce DW, et al. Sexual quality of life in women who have undergone female genital mutilation: a case-control study. BJOG 2012; 119:1606–1611.

Related topics of interest

Fertility preservation for cancer patients

Overview

As oncology treatments improve, the problems faced by cancer survivors become more important. Many survivors are young and are diagnosed and treated before they have children. Cancer and cancer treatments can significantly affect future fertility. It is therefore essential that patients are given the opportunity to discuss the effects of cancer treatments on their fertility and explore options for fertility preservation prior to treatment.

Patients in this situation are faced with two devastating diagnoses simultaneously – malignancy and future infertility, either of which can lead to significant psychological impact. Having to face both diagnoses can cause huge distress and counselling must be available. When seeing patients in this situation, it is important to consider not only how the cancer and its treatment may impact on a patient's fertility, but also how the cancer may impact on a subsequent pregnancy and how a pregnancy may impact on the underlying disease (see Topic 61). It is also important to consider the patient's prognosis and his or her support network as the welfare of a child conceived from fertility treatment must be paramount.

Male patients

Testicular cancer is the most common malignancy seen in young men. Haematological malignancies such as leukaemia and lymphomas are also seen frequently. Treatments may involve significant surgery (for testicular malignancies), chemo and radiotherapy. Systemic chemotherapy and pelvic radiotherapy may be associated with subsequent testicular failure and azoospermia. All men facing potentially sterilising therapies should be offered the opportunity to bank semen before they start treatment. A semen sample is produced, the sperm extracted and cryopreserved for the future. Samples can be legally stored for up to 55 years in the UK. When the patient returns to use the samples, they may be used for insemination. If there are additional female factors and/or the semen sample is poor quality, in vitro fertilisation (IVF) or intracytoplasmic sperm injection (ICSI) may be required.

Effects of oncology treatments on female fertility

Delay to conception

Most patients will be advised to delay conceiving for a period of time following cancer treatment. Female fecundity declines sharply in a woman's mid to late thirties and delay can significantly reduce the chance of conception. This is of particular importance following treatment for an oestrogen sensitive breast cancer as the woman will usually be placed on hormonal treatment for up to 5 years after initial treatment. If a woman is diagnosed in her mid-thirties, a 5-year delay is of huge significance.

Chemotherapy

Primordial follicles contain oocytes suspended during their first meiotic division. It takes 6–9 months for an oocyte to develop from this stage to ovulation. Chemotherapeutic agents act at the point of cellular division and hence oocytes are highly susceptible to the effects of chemotherapy. Women treated with chemotherapy are therefore at risk of oocyte damage which may ultimately result in ovarian failure. The risk of ovarian failure is higher with increased dose and duration of chemotherapy and with particular types of chemotherapeutic agent (e.g. alkylating agents are particularly toxic). It is also more likely in women with an already reduced reserve, i.e. older women. Women should be advised that menses may stop during chemotherapy, but may recover after treatment. Although some patients retain ovarian function after chemotherapy, many suffer premature ovarian failure and would need to consider treatment with donated oocytes if they wish to conceive. It is difficult to predict how individual patients will respond.

Radiotherapy

Whilst most chemotherapy treatments are administered systemically, radiotherapy is directed to a local area. Therefore, toxicity from radiotherapy is usually limited to the area treated. Pelvic radiotherapy is highly toxic to oocytes and it is extremely rare for women to retain significant ovarian reserve after such treatment. Additionally, pelvic radiotherapy is associated with uterine damage caused by fibrosis and a reduction in uterine blood flow; it is unlikely that the uterus exposed to pelvic radiotherapy would be able to support a pregnancy. Patients treated with pelvic radiotherapy need to consider fertility treatments using donated oocytes and a surrogate host.

Surgery

Obviously surgery for gynaecological malignancies can impact on a patient's chance of pregnancy in the future. Fertility options may therefore include the need for treatment with donated oocytes or a surrogate host. It is important that a patient's desire for future pregnancies is always considered and that fertility sparing treatment is performed whenever possible.

Fertility preservation options

It is crucial that young women diagnosed with a malignancy have access to a fertility specialist to discuss the effect that their cancer treatment may have on their fertility in the future and whether there is a possibility of storing genetic material, either oocytes or embryos for future use.

Oocyte cryopreservation

If a woman does not have a long term partner, she may attempt to store oocytes. Following a cycle of ovarian stimulation and oocyte

recovery (similar to that of an IVF cycle), all retrieved oocytes are cryopreserved by the process of vitrification. Vitrification freezes oocytes extremely rapidly and appears to be the optimal method. Mature oocytes are very large cells and the chromosomes within them are arranged along a spindle rather than within the nucleus. These properties make oocytes very sensitive to disruption from the freezing process. In the UK, cryopreserved oocytes can be stored for up to 55 years. When the patient returns after completion of her cancer treatment, the cryopreserved oocytes are thawed and each surviving oocyte injected with a single sperm using ICSI. Although more than 90% of oocytes survive vitrification and fertilisation rates are similar to those seen with 'fresh' oocytes, the resulting embryos tend to be of poorer quality resulting in lower pregnancy rates. More than 1000 babies have been born following oocyte cryopreservation but the technique still has a relatively poor success rate, compared to treatments using non-frozen oocytes.

Embryo cryopreservation

If the patient is in a stable relationship, the couple may wish to cryopreserve embryos instead of oocytes. The woman undergoes a cycle of ovarian stimulation and oocyte retrieval as in conventional IVF. On the day of oocyte collection, an attempt to fertilise all mature oocytes is made, either by conventional IVF or, if the sperm is of poorer quality, ICSI. The following day all fertilised oocytes are cryopreserved at the pronuclear stage and, in the UK, may be stored for up to 55 years. Embryo cryopreservation is a relatively successful procedure and follow up studies on babies born are reassuring. Approximately, 1:3 couples will conceive following embryo cryopreservation if the female partner is less than 35 years. Although more successful than oocyte cryopreservation, embryo storage should only be carried out for couples in a stable relationship as, if the couple separate, the male partner may withdraw his consent for continued storage and treatment. As a result, the embryos would have to perish.

Risks of fertility preservation treatments

Throughout, it is important that there is close communication between the fertility specialist and the clinician responsible for the patient's oncology treatment to ensure that fertility treatment does not pose significant risk.

Delay to cancer treatment

When the intention is to cryopreserve oocytes or embryos, ovarian stimulation can start at any time in the menstrual cycle as there is no need for synchronisation of the endometrium. However, ovarian stimulation takes a minimum of just over 2 weeks. It is therefore crucial that patients are referred as early as possible in their pathway to avoid delaying their oncology treatment. In some cases, such as acute leukaemia, any delay to the start of chemotherapy may be significantly detrimental and these patients are not suitable for treatment.

Risk of high circulating oestradiol during stimulation

High levels of oestradiol are seen during ovarian stimulation cycles. This could pose risk to women diagnosed with an oestrogen sensitive breast cancer. Cotreatment with Letrozole (an aromatase inhibitor) is associated with significantly lower oestradiol levels. There are no large, long term follow up studies, but early data have not demonstrated an increased risk of recurrence or disease progression in this group of patients.

Risk from oocyte retrieval

There is a potential risk for patients with ovarian malignancies following oocyte collection when there could be spill of malignant cells from the ovary into the peritoneal cavity, although in practice this is rarely thought to be significant. Discussion between the oncologist and fertility specialist is essential to minimise possible harm.

Ovarian hyperstimulation syndrome (OHSS)

OHSS is a complication seen in approximately 1% of patients undergoing a cycle of ovarian hyperstimulation for oocyte recovery. The risk is no higher in fertility preservation patients, but it is particularly important to minimise risk so that the patient is in the best position to commence her oncology treatment.

After oncology treatment

Many patients will present for fertility investigations after cancer treatment. Assessment can be carried out as for any couple. If a woman retains ovarian function after chemotherapy, she should be advised to try to conceive as soon as possible, as she has a higher risk of premature ovarian failure. Additionally investigation and treatment should be carried out without unnecessary delay. However, it is important to wait at least 9 months after the completion of treatment before assessing resultant ovarian reserve.

Further reading

Reddy J, Oktay K. Ovarian stimulation and fertility preservation with the use of aromatase inhibitors in women with breast cancer. Fertil Steril 2012; 98:1363–1369.

Jeruss JS, Woodruff TK. Preservation of fertility in patients with cancer. N Eng J Med 2009; 360:902–911.

Duncan FE, Jozefik JK, Kim AM, et al. The gynaecologist has a unique role in providing oncofertility care to young cancer patients. US Obstet Gynecol 2011; 6:24–34.

Related topics of interest

Fibroids

Overview

Fibroids, also known as myomas or leiomyomas, are the commonest benign tumour of the genital tract, being present in up to 25% of women of reproductive age. This prevalence is thought to be grossly underestimated, if the incidental diagnosis of fibroids at histology in clinically asymptomatic patients is taken into account. Fibroids arise from the myometrium and are composed of whorls of smooth muscle and connective tissue. There is a risk of sarcomatous change in 0.2%.

Classification (Figure 7)

Submucous   Project into the uterine cavity – can be polypoid, result in menorrhagia (~11%).
Intramural   Within the uterine wall; surrounded by a so-called 'false capsule' (~73%).
Subserous   Seen on the surface of the uterus – can be pedunculated (~16%).
Cervical   Associated with delivery problems and surgical removal can be fraught.
Intraligamentary   Fibroid grows within broad ligament, causes ureteric compression.
Parasitic   A fibroid attached outside the uterus, i.e. to the bladder.

Clinical features

Uterine fibroids may be completely asymptomatic in up to 50%. For others, there may be a number of presenting features. The most common symptoms tend to be abnormal bleeding, pelvic pain or abdominal bloating. Heavy menstrual bleeding or dysmenorrhoea tends to result from submucous fibroids.

Pelvic pain can be caused by pressure symptoms, which may also contribute to bladder and bowel dysfunction, or as the result of degeneration or torsion.

Other problems include subfertility and early miscarriage secondary to impaired implantation due to uterine cavity distortion from intramural fibroids.

Up to one-third of pre-existing fibroids grow during the first trimester of pregnancy. Ongoing pregnancies can be complicated by preterm labour, abruption, malpresentation, labour dystocia, caesarean section and postpartum haemorrhage. Abdominal pain is common in pregnancy and can be caused by fibroids. Pain tends to be constant and localised over the fibroid itself. Ultrasound scan (USS) may show evidence of degenerative cystic changes (red degeneration). Pain in pregnancy due to fibroids is managed with analgesia.

Aetiology

Essentially the aetiology of fibroids is unknown, although the gene coding for the mitochondrial enzyme ferrous fumatase has been thought responsible for a rare syndrome characterised by uterine fibroids and multiple cutaneous leiomyomatosis.

Deletions of chromosome 7 have been found in 50% of histolological specimens,

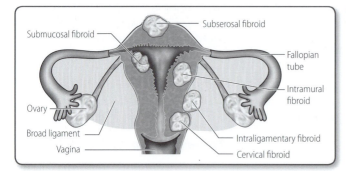

Figure 7 Classification of uterine fibroids.

although this is hypothesised to be more of a secondary event.

Fibroids are hormone dependent, with the main regulators both oestrogen and progesterone. To this extent fibroid myometrium consists of more receptors for these ovarian steroids than normal myometrium.

As a number of growth factors are responsible for mediating the action of steroid hormones on the uterus, these will also factor into fibroid growth.

There is an increased risk of fibroids with nulliparity, diabetes, hypertension, obesity, black race (more likely to have multiple, larger, more symptomatic fibroids presenting at a younger age), hereditary factors and polycystic ovarian syndrome.

Conversely, the use of the oral contraceptive pill and Depo-Provera are protective factors, as is smoking.

As one would expect with fibroids being hormonally fuelled, they tend to regress following the menopause.

Diagnosis

A thorough history and clinical examination should form the basis of any attempt at diagnosis.

USS   With expertise and the use of a vaginal probe it is possible to get an accuracy of approximately 80%. The number, size and position of fibroids should be documented, along with the overall dimensions of the uterus. Transvaginal saline infusion sonography may improve diagnostic accuracy.

Magnetic resonance imaging (MRI)   Has arguably no advantage over transvaginal USS, although may allow for better differentiation between an ovarian mass and a fibroid uterus.

Laparoscopy   Direct visualisation can be useful.

Hysteroscopy   Important in assessment of infertility and recurrent miscarriage to detect submucous fibroids, or any further intrauterine pathology.

X-ray   Calcified fibroid tissue may be visible on X-ray.

Management
Medical

It can be initiated in the primary care setting if the uterus palpates clinically, no larger than 10–12 week of gestation size.

Non-hormonal

- Non-steroidal anti-inflammatory drugs (NSAIDs) not found to be effective
- Tranexamic acid may reduce blood loss significantly by up to 50%
- Herbal preparations have not been evaluated in studies with sufficient quality or quantity. The effect of preparations such as Huoxue Sanjie and Nona Roguy is neither supported nor refuted by the data available to date

Hormonal

- Combined oral contraceptive pill (COCP) can bring about a significant reduction in blood loss if used in high doses
- Progestogens/antiprogesterones/ androgens – progestogens do not shrink fibroids, therefore their use is purely symptomatic. Long term medroxyprogesterone acetate (MPA) protects against development of fibroids. Androgens, e.g. danazol and androgenic antiprogesterone gestrinone reduce fibroid size. Mifepristone reduces heavy bleeding and improves quality of life. However, it was not found to reduce fibroid volume
- Levonorgestrel-releasing intrauterine system – not really for fibroids > 3 cm in size as there is an increased risk of expulsion (6–13% expulsion rate compared to 3% in the general population), and reduced efficacy. Its role in the management of fibroids has yet to be extensively researched
- Gonadotropin-releasing hormone (GnRH) analogues may allow shrinkage (36–49% within 3 months) such that a vaginal hysterectomy can be performed. They reduce anaemia (with increased ferritin, haemoglobin and haematocrit concentrations) and therefore the need for transfusion. Reduced intraoperative blood loss has also been reported

- Successful reduction of fibroid volume does not occur if add-back therapy is commenced simultaneously, therefore it should be delayed for 3 months. Add-back has been used successfully to treat fibroids for up to 2 years. On stopping treatment, the fibroids return within 6 months
- Reduced success rates in obese women and those with raised oestradiol levels after 3 months
- The antiprogesterone mifepristone has also been shown to decrease uterine volume and blood flow similarly to GnRH

Surgical

- Surgical treatment is classically by hysterectomy, usually by the abdominal route (**Figure 8**), although vaginal hysterectomy is advocated by some for fibroids up to 20 weeks.
- Myomectomy may conserve fertility, but the recurrence rate can be as high as 30%. The use of vasopressin has been advocated to reduce blood loss at myomectomy. Simultaneous hysterectomy is a significant risk and the patient must be warned of this.
- Laparoscopic myomectomy requires considerable skill and may be a lengthy operation. The upper limit of the fibroid is 10 mm and there should be no more than four present
- Laser/heat/cold coagulation (myolysis) has also been successfully used, where the probe is inserted into the centre of the fibroid resulting in necrosis
- Vaginal myomectomy may be possible, but again requires considerable skill
- Hysteroscopic removal with or without simultaneous endometrial ablation is an option. Pedunculated and submucous fibroids can be shaved to the level of the uterine cavity. For larger fibroids devascularisation followed by removal as a two-stage procedure may be advocated
- Laparoscopic uterine artery occlusion and temporary transvaginal uterine artery occlusion are relatively new techniques

Interventional radiology

Uterine artery embolisation (UAE):
- Performed under radiological guidance and using local anaesthesia, UAE involves catheterisation of the uterine arteries via one or both femoral arteries and injection of polyvinyl particles to embolise the uterine vascular bed
- Gradual shrinkage of fibroids with a mean of 60% at 6 months
- Complications include the formation of local haematomas, urinary retention, mild febrile reactions (postembolization syndrome), vaginal discharge and sepsis
- Randomised controlled trials (RCTs) comparing UAE, hysterectomy and myomectomy show that UAE has shorter hospital stay, faster return to work. Further intervention rates higher in UAE (23% chance of requiring further treatment a mean of 4.6 years after UAE)
- Pregnancies after UAE. Small numbers, but a number of potential complications

MRI focused ultrasound:
- Non-invasive thermal ablation device integrated with MRI system for the ablation of soft tissue. Food and Drug Administration (FDA) approved in the USA, but still under evaluation in the UK. The current National Institute for Health

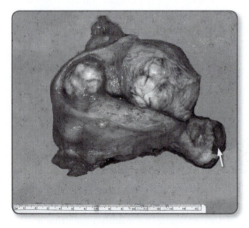

Figure 8 Hysterectomy specimen with cervix (arrow), both tubes and ovaries attached. The uterine body has been opened from fundus to endocervix to demonstrate multiple, large submucous fibroids within the uterine cavity. Photo courtesy of Mr Richard Slade.

and Clinical Excellence (NICE) guideline IPG413 suggests that current evidence is adequate, but further treatment may be required and the effect on pregnancy is unknown.

Further reading

Levy BS. Modern management of uterine fibroids. Acta Obstetricia et Gynecologica Scandinavica 2008; 87: 812–813

National Collaborating Centre for Women's and Children's Health. Heavy Menstrual Bleeding. London: National Collaborating Centre for Women's and Children's Health, 2007.

National Institute for Health and Clinical Excellence. Uterine artery embolisation for fibroids, IPG367. London: NICE, 2010.

Related topics of interest

- Hysterectomy (p. 74)
- Intermenstrual, postcoital and postmenopausal bleeding (p. 82)
- Heavy menstrual bleeding (p. 61)

Fistulae in obstetrics and gynaecology

Overview

A fistula is defined as a communication between two epithelial or endothelial surfaces. It is usually an acquired condition. Vesicovaginal fistulae (VVF) have three major causes:

- Obstetric
- Following pelvic surgery
- Radiotherapy

The most common cause of a VVF in the UK is pelvic surgery, whereas in the developing world it is obstructed labour. In the UK, there are approximately 100–120 new diagnoses of VVF per annum. In the developing world, there may be as many as 50,000–100,000 new cases each year.

Clinical features

There are early symptoms and signs of urinary tract injury which if recognised and acted upon may prevent fistula development. Persistent haematuria after pelvic surgery may be indicative of bladder injury and may warrant cystoscopic investigation. Loin pain and fever in the early postoperative period may indicate ureteric injury. Hyponatraemia may result from free spillage of urine into the peritoneal cavity, as reabsorption of water causes a decrease in serum osmolality and serum sodium. A full blood count may show an elevated white cell count with a neutrophilia. An urgent CT urogram and urology opinion should be sought if there are concerns about the integrity of the urinary tract. If these early signs and symptoms are missed then patients may present at a later date with constant leakage of urine due to the formation of a fistula.

Insensible, unprovoked or constant urinary leakage is the classical presentation of a urogenital fistula. A woman who develops leakage of urine after any pelvic surgical intervention should be considered to have a fistula until proven otherwise. Early prolonged catheterisation, for 6–12 weeks, may allow a small fistula to heal spontaneously.

Aetiology

Nearly all fistulae in the UK are iatrogenic in origin. Most cases of surgical damage to the urinary tract occur in patients with abnormal pelvic anatomy, e.g. those with congenital anomalies, dense adhesions, endometriosis, malignancy, large pelvic masses or previous radiotherapy. The need to control severe haemorrhage at, e.g. emergency caesarean hysterectomy, also increases the risk of injury. The incidence of fistulae following hysterectomy in the UK is approximately 1 in 780 cases; however, the incidence varies depending on the type of hysterectomy performed.

- 1 in 3861 – Vaginal hysterectomy
- 1 in 2279 – Subtotal hysterectomy
- 1 in 540 – Benign abdominal hysterectomy
- 1 in 100 – Radical hysterectomy

If bladder damage is noted at the time of surgery, it should be repaired with a 3/0 polyglycolic acid suture. This may be done with a single or double suture layer. It should be followed by 7–10 days free urinary drainage via a catheter. After the catheter has been removed, if the patient is wet, a methylene blue dye test should be performed to exclude a fistula.

If ureteric damage is suspected intraoperatively, an urologist should be called to evaluate the ureter. If injury is confirmed, ureteric repair followed by short term (6 weeks) ureteric catheterisation with a double J stent may be all that is required. Other injuries may warrant ureteric reimplantation, particularly if a large portion of the ureter has been damaged or excised.

Diagnosis

It is essential to have a high index of clinical suspicion for possible urinary fistulae following complex pelvic surgery.

Most of the VVF can be diagnosed by observing the anterior vaginal wall whilst filling the bladder with a solution of dilute methylene blue dye. If a VVF is present, blue dye will be seen in the vagina. If clear fluid, instead of blue, is seen in the vagina, a ureteric injury and an ureterovaginal fistula is more likely.

Occasionally, if the leakage of urine is intermittent, a 3 swab test is required to detect the fistula. Three cotton wool balls are inserted into the vagina and the bladder is filled with methylene blue. These are removed after 30-60 minutes, prior to micturition. If the cephalid cotton wool ball is stained blue and the caudal one is not, then a fistula must be present.

Once the presence of a fistula has been confirmed it is advisable to perform a CT urogram to establish that there has not been concurrent injury to the upper urinary tracts. The CT urogram will demonstrate the level of ureteric obstruction and/or injury. There is currently no agreed classification system for the VVF.

Management

If the VVF is small and diagnosed soon after the original surgery, conservative management with free catheter drainage for up to 12 weeks may allow the fistulous tract to close.

Surgical repair is usually performed as a planned procedure about 8–12 weeks after the initial surgery that caused the VVF. This allows postsurgical inflammation to resolve. The repair of a VVF should be performed by an experienced surgeon, as the chances of success are greatest with the first attempt. There should be adequate exposure, careful dissection of the fistulous tract, accurate suturing of the bladder without tension in one or two layers, followed by closure of the vagina. The repair is checked with a small volume of methylene blue to confirm that it is watertight. Continuous drainage of the bladder is essential with a urethral and/or suprapubic catheter postoperatively.

Most of the VVF can be repaired vaginally, some require an abdominal approach and some can be repaired laparoscopically. Occasionally, an interposing graft of fat is used between the bladder and vagina if tissue viability is thought to be poor. The fat can be obtained from the labia majora, a Martius graft if a vaginal approach is being used, or from the omentum if the procedure is performed abdominally. The most important aspect of management following the repair is to ensure the bladder remains empty for at least 7 days to avoid tension on the suture line. The duration of catheterisation following repair of a fistula is not evidence-based and practice varies from 7–28 days.

There is currently inadequate evidence about the role of prolonged courses of antibiotics following VVF repair.

Following radiotherapy some fistulae may be inoperable due to the degree of tissue damage and may require urinary diversion.

Further reading

Hilton P, Cromwell D. The risk of vesicovaginal and urethrovaginal fistula after hysterectomy performed in the English National Health Service—a retrospective cohort study examining patterns of care between 2000 and 2008. BJOG 2012; 119:1447–1454.

Clement KM, Hilton P. Diagnosis and management of vesicovaginal fistulae. The Obstetrician & Gynaecologist 2001; 3:173–178.

Kelly J. Repair of obstetric fistulae: review from an overseas perspective. The Obstetrician & Gynaecologist 2002; 4:205–211.

Related topics of interest

Forensic gynaecology

Overview

Sexual violence is a common but often hidden problem. Although women and girls are more at risk, men and boys can also be victims. Figures from surveys such as the British Crime Survey indicate a high prevalence both for child sexual abuse and abuse against adults. Each year, over one million women suffer domestic abuse, over 300,000 women are sexually assaulted and 60,000 women are raped.

Sexual violence can have a huge impact on both immediate and long term physical and psychological wellbeing.

Doctors should know how to respond to a direct disclosure and perhaps more importantly they should be alert to the possibility of sexual violence as the root of other presentations, e.g. chronic pelvic pain, sexually transmitted infections, requests for emergency contraception, unplanned pregnancy, and mental health problems including depression, self-harm, and substance misuse.

Contrary to popular belief, stranger assaults are not the norm and most victims will be attacked by someone known to them including family members, partners, ex-partners, acquaintances and friends.

History and examination

Wherever possible victims of rape or serious sexual assault should be seen in a dedicated unit, such as a Sexual Assault Referral Centre (SARC) by a forensic physician with the appropriate skills and experiences.

The initial assessment should cover a number of areas including:

- Safety issues
  - Are there any immediate safety concerns for the patient, third parties, such as dependent children, health care workers involved?
- Therapeutic needs
  - Emergency contraception, pregnancy testing

  - Postexposure prophylaxis for HIV, hepatitis B
  - Screening for sexually transmitted infections
  - Are there injuries that need assessing and treating?
- Psychological needs
  - Mental capacity assessment
  - Mental health assessment, risk of self-harm, post-traumatic stress disorder
  - Vicarious trauma to those caring for the victim
- Forensic considerations
  - Documentation of allegations
  - Is there forensic evidence, such as trace evidence, e.g. DNA, that could be obtained?
  - Identification and documentation of injuries
  - All of the above needs to be collected in a manner that would make it admissible to any subsequent court process
- Legal considerations
  - Does the victim wish to involve the police?
  - Does the doctor have a statutory and/or ethical duty to involve police or social care?
  - Has the victim the capacity to consent to a forensic examination and if not, does the best interest arguments apply?
  - What are the limitations to confidentiality regarding information gathered?
  - Are there safeguarding duties?

History taking should be mindful of the above. Record keeping must reflect the high likelihood of future legal scrutiny and therefore be contemporaneous, comprehensive and comprehensible. Objective findings must be clearly separated from subjective opinion.

Regarding the actual allegations it is important that leading questions are not asked.

Should direct questions about the nature and extent of the sexual acts be necessary, both questions and answers should be recorded verbatim, with careful recording of who provided the information and who else was present at that time.

The Faculty of Forensic and Legal Medicine has developed proformas as an aide-memoire for this purpose.

Although it is vital that the patient is treated with great respect and sensitivity, equally the doctor must be independent and open-minded.

Information that will help put forensic findings into context, e.g. time passed, actions since assault, medication, etc. should be gathered.

Obtaining evidence

Forensic evidence may take various forms, e.g.
- The allegations as disclosed by the patient
- Physical findings such as injuries
- Forensic samples that might link the victim to the suspect or crime scene, e.g. toxicology, DNA from saliva, semen, blood, DNA from products of conception.

Most rape victims, even if examined within hours of the assault, will have either no injuries or only a few minor ones that would rapidly heal leaving no trace. Of course there will be some who sustain life-threatening injuries but these are rare.

Injuries, if present, should be carefully documented including precise description such as type, size, shape, depth, position from a fixed bony point, swelling, evidence of healing, etc.

If possible, injury descriptions should be accompanied by line drawings, body maps and photographs.

The Faculty of Forensic and Legal Medicine produces 'Recommendations for the Collection of Forensic Specimens from Complainants and Suspects', a document which is updated every 6 months. These set out what samples may be useful, the time frames in which they should be taken, and how they should be collected and stored.

Samples must be taken and stored in a way that minimises risk of cross contamination and allows any results to be admissible to court, e.g. clear record of the chain of evidence.

Management

Best management will include:
- Making health service provision such that it provides opportunities for disclosure. Remember domestic abuse may include rape and sexual assault, both frequently kept secret.
- Appropriate response from the clinician when disclosure made, e.g. non-judgemental, avoid open disbelief.
- Assess need for immediate intervention
- Awareness of appropriate local specialised services
- Provide victim with options and help facilitate any referrals
- Excellent record keeping
- Awareness of safeguarding responsibilities
- Patient feedback
- Awareness training of staff, including prevalence, signs and symptoms, risk factors, local services

Legal issues

The Sexual Offences Act 2003 will be the legislation covering most of the sexual allegations.

Other legal considerations might include The Mental Capacity Act 2005 and 2007, Data Protection Act 1998, and The Children Act 2004.

Forensic medicine is the interface between medicine and the law. It can often throw up ethical dilemmas such as the balance between autonomy of the individual versus public interest and protection of others.

When facing difficult decisions, doctors are urged to seek early advice from senior colleagues, safeguarding teams, Caldicott Guardians and medical defence organisations, and as always keep good records of such discussions and subsequent action plans.

Safeguarding

As discussed above, safeguarding issues are common in patients of sexual violence. Safeguarding issues may not always be obvious.

Consider if the patient is:
- A child who is being abused
- Are there other children at risk?

- An adult but with dependent children who are at risk themselves of abuse or suffering as a result of witnessing the abuse
- A vulnerable adult
- Given the details of the assailant and abuse, are there others at risk, e.g.

the assailant is in a position of care, custody or control such as a care worker, teacher, etc.

Know your local safeguarding procedures. If in doubt about a case seek advice.

Further reading

General Medical Council. Protecting children and young people: The responsibilities of all doctors. London: GMC, 2012.

The Physical Signs of Child Sexual Abuse. An evidence-based review and guidance for best practice. London: Royal College of Paediatrics and Child Health, 2008.

Eddy JW, James HM. Forensic gynaecological examination for beginners: management of women presenting at A&E. The Obstetrician & Gynaecologist 2005; 7:82–88.

Related topics of interest

- Paediatric gynaecology (p. 108)
- Termination of pregnancy (p. 146)
- Sexually transmitted infection (p. 135)

Genital prolapse

Overview

Pelvic organ prolapse (POP) is common. Approximately, 1 in 10 women will undergo surgery for prolapse or incontinence at some time in their lives. Prolapse can have a significant affect on a woman's quality of life.

Clinical features

The majority (80%) of patients present complaining of 'something coming down', a lump or a bulge. Prolapse can also cause symptoms that affect bladder, bowel and sexual function, as summarised in **Table 8**. With the exception of vaginal bulge, the extent of anatomical prolapse does not correlate well with symptoms. It is therefore important to consider carefully the symptoms that a patient attributes to her prolapse and whether or not these are likely to be altered by treatment.

Aetiology

The pathophysiology of POP is believed to be multifactorial. Childbirth and ageing are important contributors. There may also be a significant heritable contribution to POP.

The relative role of connective tissue, muscles and neurovascular tissue in maintaining normal pelvic floor anatomy remains controversial. DeLancey describes three levels of support for the pelvic organs. Level I support, the upper vagina and uterus, is suspensory and is provided by the uterosacral and cardinal ligaments. Level 2, the mid portion of the vagina, is attached by endopelvic fascia to the pelvic sidewall along the 'white line', which is the arcus tendineus fascia pelvis. This attachment stretches the vagina between the bladder and rectum. Level 3, the distal vagina, is directly attached to surrounding structures: the urethra anteriorly, the perineal body posteriorly and the levator muscles laterally.

Diagnosis

Prolapse is diagnosed on clinical examination during Valsalva or cough. It may be necessary to examine the patient standing to demonstrate the maximum extent of the prolapse. Common terms used to describe prolapse clinically are:

- Cystocele – Prolapse of the bladder base or anterior vaginal wall
- Enterocele – Hernia and prolapse of the Pouch of Douglas
- Rectocele – Prolapse of the rectum or posterior vaginal wall
- Uterine prolapse – Descent of the uterus
- Vault prolapse: Vault descent following a previous hysterectomy
- Procidentia – Complete prolapse of the uterus and vaginal walls

These terms do not quantify the extent of prolapse and clinicians should use the pelvic organ prolapse quantification (POP-Q) system, which is reproducible and standardised and recommended by the International Association of Urogynaecologists (IUGA) **(Figure 9)**.

Table 8 Symptoms of prolapse			
Urinary symptoms	**Bowel symptoms**	**Sexual symptoms**	**Other symptoms**
Incomplete emptying	Incomplete emptying	Obstructive	Lump
Digitate to void	Digitate to defecate Anal/vaginal/perineal	Reduced sensation	Bulge
Frequency micturition	Difficult defecation	Reduced libido	Something coming down
Urgency to void	Anal incontinence	Body image	Dragging
Urinary incontinence		Pain	Backache
Recurrent urinary tract infection			Vaginal bleeding

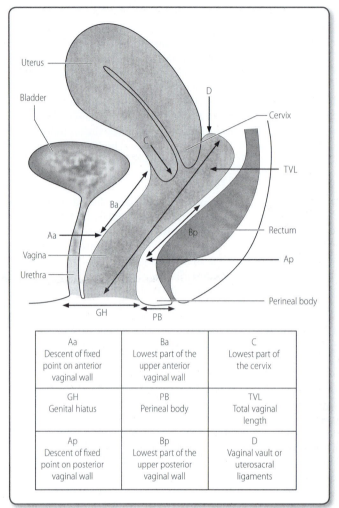

Figure 9 The pelvic organ prolapse quantification (POP-Q) system.

Aa Descent of fixed point on anterior vaginal wall	Ba Lowest part of the upper anterior vaginal wall	C Lowest part of the cervix
GH Genital hiatus	PB Perineal body	TVL Total vaginal length
Ap Descent of fixed point on posterior vaginal wall	Bp Lowest part of the upper posterior vaginal wall	D Vaginal vault or uterosacral ligaments

Management

Prevention   It is not possible to predict who will develop prolapse following vaginal delivery. Lifestyle changes to avoid heavy lifting, stopping smoking and avoiding obesity may reduce the risk of prolapse. Regular pelvic floor exercises may reduce the risk of prolapse.

Conservative treatment

- Pessary – Ring shelf, gellhorn, schatz and cube pessaries are all used to treat prolapse. Some clinicians use pessaries as the first line treatment of all prolapses. Silicone pessaries are available which can be inserted on a daily basis. Pessaries can

cause increased vaginal discharge. They can also cause ulceration and bleeding but these symptoms often settle if the pessary is removed for a few weeks and oestrogen cream is inserted into the vagina. Rarely, they can erode through into the rectum, bladder or urethra. This is more common if a pessary is neglected and not changed every 6 months

- Physiotherapy – Pelvic floor exercises may improve mild prolapse symptoms if the leading edge of the prolapse is not beyond the hymen
- Oestrogen – Vaginal oestrogen pessaries or cream can improve the symptoms of mild

prolapse. There is evidence that low dose regime 10 μg twice weekly appears to be safe for up to 12 months in women who have a uterus

Surgery There are many different operations available to treat prolapse depending on the anatomical site affected and whether it is a primary or secondary repair.

Traditionally

- A vaginal hysterectomy with vault support using the transverse cervical and uterosacral ligaments and obliteration of the space between the uterosacral ligaments to prevent enterocele formation has been used to treat uterine prolapse
- Anterior and posterior colporrhapy (vaginal repair) are used in isolation when anterior or posterior wall prolapse occurs without uterine prolapse
- A Manchester repair produces uterine elevation by approximating the shortened uterosacral ligaments anterior to the cervix and suturing them to the cervical stump following its partial amputation; it is combined with an anterior repair. It is a traditional procedure used if the patient wishes to retain her uterus. It is associated with a risk of either cervical stenosis or cervical incompetence. It is being superseded now by the sacrohysteropexy, in which the uterus is suspended to the anterior surface of the spine at the level of the 5th lumbar vertebra using polypropylene mesh

- Colpocleisis is an operation for procidentia or complete vault eversion. It is usually reserved for the frail elderly, who are certain they no longer require their vagina for coitus. In this procedure apposition of the anterior and posterior vaginal walls occurs, allowing two narrow lateral canals to exist
- Posthysterectomy vaginal vault prolapse can be treated by sacrocolpopexy using a polypropylene mesh to attach the vagina to the anterior surface of the spine. This procedure is often performed laparoscopically. An alternative is transvaginal fixation of the vault to the sacrospinous ligament

Other procedures

- Recently many different commercial kits have been produced for vaginal mesh repairs using type 1 polypropylene mesh. The role of these remains controversial and there is currently a large multicentre randomised controlled trial, PROSPECT, being performed in the UK to evaluate these procedures
- Uterine preservation surgery for uterine prolapse in the form of laparoscopic sacrohysteropexy or vaginal sacrospinous hysteropexy is another controversial aspect of the surgical management of prolapse

Further reading

DeLancey JO. Anatomic aspects of vaginal eversion after hysterectomy. Am J Obstet Gynecol 1992; 166:1717–1724.

Reid FM. Assessment of pelvic organ prolapse. Obstetrics, Gynaecology and Reproductive Medicine 2011; 21:190–197.

Bump RC, Mattisson A, Bo K, et al. The Standardization of terminology for female pelvic organ prolapse and pelvic floor dysfunction. Am J Obstet Gynecol 1996; 175:10–17.

Reid F, Smith T. Anterior vaginal repair. The Obstetrician & Gynaecologist 2012; 14:137–141.

Related topics of interest

Gestational trophoblastic disease

Overview

- Gestational trophoblastic disease comprises a spectrum of conditions in which abnormal proliferation of trophoblastic tissue occurs (**Table 9**)
- The overall prevalence in the UK is 0.7–1.0 per 1000 pregnancies. In other areas of the world, notably in Southeast Asia, the incidence is much higher
- The risk of developing the disease is greater at the extremes of reproductive life, increasing 6-fold before age 15 years and 26-fold after age 45 years
- Other predisposing factors include blood groups (higher if partners have different A and B groups and if the mother is group B or AB)

Clinical features

- Vaginal bleeding occurring between 6–16 weeks of gestation is the predominant symptom and occurs in 80–90% of complete hydatidiform moles and 75% of partial hydatidiform moles
- The classical signs associated with complete hydatidiform moles, including an enlarged uterus greater than that of the gestational age, hyperemesis, hyperthyroidism and pregnancy induced hypertension in the first and second trimester, occur less frequently with the widespread use of ultrasound facilitating earlier diagnosis
- The majority of partial hydatiform moles are only recognised histologically as they can often mimic incomplete miscarriages
- Bilateral theca lutein cysts are seen in 15% of complete hydatiform moles but occur infrequently in partial hydatiform moles
- Gestational trophoblastic neoplasia (i.e. invasive moles, choriocarcinomas, placental site tumours) have a variable presentation depending on type and extent of disease

Table 9 The spectrum of gestational trophoblastic neoplastic diseases			
Gestational trophoblastic disease	Aetiology	Histological features	Risk of progression
Complete hydatidiform mole	90% 46XX resulting from duplication of haploid sperm (23X) 10% arise from the fertilisation of an empty ovum with two sperm	Hydropic avascular villi, diffuse hyperplasia of syncytio and cytotrophoblast, absence of fetal tissue	15% progress to gestational trophoblastic neoplasia
Partial hydatidiform mole	Triploid (69XXY, XYY, XXX) arise from the fertilisation of a normal egg with two sperm	Oedematous villi of varying sizes and shapes, stromal inclusions, focal hyperplasia of trophoblast. Presence of fetal tissue	<5% progress to neoplasia
Invasive mole	Invasion of the myometrium by a hydatidiform mole	Invasion of myometrium by tissue with features as above	15% metastasise to lung/vagina
Choriocarcinoma	Can result from any type of pregnancy (25% from miscarriage/ectopic, 25% from normal pregnancy, 50% from molar pregnancy)	Abnormal trophoblastic hyperplasia and anaplasia, absent villi, prominent haemorrhage and necrosis	Vascular spread to lungs/liver/brain
Placental site tumour	Usually arise from non-molar pregnancies	Cords of intermediate trophoblast invading myometrium, absence of villi. Positive for human placental lactogen	Lymphatic spread

- Postmolar neoplasia presents with irregular bleeding following evacuation of a molar pregnancy
- Gestational trophoblastic neoplasia following a non-molar pregnancy must be considered in women presenting with late secondary postpartum haemorrhage
- Metastatic disease may present with pelvic pain, abnormal vaginal or rectal bleeding, haemoptysis, dyspnoea or bizarre neurological symptoms

Aetiology

Gestational trophoblastic disease arises from trophoblastic tissue. Normal trophoblast comprises three types of cell: syncytiotrophoblast, cytotrophoblast and intermediate trophoblast. Gestational trophoblastic disease can arise from any of these three cell types and can be classified as complete and partial hydatidiform mole, invasive mole, gestational choriocarcinoma and placental site tumour.

Diagnosis

Diagnosis preoperatively is predominantly by ultrasonography and confirmed histopathologically.

- Complete hydatidiform moles are characterised by a 'snowstorm' pattern ultrasonographically which consist of multiple cystic anechoic areas within the placental mass. The gestational sac is anembryonic
- Partial hydatiform moles are distinguished by the presence of fetal tissue within a gestational sac which has a greater transverse to anterior posterior diameter and the presence of more focal areas of cystic tissue
- Ultrasonographic diagnosis is supplemented by human chorionic gonadotropin (hCG) measurements which may help to distinguish retained products of conception and missed miscarriage from early molar pregnancies
- Over 50% of complete hydatiform moles will have hCG levels greater than 100,000 IU/L

Management
Initial management

- Suction curettage is the recommended first line management for suspected complete and partial hydatiform moles. Medical evacuation should only be considered where the fetal parts may limit surgical management
- Although excessive bleeding is relatively common with surgical management of molar pregnancies, oxytocics should not be used routinely. Oxytocics are thought to encourage the dissemination of trophoblastic cells and their use may be associated with a need for future chemotherapy

Follow-up

- All women with confirmed gestational trophoblastic disease should be referred and registered with the nearest regional trophoblastic screening centre. Follow-up consists of blood and urinary hCG measurements
- Women in whom hCG levels normalise within 42 days are followed up for 6 months from the date of their surgery whereas women in whom hCG levels do not return to normal within 42 days are followed up for 6 months following the normalisation of the hCG levels
- Women with gestational trophoblastic disease should be asked to notify their regional centre at the end of all subsequent pregnancies regardless of the outcome to exclude disease recurrence

Chemotherapy

- 15% of patients with complete hydatidiform moles and 0.5% of patients with partial hydatidiform moles will require chemotherapy
- Cure rates are in the region of 95–100%
- Patients are stratified into low and high risk according to the International Federation of Gynecology and Obstetrics 2000 scoring system based on prognostic factors such as age, interval and features of the antecedent pregnancy, e.g. a mole, abortion or full-term delivery, the level of βhCG, the size of the largest tumour mass

and the site, number of metastases and the need for previous chemotherapy
- Single-agent therapy is employed in low risk patients. The drug of choice is methotrexate with folinic acid rescue
- In high risk patients a combination of methotrexate, etoposide, actinomycin D, vincristine and cyclophosphamide are used
- Treatment is continued for 6 weeks after the hCG has normalised

Contraception and future pregnancy

- Women should be advised to use barrier contraception during follow-up. The combined oral contraceptive pill and intrauterine devices should only be considered after the hCG has returned to normal
- Women with gestational trophoblastic disease should not conceive until their follow-up is complete. Those who have received chemotherapy should not conceive for 12 months following the completion of treatment
- However, the risk of recurrence is low (1%). 98% of patients will not have a further molar pregnancy. Their risk of obstetric complication is unchanged following a molar pregnancy

Further reading

RCOG Green-top Guideline No. 38. The management of gestational trophoblastic disease. London: ROCOG, 2010.

Lurain J. Gestational trophoblastic disease I: epidemiology, pathology, clinical presentation and diagnosis of gestational trophoblastic disease, and management of hydatidiform mole. American Journal of Obstetrics and Gynecology 2010; 203:531–539.

Savage P. Molar pregnancy. The Obstetrician & Gynaecologist 2008; 10:3–8.

Related topics of interest

- Miscarriage (p. 94)
- Recurrent miscarriage (p. 129)
- Chemotherapy (p. 20)

Heavy menstrual bleeding

Overview

The 1997 evidence-based guideline commissioned by National Institute for Clinical Excellence (NICE) and undertaken by the National Collaborating Centre for Women's and Children's Health favoured the term heavy menstrual bleeding (HMB) over menorrhagia. HMB should be considered as excessive menstrual blood loss which interferes with the woman's physical, emotional, social and material quality of life, occurring either alone or in combination with other symptoms. The former definition of blood loss > 80 mL per cycle has been found to be impractical for clinical practice and should be confined to use as an adjunct to research. Since the early 1990s the use of hysterectomy as first line treatment has declined as more conservative options become available.

Clinical features

Women with heavy periods are often troubled by a number of symptoms that impact on daily life. As well as heavy bleeding, women may report pain, bloating, mood changes and tiredness as additional factors that restrict their functional capacity at this time. There may be underlying social or psychological issues.

Aetiology

Heavy menstrual bleeding may be associated with pelvic pathology as well as certain endocrine and medical disorders, but in the majority of cases, no obvious underlying pathology is seen.
1. Local pelvic pathology
- Fibroids (in about 30%)
- Endometriosis
- Pelvic inflammatory disease
- Endometrial polyps
- Adenomyosis
- Carcinoma of uterus/cervix/ovary
2. General medical causes
- Hypothyroidism/hyperthyroidism
- Coagulation disorders: von Willebrand's disease (in 5–20%)/idiopathic thrombocytopenia (ITP)
3. Iatrogenic causes
- Intrauterine contraceptive devices
- Progesterone only contraception
- Anticoagulant therapy

Diagnosis

A thorough history and examination should form the basis for a diagnosis of HMB. This should ideally have been undertaken in the primary care setting.

If the history suggests HMB but with no obvious underlying abnormality, then treatment can be commenced in the primary care setting without the need for examination [unless management with the levonorgestrel-releasing intrauterine system (LNG-IUS) is being considered].

If there is a suspicion of a structural or histological abnormality, pelvic examination and further investigations are warranted.

Direct measurement of blood loss using alkaline haematin, or indirect assessment using pictorial charts is not routinely recommended.

Investigations may include:
- Full blood count
- Thyroid testing only if clinically indicated
- Consider testing for coagulopathies if there is a family history, or heavy bleeding from menarche
- Ultrasound scan (USS) is the first line diagnostic imaging of choice
- Hysteroscopy/magnetic resonance imaging (MRI)/saline infusion sonography are not first line investigations, but may provide a useful adjunct if USS is inconclusive
- Endometrial sampling should be taken to exclude endometrial carcinoma or atypical hyperplasia for those > 45 years of age, or those with persistent intermenstrual bleeding or initial treatment failure

Management

Should there be an underlying structural, histological or endocrine cause for HMB, then treatment is aimed at addressing this. In around 50%, however, there is no obvious explanation for their HMB. For management of HMB associated with fibroids see the corresponding topic.

Medical treatment

Suitable where there is no structural or histological abnormality or for fibroids < 3 cm. It is recommended that the following be used in order.

- LNG-IUS is now considered first line management
- Antifibrinolytic agents such as Tranexamic acid reduce blood loss by around 50% (stop if no improvement within three cycles), non-steroidal anti-inflammatory drugs (where there is coexisting dysmenorrhoea), combined oral contraceptives
- Norethisterone 15 mg daily (5 mg thrice daily, day 5–26 of cycle) or injectable long-acting progestogens
- Danazol is no longer recommended
- Gonadotropin-releasing hormone analogues are more likely to be used to shrink fibroids prior to surgery. Their cost, side effects and recurrence rate on cessation have seen them used less frequently as medical management
- It is estimated that 20–40% require surgical intervention following initial attempts at medical management

Endometrial ablation

- The aim of endometrial ablation (and resection) is to remove the part of the uterus that bleeds abnormally and allow the lining of the uterus to be replaced by fibrous tissue. Endometrial ablation may be suitable for those with a uterus < 10 cm size and also those with fibroids < 3 cm, where the patient considers their family to be complete. Adequate contraception should be ensured postprocedure. Relatively new ablative techniques are associated with reduced hospital stay and a faster recovery time. Even if these techniques are unsuccessful, the recourse to hysterectomy is available. With this in mind, it is imperative if the patient is anaesthetised for the ablation that

suitability for a vaginal hysterectomy is assessed. Success rates approaching 80% have been quoted
- Second generation techniques are recommended:
  - Impedance-controlled bipolar radiofrequency ablation (e.g. Novasure)
  - Fluid filled thermal balloon endometrial ablation (e.g. Thermachoice)
  - Microwave endometrial ablation (e.g. Microsulis)

All of these techniques are suitable as outpatient or day-case procedures. Specific contraindications include: large/irregular uterine cavities (balloon ablation), latex allergy (balloon ablation), and uterine wall thickness < 8 mm (microwave ablation). Risks include: uterine perforation, intra-abdominal injury, infection, visceral burn and pelvic pain

- Pregnancy after endometrial ablation: Although successful pregnancies have been reported, most opinion is that pregnancy after such procedures is unlikely, with an increased risk of miscarriage, uterine rupture and placenta accreta.
  Some 6% of patients who have undergone microwave endometrial ablation and 1–10% of those who have undergone balloon ablation ultimately require a hysterectomy.

Endometrial resection

This was initially described by Neuwirth for resection of submucous fibroids. De Cherney first used the technique for intractable menstrual bleeding. These techniques appear to have been superseded by the newer ablative techniques described above. Transcervical resection of the endometrium (TCRE):

- Performed under direct vision and can be undertaken as a day case
- Purely for heavy menstrual bleeding
- Uterus size < 10 cm
- Family complete (ensure ongoing contraception)

Surgery

Hysterectomy is not a first line treatment for HMB. If previous treatments have failed, are contraindicated, or have been refused, then it can be considered, as long as the patient has been fully counselled as to the potential complications.

- Hysterectomy should be performed vaginally if possible

- Laparoscopic assisted hysterectomy for those with associated co-morbidities
- Oophorectomy should not be routinely performed

Further reading

National Collaborating Centre for Women's and Children's Health. Heavy Menstrual Bleeding. London: NICE, 2007.

Justin W, et al. Current minimal access techniques in the treatment of heavy menstrual bleeding. The Obstetrician & Gynaecologist 2007; 9:223–232.

Carey MS, Allen RH. Non-contraceptive uses and benefits of combined oral contraception. The Obstetrician & Gynaecologist 2012; 14:223–228.

Related topics of interest

Hirsutism

Overview

Hirsutism is a common clinical problem of excess hair growth in a male distribution in women. It is characterised by the presence of increased terminal hair growth in androgen-dependent areas of skin, and usually results from relatively benign disorders including polycystic ovarian syndrome (PCOS), which is the most frequent association. It is important to diagnose hirsutism and its possible underlying causes, via detailed clinical history, physical examination and laboratory tests including hormone levels. When hirsutism is not related to medication use, evaluation is focused on testing for endocrine-related disease and rare but life-threatening tumours. Benign causes of hirsutism often begin around puberty and progress slowly, whereas rare androgen-secreting neoplasms can have sudden onset hirsutism, progress rapidly, and are associated with other clinical signs of virilisation and defeminisation. Treatment of hirsutism often involves both cosmetic treatments such as waxing, shaving and light therapy and systemic treatments. Systemic treatments are targeted at reducing the production and bioavailability of testosterone, as well as blocking target tissue androgen action, and include oral contraceptives, cyproterone acetate and metformin.

Clinical features

Hirsutism affects terminal hairs which depend on androgen, and are curly and pigmented. By contrast, vellus hair, which is androgen-independent, is fine, soft and lightly pigmented. Because small amounts of terminal hair are normal in women, quantitation of the hair growth is important. The gold standard method for the evaluation of hirsutism is the modified Ferriman and Gallwey scale proposed by Hatch et al. (1981) where hair growth is assessed in each of nine androgen-sensitive areas: upper lip, chin, chest, upper and lower back, upper and lower abdomen, arm, forearm, thigh and lower leg, and graded for hair coarseness (**Figure 21.1**).

The scores derived from this method should be interpreted according to the race of the patient (since terminal body hair growth has substantial racial and ethnic variability), and time since hair removal techniques have been used.

Some women may have additional signs of hyperandrogenism, including oily skin and acne, deeper masculine voice, well-developed musculature, enlargement of the clitoris, and oliomenorrhoea or amenorrhoea. There can also be psychological changes such as increased aggression or libido. These features are associated with virilisation, and the more of these that are found, the higher the probability of an underlying serious cause of hirsutism such as a tumour.

Women with benign causes of hirsutism such as PCOS are usually obese. This condition is discussed in Topic 36. A thorough abdominal and pelvic examination of hirsute women should always be performed as it may occasionally reveal androgen-secreting adrenal or ovarian tumours. Other clinical features will depend on the underlying cause of the hirsuitism which are numerous and listed below.

Aetiology

Hirsutism is thought to be caused by an underlying increase in androgen production. In response to the increased levels of androgens during puberty, the growth of hair in pubic and axillary regions of women is stimulated, resulting in terminal hairs that are larger, curlier and darker then prepubertal vellus hairs. Similarly, the development of facial hair and male-pattern body hair in men is also attributed to androgen stimulation. Hirsutism is thought to reflect the interaction between circulating and local androgen concentrations and the sensitivity of hair follicles to these androgens. Hirsutism severity, however, does not correlate well with circulating androgen concentration, and many women with hirsutism have normal androgen concentrations. These women are likely to have hair follicles with increased sensitivity to circulating androgens.

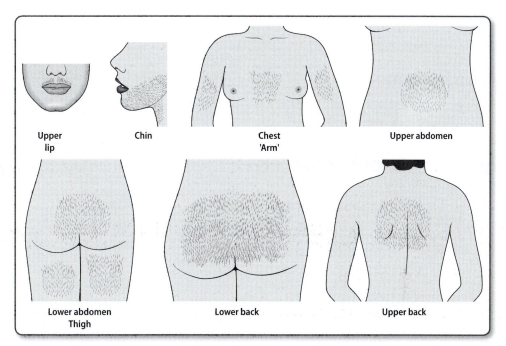

Figure 21.1 Schematic representations of the nine body areas assessed by the modified Ferriman and Gallwey scale for hirsutism showing the distribution corresponding to the greatest score for each area.

Causes of hirsutism include:

- Racial
- Familial
- Idiopathic
- Physiological – puberty, pregnancy, menopause
- Anorexia nervosa
- Drugs – dilantin, diazoxide, steroids, danazol
- Traumatic
- Ovarian – PCOS, hyperthecosis, virilising tumours
- Adrenal – carcinoma, hyperplasia
- Thyroid disease
- Acromegaly
- Cushing syndrome
- Turner syndrome
- Porphyria
- Central nervous system linked – multiple sclerosis, encephalitis

Diagnosis

Diagnosis of hirsutism is complex and involves:

Detailed history and examination Using photography where possible.

Investigations The main androgens measured are dehydroepiandrosterone (DHEA), dehydroepiandrosterone sulphate (DHEAS), androstenedione and testosterone. In the female, androgens come from either the ovary or the adrenal gland. Androgen production is subject to diurnal rhythm, linked to the production and metabolism of cortisol. There is much debate as to the final common source of excess androgens in hirsute women, but it is generally believed to be ovarian in origin. The ovary is under luteinising hormone (LH) control, so PCOS leads to elevated androstenedione and testosterone levels which commonly result in hirsutism.

If an early morning total testosterone level is moderately elevated, it should be followed by a plasma free testosterone level. If total testosterone level is greater than 200 ng/dL (6.94 nmol/L) this should prompt evaluation for an androgen-secreting tumour. Further investigations should be guided by history and examination, and may include thyroid function tests, prolactin levels, and corticotropin stimulation tests.

Management

Treatment of hirsutism will depend on the underlying cause and appropriate referral and treatments should be instigated for endocrine disease and tumours.

For patients with findings indicating a benign cause of hirsutism, such as PCOS, the most effective strategy is to combine systemic therapy, which has a slow onset of effectiveness, with cosmetic treatments which include shaving, plucking, waxing, depilatory creams and laser hair removal. Shaving is quick, inexpensive and effective but needs to be repeated often, whereas the other methods generally give longer-lasting hair free intervals.

Systemic therapies for hirsutism work by either decreasing ovarian or adrenal androgen production, or by inhibition of androgen action in the skin. For patients who are not planning a pregnancy, first line pharmacologic treatment should include oral contraceptives. Other therapies include topical eflornithine, antiandrogens (androgen receptor blockers and 5α-reductase inhibitors), glucocorticoids, cyproterone acetate and insulin sensitisers (metformin and rosiglitazone).

Further reading

Hatch R, Rosenfield RL, Kim MH, et al. Hirsutism: Implications, etiology and management. Am J Obstet Gynecol 1981; 140: 815–30.

Escobar-Morreale HF, et al. Epidemiology, diagnosis and management of hirsutism: a consensus statement by the Androgen Excess and Polycystic Ovary Syndrome Society. Human Reproduction Update 2012; 18:146–170.

Paparodis R, Dunaif A. The hirsute woman: challenges in evaluation and management. Endocrine Practice 2011;17:807–818.

Shah D, Patel S. Hirsutism. Gynecol Endocrinol 2009; 25:140–148.

Related topics of interest

Human papillomavirus vaccination

Overview

Human papillomavirus (HPV) infection is a prerequisite for the development of cervical malignancy. HPV is a DNA virus which targets epithelial cells, and high risk genotypes 16, 18, 31, 33, 35 and 45, amongst others, can lead to cervical cancer, as well as anogenital, and head and neck cancers. Low risk genotypes such as 6 and 11 can cause condyloma acuminata (genital warts) in men and women, and respiratory papillomatosis which can affect both adults and children. The main burden of HPV-related disease is from cervical cancer.

It is estimated that around 80% of sexually active women will be infected with HPV in their lifetime, but most infections are transient and 90% of women will clear the infection within 2 years. Genital tract HPV infection is primarily acquired through sexual contact. Persistence of infection depends upon failure of the host immune system to adequately respond to the virus via the cell-mediated adaptive immune system. Long term immunosuppression (e.g. as a result of HIV infection) is associated with an increased incidence of HPV-associated warts, cervical intraepithelial neoplasia (CIN) and cervical cancer. Smoking is also a risk factor, since cigarette smoke suppresses effective local immunity within the cervix. Most persistent HPV infections cause low grade CIN, of which 60% will regress spontaneously and 10% will progress to high grade disease. The advent of a computerised call–recall system for cervical screening in the UK in the 1980s has halved mortality from cervical cancer, and it has been estimated that the current screening programme will prevent 70% of cancer deaths. However, the greatest burden of cervical cancer is seen in developing countries that do not have the resources or facilities to roll out screening programmes or manage preinvasive cervical disease.

Vaccines

There are currently two types of commercially available HPV vaccines. Bivalent Cervarix protects against HPV 16 and 18 and quadrivalent Gardasil protects against HPV 16, 18, 6 and 11. As 70% of cervical cancers are caused by HPV 16 and 18, a widely adopted vaccination programme will significantly reduce the incidence of invasive cervical disease as well as premalignant lesions, although the proportion of the latter caused by HPV 16 and 18 is much lower.

The UK HPV vaccination programme started in September 2008 with all 12–13 year-old girls being offered the vaccine. A catch-up programme was also initiated, with 13–18 year-old girls being offered the vaccine over that and the following two academic years. An accelerated catch-up programme was announced in December 2008 so that all girls born on or after 1 September 1990 could be protected before the end of the academic year 2009 or 2010. Now all girls in years 8 (age 12–13 years) are offered the vaccine as part of the National Vaccination Programme, and since September 2012 have received the quadrivalent vaccine (the bivalent vaccine was used before then). Three intramuscular injections are given within a 12-month period, the second being at least 4 weeks from the first, and the third at least 12 weeks from the second. Boys are not routinely vaccinated, but the vaccine may be purchased and administered privately.

Mechanism of action

HPV infects basal epithelial cells which then migrate through the various layers of the epithelium as they mature, until they are sloughed from the surface. New infectious viral particles (virions) are produced only in the most superficial epithelial cells at the end of a maturation process that takes several weeks to complete. The papillomavirus encodes six early functional proteins (E1, 2, 4,

5, 6, 7) and two late structural proteins (L1 and 2). E1 and 2 control viral replication, E6 and 7 are oncoproteins which interact with p53 and retinoblastoma genes. In combination they create a pro-proliferative environment which lacks the normal checks on cell cycle control.

Prophylactic HPV vaccines induce high titres of antibodies to HPV with the aim of preventing infection. The L1 capsid protein has the ability to assemble into virus-like particles (VLPs) in the absence of other HPV gene products, and these VLPs are morphologically identical to HPV but lack the infectivity as they lack the viral genome. Clinical trials have shown that the vaccines result in antibody titres at least 40 times greater than those induced by natural infection.

Efficacy

When given to previously unexposed individuals, both the bivalent and the quadrivalent vaccines are highly effective at preventing new HPV 16 and 18 infections. Efficacy of the vaccine has been demonstrated up to at least 10 years with longer term follow-up studies ongoing. Both vaccines result in high titres of virus-neutralising HPV 16 and 18-specific antibodies. Neither vaccine is designed to treat established infection or eradicate premalignant or malignant disease. Therefore, vaccination should be administered prior to the onset of sexual activity, where possible. There is some evidence for cross protection with other, similar, high risk HPV types (e.g. 31, 33, 45, 51), particularly with the bivalent vaccine, although the strength and duration of protection resulting from this is unknown. In Australia, where uptake of the quadrivalent vaccine by girls and young women tops 80%, a dramatic reduction in the incidence of genital warts has been observed, not only in young women (by 73%), but also in young men (by 44%) who are not part of the free vaccination programme. These findings suggest that mass vaccination of girls provides substantial herd immunity.

Side effects

The Food and Drug Administration (FDA) and the Medicines and Healthcare products Regulatory Agency (MHRA) continue to endorse the safety profile of Gardasil, which is currently in widespread use in the UK and the USA. **Table 10** documents common and serious side effects of the vaccine.

Challenges

Women who are unvaccinated, or imperfectly vaccinated (i.e. those who received one or two of the three vaccine doses) will still need to undergo frequent cervical screening, although identifying these women may be logistically challenging. Emerging evidence suggests that two (or one) doses of vaccine may be as effective as three. Screening is still required for vaccinated women as they will continue to be at risk from other HPV types which can cause cervical cancer. It remains to be seen whether vaccination will adversely affect the uptake of cervical screening. It is unknown at present whether the natural spectrum of HPV subtypes will be affected by widespread introduction of vaccines targeting the most common oncogenic subtypes. Studies are needed to see whether screening intervals for vaccinated women can safely be extended.

Vaccination programmes are aimed at young adolescents and require parental consent, and as such require sensitive and targeted education programmes to reassure parents of the safety of the vaccines as well as

Table 10 Adverse effects of human papillomavirus vaccine		
Very common	>1:10	Injection site problems Headaches
Common	>1:100	Fever Nausea Limb pain
Rare	>1:10,000	Urticaria
Very rare	<1:10,000	Bronchospasm

address parental concerns that vaccination may increase promiscuity.

Future directions

Those who stand to benefit the most from HPV vaccination live in countries least able to afford it, and it is important to continue to endeavour to make the vaccine accessible to developing countries.

Follow up studies continue to assess long term efficacy of HPV vaccination, both in terms of antibody titres and clinical protection.

A large proportion of women have already been exposed to and infected with HPV. Further information is needed to address the possibility of a therapeutic vaccination in these women, or the effectiveness of vaccination in sexually active women who may be infected with other HPV types.

Further reading

Crosbie EJ, Kitchener HC. Vaccination against cervical cancer. Scientific Advisory Committee Opinion Paper 9. London: Royal College of Obstetricians and Gynaecologists, 2007.
Crosbie EJ, Brabin L. Cervical cancer: problem solved? Vaccinating girls against human papillomavirus. BJOG 2010; 117:137–42.

Crosbie EJ, Einstein M, Franceschi S, et al. Human papillomavirus and cervical cancer. Lancet 2013: Epub ahead of print.

Related topics of interest

• Cervical screening (p. 16)
• Cervical cancer (p. 12)

• Sexually transmitted infection (p. 135)

Hyperemesis gravidarum

Overview

Up to 50–90% of pregnancies are affected by nausea and vomiting. Symptoms usually start at 6–8 weeks of gestation, peak at 9–11 weeks and resolve by 16 weeks. Only a minority of women have symptoms beyond 20 weeks of gestation.

'Morning sickness' is a misnomer: just 15% of women have symptoms exclusively in the mornings. Most experience episodic or persistent nausea and vomiting throughout the day. Mild symptoms are most common but in 35% of cases, symptoms are clinically significant, resulting in the need for time off work and negatively impacting on family relationships and a woman's quality of life. Many women describe the nausea as intolerable, making them unable to cook, shop, eat or function normally, for fear of vomiting.

Approximately 1% of pregnant women have such severe nausea and vomiting that they require hospital admission for intravenous rehydration and correction of electrolyte imbalance: this condition is called hyperemesis gravidarum.

Aetiology

The aetiology of hyperemesis gravidarum is incompletely understood, but genetic, hormonal, gastrointestinal and psychosocial factors may all contribute.

- Genetic factors
  - There is a 3-fold increased risk of hyperemesis in women born to mothers who also experienced hyperemesis in pregnancy
  - Hyperemesis tends to recur in subsequent pregnancies
- Hormonal factors
  - Symptoms are caused by placental human chorionic gonadotrophin (hCG) levels
    - hCG stimulates ovarian production of oestrogen, which is known to cause nausea and vomiting
    - Symptoms peak at 9 weeks, coinciding with the peak of placental hCG production
    - Hyperemesis is more common where hCG levels are highest (e.g. in multiple and molar pregnancies)
    - There is cross reactivity with the thyroid stimulating hormone (TSH) receptor due to the structural similarity between hCG and TSH. Up to 60% women with hyperemesis experience transient hyperthyroidism
    - Hyperemesis is more common in non-smokers (due to larger placental volume and higher hCG levels)
- Gastrointestinal
  - Pregnancy-induced progesterone-mediated relaxation of smooth muscle results in reduced oesophageal pressure and delayed stomach emptying, which lowers the threshold for vomiting
  - 80% of women with hyperemesis are seropositive for helicobacter pylori, which is thought to play a role in this condition
- Psychosocial
  - Risk factors include: young age, first pregnancy, poor socioeconomic background, low education levels, poor communication with partner, home life stress
  - There is an increased risk of hyperemesis in women with a history of eating disorders
- Other factors
  - There is an increased risk of hyperemesis in women with pre-existing diabetes, hyperthyroidism, psychiatric illness and gastrointestinal disorders
  - Vitamin B deficiency may be important (use of multivitamins/vitamin B6 supplements reduces symptoms of nausea and vomiting)

Clinical features

These include:
- Persistent vomiting, with onset in the first trimester of pregnancy
- Inability to tolerate oral fluids or diet

- Ptyalism (inability to swallow saliva) and spitting
- Electrolyte imbalance (e.g. hypokalaemia)
- Ketosis
- Dehydration, tachycardia and postural hypotension
- Weight loss > 5% of pre-pregnancy weight
- The need for hospital admission for rehydration and correction of electrolyte imbalance

Severe untreated hyperemesis may cause maternal and fetal complications. Maternal complications include:

- Malnutrition
  - Severe weight loss (10–20% body weight), wasting and weakness
  - Vitamin B1 deficiency, which can cause Wernicke's encephalopathy (triad of ophthalmoplegia, ataxia and confusion) and Korsakoff's psychosis (confabulation, inability to learn, anterograde amnesia)
  - Vitamin B6 and B12 deficiencies, which cause anaemia and peripheral neuropathy
- Dehydration and electrolyte imbalance
  - Hypokalaemia (causes muscle weakness and cardiac arrhythmias)
  - Hyponatraemia (plasma sodium < 120 mmol/L), leading to lethargy, confusion, seizures and respiratory arrest
- Mallory–Weiss tears (from repeated retching)

Fetal complications include:

  - Intrauterine growth restriction and low birth weight
  - Prematurity

Diagnosis

Hyperemesis is a diagnosis of exclusion. Rule out other causes of nausea and vomiting first (Table 11).

The history should establish when the symptoms started since pre-pregnancy nausea and vomiting suggests a different cause. Abdominal pain is not usually a feature. Signs of dehydration are likely to be observed, including tachycardia and postural hypotension.

Table 11 Differential diagnosis of nausea and vomiting in pregnancy

System	Disorder
Genitourinary	Urinary tract infection, pyelonephritis
Gastrointestinal	Appendicitis, pancreatitis, cholecystitis Peptic ulcer, gastritis
Neurological	Migraine Diseases of the central nervous system
Metabolic and endocrine disease	Thyrotoxicosis, Addison's disease Hypercalcaemia, uraemia
Middle ear problems	Vestibular dysfunction, Ménière's disease, labyrinthitis
Drugs	Opioids, iron
Psychological	Bulimia nervosa
Pregnancy-related conditions	Molar pregnancy Pre-eclampsia, acute fatty liver of pregnancy

Adapted from Jarvis S and Nelson-Piercy C. Management of nausea and vomiting in pregnancy. BMJ 2011; 342:3606.

Urinalysis will show increased urine specific gravity and ketonuria. A midstream specimen of urine should be sent for culture and sensitivities to exclude a urinary tract infection.

Blood biochemistry may indicate hyponatraemia, hypokalaemia and low serum urea. A metabolic alkalosis results from excessive loss of H^+ in vomitus; a metabolic acidosis indicates severe hyperemesis.

Biochemical hyperthyroidism (raised T4 and suppressed TSH) due to cross reactivity between hCG and the TSH receptor, are typical and establish the severity of the condition. Whilst rare, Graves's disease can present for the first time in pregnancy, so clinical signs of thyrotoxicosis (e.g. goitre, eyelid lag, exophthalmia) must be sought. Abnormal liver function tests are commonly seen, particularly raised serum aminotransferase and bilirubin, although frank jaundice is rare.

A pelvic ultrasound scan will exclude molar or multiple pregnancies.

Management

Simple measures for the treatment of mild nausea and vomiting in pregnancy include:

- Avoidance of odours or foods that trigger nausea
- Small, regular amounts of bland, dry, carbohydrate foods (e.g. crackers) throughout the day, with fluids between meals
- Ginger has been shown to reduce nausea and vomiting in early pregnancy
- Antiemetics may be necessary where simple measures fail

Inability to tolerate oral fluids and significant ketonuria usually trigger hospital admission. The principles of inpatient care include:

- Intravenous rehydration with normal saline supplemented with potassium chloride, or Hartmann's solution. It should be noted that:
  - Intravenous dextrose can precipitate Wernicke's encephalopathy and should never be used
  - Hyponatraemia must be corrected slowly; double strength saline should never be used as the rapid correction of hyponatraemia can cause central pontine myelinolysis (characterised by spastic quadriparesis, pseudobulbar palsy and impaired consciousness)
- Vitamin supplementation
  - Folic acid 400 µg daily (to reduce the risk of fetal neural tube defects)
  - Thiamine 50 mg three times daily (to reduce risk of Wernicke's encephalopathy)
  - Pyridoxine (vitamin B6). This is first line treatment of nausea and vomiting in pregnancy in the USA in combination with doxylamine (an antihistamine antiemetic). Randomized controlled trials (RCTs) have shown a 70% reduction in symptoms with its use. Fears about the possible teratogenic effects of this combination of drugs have made its use unpopular in the UK, although the evidence for teratogenicity is weak
- Thromboprophylaxis: thromboembolic deterrant stockings and low molecular weight heparin (e.g. enoxaparin 40 mg daily) to counteract the thrombophilic effects of dehydration and bed rest
- Antiemetics
  - Antiemetics are safe for use in pregnancy but women may need reassurance. Standard antiemetic regimes are shown in **Table 12**
  - There is no evidence for superiority of one antiemetic over another
  - Combinations of antiemetics may be required in intractable cases
  - Proton pump inhibitors (e.g. omeprazole) and H_2 antagonists (e.g. ranitidine) are safe to use in pregnancy and are recommended where gastro-oesophageal reflux is a feature
- Steroids may be helpful in severe, refractory hyperemesis. Small RCTs have shown dramatic and complete responses

Table 12 Antiemetic regimes for the treatment of hyperemesis gravidarum				
Class of drug	Example	Dose	Route of administration	Side effects
H_1 receptor (histamine) antagonist	Cyclizine	50 mg TDS	PO, IM, IV	Drowsiness
Dopamine antagonist	Metoclopramide	10 mg TDS	PO, IM, IV	Drowsiness
	Domperidone	10 mg QID 30–60 mg TDS	PO PR	Extrapyramidal effects and oculogyric crises
Phenothiazines Dopamine antagonists	Prochlorperazine (Stemetil)	5 mg TDS 12.5 mg TDS 25 mg OD 3–6 mg BD	PO IM, IV PR buccal	Drowsiness Extrapyramidal effects and oculogyric crises
	Promethazine	25 mg nocte	PO	
	Chlorpromazine	10–25 mg TDS	PO	
Selective $5HT_3$ receptor antagonist	Ondansetron	4–8 mg TDS	PO, IM, slow IV infusion	Constipation

in some women. The standard regime is 100 mg IV hydrocortisone twice daily followed by 40 mg oral prednisolone if clinically effective. This can be tapered down until the lowest dose that suppresses symptoms is achieved. There are no reported adverse effects on the fetus (who receives 10% of the maternal dose because prednisolone is metabolised by the placenta) but long term use should prompt screening for urinary infections and gestational diabetes.

- Total parenteral nutrition (TPN) may be life saving. Its use is reserved for intractable vomiting not effectively treated by optimal rehydration, antiemetic therapy and a trial of corticosteroids. Risks include line sepsis, bacterial endocarditis, pneumonia and steatohepatitis.
- Termination of pregnancy at maternal request has been reported
- Psychological support

Further reading

Jarvis S, Nelson-Piercy C. Management of nausea and vomiting in pregnancy. BMJ 2011; 342:3606.

Niebyl JR. Nausea and vomiting in pregnancy. N Engl J Med 2010; 363:1544–1550.

Neill AM, Nelson-Piercy C. Hyperemesis gravidarum. The Obstetrician & Gynaecologist 2003; 5:204–207.

Related topics of interest

- Gestational trophoblastic disease (p. 58)
- Multiple pregnancy (p. 265)
- Thyroid and pregnancy (p. 329)

Hysterectomy

Overview

The first hysterectomy is thought to have been performed by mistake by a GB Paletta who, on intending to perform cervical amputation, removed the entire uterus. His assistant that day in Milan 1812 went on to undertake the first deliberate vaginal hysterectomy some 10 years later. His name was DB Monteggia. The first abdominal hysterectomy was carried out by Charles Clay in Manchester in 1844.

Approximately 50,000 hysterectomies were performed in the UK in 2010. The vast majority of these were performed abdominally (70–90%), with vaginal hysterectomy (10–30%) and laparoscopic hysterectomy (< 5%) some way behind. Ovarian removal at the time of hysterectomy is contentious: unnecessary removal of normal organs versus prophylaxis against malignant change. A total of 95–99% of ovaries can also be removed vaginally if so required. There is still a definite mortality rate from hysterectomy, so other treatments should be considered. Hysterectomy rates have been steadily dropping over recent years, reflecting improved uterine-sparing treatments for dysfunctional uterine bleeding (e.g. Mirena coil, endometrial ablation).

Abdominal hysterectomy

Indications for abdominal hysterectomy include:
- Fibroids > 14 weeks size
- Concurrent ovarian pathology where ovarian removal is predicted
- No descent on examination (nulliparous)
- Laparotomy indicated
- Malignancy

Technique

Techniques will understandably vary between individual surgeons. The following steps provide a generalised overview (**Figure 10**).

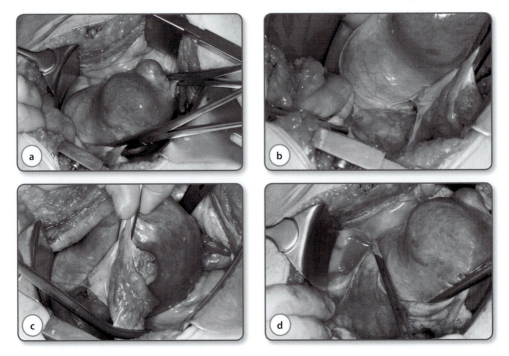

Figure 10 Total abdominal hysterectomy and bilateral salpingo-oophorectomy for fibroids. *Continued...*

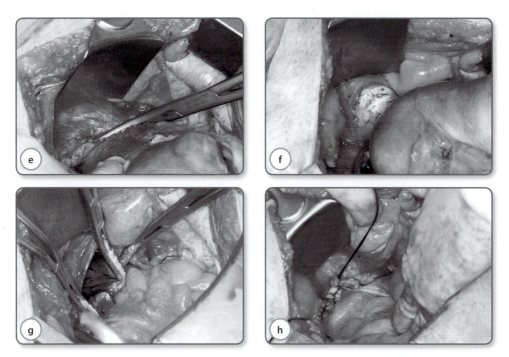

Figure 10 Total abdominal hysterectomy and bilateral salpingo-oophorectomy for fibroids (a) The abdomen is opened, the bowel packed away and the uterus is put under traction using long straight clamps. (b) The round ligaments are clamped and cut, allowing the broad ligament to be opened. The ureters can now be identified and their integrity protected. (c) Windows are made in the posterior leaf of the broad ligament to isolate the infundibulopelvic ligaments, which are then clamped, cut and ligated. (d) The uterovesical fold of peritoneum is opened and the bladder deflected caudally. (e) The uterine pedicles are clamped and cut on both sides. The bladder is gently dissected caudally to reveal the white muscular tube of the vagina. (f) The vagina is opened in the midline (vaginal mucosa stained with methylene blue for ease of identification). (g) The vaginal angles are secured with heavy curved Slade–Ellis dog-leg clamps and the hysterectomy is completed. (h) The vagina is closed with continuous locking sutures. The pedicles are checked and haemostasis confirmed. The abdomen is closed in layers. Photos courtesy of Mr Richard Slade.

Incision

- Transverse lower abdominal incision preferable, both in terms of postoperative pain and recovery
- Consider midline or paramedian if better access is required

Procedure

- Inspection of abdominal contents once peritoneal cavity entered
- Trendelenberg position
- Bowel packed away
- Secure uterus
- Identify round ligaments – these run from uterine cornu to the pelvic side wall
- Round ligaments clamped and incised to open the broad ligament. Round ligaments are tied
- Anterior leaf of the broad ligament opened inferomedially to reach the bladder peritoneum
- Posterior leaf of the broad ligament opened
- The path of the ureters is identified to avoid accidental damage
- The avascular portion of the posterior leaf of the broad ligament is tented and bluntly entered to provide a window
- If the ovary and fallopian tube are to be removed then the window formed in

the posterior leaf of the broad ligament isolates the infundibulo-pelvic ligament, which can be clamped and divided
- If the ovary and fallopian tube are to be conserved, then clamps are placed across the fallopian tube and utero-ovarian ligament close to the uterus
- Deflection of the bladder inferiorly and away from the operative site (ensuring that the ureters follow) is achieved by elevation of the uterovesical fold and incising through the peritoneum
- Uterine artery pedicles are taken at the cervicouterine junction and can incorporate the uterosacral ligaments posteriorly. The pedicles are transfixed and cut
- Cardinal ligaments can be divided medially to the previous ligated uterine arteries
- Vagina opened in the midline below the level of the cervix and clamps passed both sides from front to back. The vagina can be transected above these clamps and the specimen removed
- The position of the vaginal clamps allows for the vaginal angles to be safely transfixed
- The central part of the vagina can be closed, using either a continuous or mattress suture. By incorporating the peritoneal edge into this closure, haemostasis can be insured
- Pedicles checked for haemostasis
- The peritoneum does not need to be closed
- Rectus sheath with one vicryl suture (low transverse incision) or mass closure using Loop Polydioxanone (midline incision)
- Skin (subcuticular 3/0 monocryl, interrupted prolene or staples)

Vaginal hysterectomy

Less commonly performed than its abdominal counterpart, although it is the operation of choice for the following:
- Menorrhagia with adequate descent (multiparous)
- Prolapse
- Menorrhagia with concurrent prolapse

Vaginal hysterectomy is the treatment of choice for prolapse, particularly procidentia. Its use for the management of menstrual abnormalities appears to be gaining favour once more. Once a woman has had a single normal delivery it is usually possible to perform a vaginal hysterectomy. Mortality is similar to abdominal hysterectomy.

Technique

Techniques will understandably vary between individual surgeons. The following steps provide a generalised overview.

Examination under anaesthesia
- Vaginal capacity/introital access
- Cervix accessible: a cervix flush with the vaginal vault may make the procedure difficult
- Mobility of cervix and descent. If the uterus is fixed, e.g. from endometriosis or adhesions, the vaginal route is not advised
- Pouch of Douglas free from scarring
- Access to uterosacral ligaments
- Uterine size and volume

Preparation
- Empty bladder: some do not advocate the use of a catheter as the bladder may be easier to identify
- Local infiltration in the form of simple saline or anaesthetic such as lignocaine/bupivacaine +/– adrenaline may help in preventing bleeding and in the identification of tissue planes

Cervical incision
- Cervix on traction
- Gap between the rugae of the anterior vaginal wall and smooth cervix identified
- Lift anterior vaginal wall to show pubocervical ligament
- Full thickness incision at this point to enter plane between bladder and cervix
- Posterior incision at the cul-de-sac base

Posterior peritoneal entry
- Peritoneum should be easily visualised posteriorly providing the initial incision has been made at the correct level and depth
- The cul-de-sac should be explored once the peritoneum has been opened to check for any adhesions or masses

Uterosacral ligaments

- Identified, clamped, cut and tied
- The clamp will be close to the cervix if no prolapse is present
- This tissue is used to provide vaginal support at the end of the procedure

Anterior peritoneal entry

- Once the vagina has been incised, the bladder can be reflected with a mixture of blunt and sharp dissection, made easier by ensuring that the correct tissue plane has been entered
- By dividing the uterosacral ligaments, the subsequent descent may facilitate easier anterior dissection
- Adequate refection of the bladder ensures that the ureters are kept free and away from the operative field
- Anterior peritoneum is entered

Uterine arteries

- This pedicle contains the uterine vessels as well as the upper cardinal ligament

Delivery of the uterus

- Infundibulopelvic ligament is identified, clamped, cut and tied
- Failure to deliver the uterus should arouse suspicion of additional pathologies such as fibroids or adhesions

Closure of the peritoneum

- May increase the risk of ureteric injury
- Closure results in exteriorisation of the pedicles, thus any bleeding would be per vaginum and easily recognised
- Can be difficult and cause unwanted bleeding
- Possible to incorporate the peritoneum into the skin closure

Vaginal support

- Traditionally the vault is supported by using the uterosacral pedicles, tied together in the midline
- Obliteration of the cul-de-sac is standard

Laparoscopic techniques for hysterectomy

Consists of:
- Laparoscopically assisted vaginal hysterectomy
- Laparoscopic hysterectomy
- Laparoscopic supracervical hysterectomy
- Total laparoscopic hysterectomy
- Laparoscopic radical hysterectomy

The current evidence regarding the safety and efficacy of these techniques has been sufficient to advocate their usage. However, advanced laparoscopic skills are required which are outwith the scope of normal training.

Advantages

- Reduced length of hospital stay of 1-2 days when compared with abdominal hysterectomy. This will therefore have cost implications
- Increased speed of return to normal activities when compared with abdominal hysterectomy
- Smaller incisions
- Less postoperative pain

Disadvantages

- There would appear to be an increased risk of damage to the urinary tract
- Increased risk of bleeding
- Up to 7% conversion rate to abdominal hysterectomy in a woman with a normal body mass index (as high as 20–25% in a morbidly obese woman)
- Port site hernias
- Longer operating time, therefore increased exposure to anaesthesia
- Increased cost of procedure (although offset by shorter hospital stay)

Laparoscopic versus abdominal versus vaginal hysterectomy

- Postoperative infection rates – 18% abdominal hysterectomy, 15% laparoscopic hysterectomy, 14% vaginal hysterectomy
- Mean length of hospital stay – 1.6 days laparoscopic hysterectomy, 2.2 days vaginal hysterectomy, 3.7 days abdominal hysterectomy.
- No overall difference in cost between abdominal hysterectomy and laparoscopic hysterectomy. However, significantly lower overall cost for vaginal hysterectomy when compared with the other two methods.

Further reading

Nieboer TE, Johnson N, Lethaby A, et al. Surgical approach to hysterectomy for benign gynaecological disease. Cochrane Database of Systematic Reviews, 2009; (3) CD003677.

Maxwell DJ. Surgical Techniques in Obstetrics and Gynaecology. London: Churchill Livingstone, 2004.

National Institute for Health and Clinical Excellence. Laparoscopic techniques for hysterectomy: guidance. London: NICE, 2007; IPG239.

Related topics of interest

- Fibroids (p. 46)
- Intermenstrual, postcoital and postmenopausal bleeding (p. 82)
- Heavy menstrual bleeding (p. 61)

Imaging in gynaecology

Overview

Imaging is an important diagnostic tool in gynaecology. The widespread adoption of ultrasound into gynaecological practice has facilitated the development of a range of one-stop clinics. Its growing importance has been reflected in the addition of this skill as a compulsory element of training in gynaecology.

Uses of imaging

Early pregnancy

Transabdominal and transvaginal pelvic ultrasound have revolutionised early pregnancy care. Ectopic pregnancies as well as failing pregnancies can be differentiated from gynaecological and non-gynaecological causes of pain and bleeding, allowing early medical and surgical management to be instigated where appropriate. However, as patients are presenting earlier to early pregnancy units, the diagnosis of pregnancy of unknown location (PUL) has become common, necessitating additional blood tests and further scans.

Benign gynaecology

Ultrasound has a key role in assessing benign uterine pathology including fibroids, uterine anomalies, endometrial polyps and ovarian cysts.

Fertility

Ultrasound is important to identify structural anomalies and pathologies within the reproductive tract in the initial work-up of patients with subfertility and recurrent miscarriage. Tubal patency can be assessed non-invasively either ultrasonographically by HyCosy or fluoroscopically by hysterosalpingogram. Ultrasonography is also used to track follicles and assist in egg collection in patients undergoing fertility treatments.

Gynaecological oncology

Ultrasound is important in the initial assessment of patients with symptoms which may be consistent with an increased risk of ovarian or endometrial cancer. Patients with suspected ovarian cancer are managed according to their Risk of Malignancy Index which is based on ultrasonography, patient factors and serum markers. Patients with postmenopausal bleeding are stratified according to the thickness of the endometrium into those requiring further investigation for endometrial malignancy (endometrial thickness greater than 4 mm) and those where malignancy is unlikely. In patients where malignancy has been diagnosed, further imaging is needed to help plan the management, stage disease and monitor disease response/identify progression.

Urogynaecology

Although imaging is of lesser importance in the management of urogynaecological conditions, endoanal ultrasound has a role in the assessment of patients following obstetric anal sphincter injury, whereas fluoroscopy may be of use in assessing fistulae.

Imaging modalities

Ultrasonography

Principles

- In ultrasonography piezoelectric crystals within the transducer are used to convert electrical energy into high frequency sound waves. Tissues scatter, reflect and absorb these waves to varying degrees. The returning sound waves are detected and analysed to give a two-dimensional real time image of the tissue (B-mode imaging)
- Transvaginal probes utilise higher frequencies (5–7.5 MHz) to give better resolution (meaning that they are better able to distinguish two targets closer together). This comes at the expense of a narrower beam width and decreased penetration
- Transabdominal probes work at lower frequencies (3–5 MHz) and are able to visualise deeper structures but with poorer resolution

Image quality and enhancement

- Image quality can be optimised by altering the gain (sensitivity of the probe to echoes), time gain compensation (adjustment for acoustic loss in parts of the field), focal zone, depth and zoom
- Different types of tissue can cause imaging artefacts. Bone causes acoustic shadowing. Abdominal wall fat causes attenuation

Safety

- Theoretically, high levels of ultrasound may cause tissue damage by heating, cavitation and streaming of fluid. Prolonged exposure times and prolonged use of high energies, e.g. in colour flow Doppler imaging, should be avoided especially in early pregnancy scanning

Magnetic resonance imaging

Principles

- Magnetic resonance imaging (MRI) is a non-ionising imaging modality. MRI scanners detect the radiofrequency emitted by hydrogen nuclei as they return to equilibrium after being exposed to variations within the electromagnetic field of the scanner. The detected radiofrequencies and the magnetic field strength at a given position can be used to map the position of the protons using a process called inverse Fourier transformation
- MRI provides good soft tissue contrast and is of particular use in imaging the pelvis, especially delineating perineal, vaginal, cervical, uterine and adnexal pathologies

Image quality and enhancement

- Different acquisition techniques can be used to highlight tissues of interest
- MRI contrast agents may be of use to enhance the contrast of different structures. Commonly used agents such as gadolinium are thought to be safer than the iodinated contrast agents used in computed tomography (CT) and angiography. They are less associated with anaphylactoid reaction and have less nephrotoxicity

Safety and limitations

- Patients with implants/foreign bodies that contain ferromagnetic material should not undergo MRI as they may be at risk of injury due to the movement of the object within the magnetic field or thermal heating injury
- Claustrophobia and patient habitus may limit the ability to perform a scan
- MRI is thought to be safe in pregnancy. However, contrast agents are contraindicated
- Lactating women should be reassured that the use of gadolinium is safe in breastfeeding

Ionising modalities

- Plain X-ray and fluoroscopy which utilises X-rays to produce real time images are used in a small number of limited indications in gynaecology, e.g. assessment of tubal patency, locating lost intrauterine devices, assessing for fistulae
- CT which uses computer processing of X-rays to generate 'slice views' is commonly used to assess the extent of distant spread in gynaecological malignancies
- Nuclear medicine imaging, e.g. positron emission tomography (PET) and lymphoscintigraphy, utilise radioactive substances in the form of radiopharmaceuticals to map 'hotspots' of cellular activity based on the uptake of these isotopes differentially by diseased/target tissue, e.g. metastases in cervix cancer, identification of sentinel lymph nodes in vulval cancer

Principles

- X-ray images are generated by placing the patient between the X-ray source and its detector and are dependent on different tissues impeding the passage of X-ray photons to different degrees
- Unlike X-rays where there is an external source, nuclear medicine imaging relies on the detection of gamma rays from injected radioisotopes

Image quality and enhancement

- Image artefact can occur where patients have metallic implants
- Iodinated contrast agents can be used to enhance vascular structures and hollow viscera
- Superimposing CT/MRI with nuclear medicine scans allows the localisation of 'hotspots'

Safety

- Ionising radiation can cause harm at a cellular level by disrupting DNA leading to effects on cell division and replication
- Diagnostic imaging techniques vary in the amount of ionising radiation delivered
- To reduce the risk to patients and staff the use of ionising radiation should be justified, optimised to ensure the lowest reasonable achievable dose is given and upper dose limits set by regulatory agencies adhered to
- Breast tissue in pregnant women and those within a month of delivery is more sensitive to the carcinogenic effects of ionising radiation, and therefore CT imaging of the chest should be minimised in this period
- The risk of miscarriage, malformation, growth or mental retardation in the fetus of women undergoing diagnostic imaging in pregnancy is negligible when exposed to 50 mGy or less. The majority of diagnostic procedures confer far less than this level
- For the majority of diagnostic procedures the risk of childhood cancers from fetal radiation exposure is very low (< 1 in 10,000). Exposure to higher dose procedures (i.e. exposures of 1–10 mGy) such as CT of the abdomen and pelvis may result in the doubling of the rate of childhood cancers. However, the absolute rate of childhood cancers remains low (1 in 200) thus such interventions should be carried out if its avoidance would otherwise be detrimental to the mother's immediate health
- Fetal radiation exposure can be reduced by adjusting acquisition protocols and the use of abdominal shielding
- The use of iodinated contrast agents should be avoided in pregnancy but is safe in breastfeeding women as very little appears in breast milk and moreover very little is absorbed by the infant

Further reading

Eskandar O, Eckford S, Watkinson T. Safety of diagnostic imaging in pregnancy. Part 1: X-ray, nuclear medicine investigations, computed tomography and contrast media. The Obstetrician & Gynaecologist 2010; 12:71–78.

Eskandar O, Eckford S, Watkinson T. Safety of diagnostic imaging in pregnancy. Part 2: magnetic resonance imaging, ultrasound scanning and Doppler assessment. The Obstetrician & Gynaecologist 2010; 12:171–177.

Dodge JE, Covens AL, Lacchetti C, et al. Gynecology Cancer Disease Site Group. Preoperative identification of a suspicious adnexal mass: a systematic review and meta-analysis. Gynecol Oncol 2012; 126:157–166.

Related topics of interest

- Abnormality of the genital tract (p. 1)
- Ovarian cancer (p. 97)
- Ovarian cysts (p. 104)

Intermenstrual, postcoital and postmenopausal bleeding

Overview

Abnormal uterine bleeding, including intermenstrual, postcoital and postmenopausal bleeding, is often due to benign causes, although more serious pathologies such as carcinoma need to be excluded. Often no obvious cause can be found, and reassurance and symptomatic treatment may be all that is required once investigations have been concluded.

Clinical features

Intermenstrual and postcoital bleeding often coexist. They may result from physiological changes secondary to the influence of endogenous or exogenous hormones and only rarely reflect an underlying carcinoma of the uterus or cervix. Most postmenopausal bleeds result from atrophic changes to the urogenital tract. Only 10% are due to malignancy.

Aetiology

Intermenstrual bleeding can be caused by:
- Physiological changes. Mid-cycle bleeding is due to the oestradiol surge
- Hormonal imbalance, e.g. on progesterone-only or low-dose oestrogen contraceptive pills (particularly if the patient has forgotten to take some)
- Infection, e.g. chlamydia, vaginitis associated with trichomoniasis or candidiasis, condylomata acuminate
- Benign tumours, e.g. endometrial or cervical polyps, fibroids, vaginal or cervical adenosis
- Malignant tumours, e.g. endometrial, cervical, vaginal (rare) or vulval cancer
- Drugs, e.g. antipsychotics, anticoagulants, corticosteroids, antiepileptics or antibiotics [if taken together with the combined oral contraceptive (COC)]

Postcoital bleeding can be caused by:
- Infection
  - Cervicitis from chlamydia or gonorrhoea
  - Vaginitis due to trichomonas or candidiasis

  - Endometritis in the presence of an intrauterine contraceptive device (IUCD)
- Benign cervical conditions, e.g. ectopy, polyps or fibroids
- Cervical cancer

Postmenopausal bleeding can be caused by:
- Atrophic vaginitis
- Endometrial or cervical polyps
- Endometrial, cervical, vaginal or vulval cancer

Diagnosis

A thorough history and examination should be undertaken. The history needs to take into account the patient's age, menstrual history, sexual history (as appropriate) as well as addressing more specific issues, such as:

History
- Time interval from the onset of symptoms to presentation, the frequency and amount of bleeding
- The period of amenorrhoea if postmenopausal, as this is related to an increased incidence of carcinoma of the corpus uteri
- Exogenous hormone therapy in the form of oral contraception or hormone replacement therapy
- The presence of vaginal discharge (associated with secondary infection of a cervical ectropion or carcinoma)
- Rarely there may be a history of a bleeding disorder or of trauma
- Coexistent medical conditions such as diabetes or tamoxifen use
- Any previous history of abnormal cervical smears
- Pain, fever or changes in bladder/bowel function might suggest an underlying infective process such as a pyometra

Examination
- A general physical examination should be undertaken, noting the patient's general condition, signs of metastatic cancer, e.g. left supraclavicular lymphadenopathy,

or other factors such as obesity that may point towards a possible underlying cause
- Any atrophic change of the urogenital tract should be noted
- Inspection of the vulva and vagina for atrophic change, vulval dermatoses, vulval or vaginal ulcers or suspicious nodules
- Inspection and palpation of the cervix to assess normality of the ectocervix, contact bleeding and cervical tenderness, friability of tissue, presence of ulceration or cervical polyp
- Bimanual examination provides an assessment of the uterus and adnexae followed by a rectal examination if there is suspicion of malignancy, or if there is a possibility that the bleeding could be from the gastrointestinal tract

Investigations

The bleeding pattern will obviously dictate the relevant investigation pathway to follow.

Intermenstrual bleeding

- Pregnancy test
- Triple swabs
- Cervical smear (if due)
- Colposcopy for all suspicious cervical features at speculum examination
- Transvaginal ultrasonography to exclude endometrial polyps
- Hysteroscopy and endometrial biopsy for persistent intermenstrual bleeding in order to exclude endometrial carcinoma or atypical hyperplasia. Hysteroscopy can detect up to 95% of intrauterine abnormalities
- Mid-cycle bleeding is physiological and requires no further investigation

Postcoital bleeding

- As for intermenstrual bleeding

Postmenopausal bleeding

These patients should be investigated as a matter of urgency. 10% of women who present with postmenopausal bleeding will have an underlying malignancy. Most gynaecological departments offer a dedicated service with direct referral access to general practitioners. Often this can be in the form of a 'one-stop' clinic, where patients can be seen, investigated and, in most cases, reassured and discharged the same day.

- Transvaginal ultrasonography for endometrial thickness. If < 5 mm, no further intervention is required. If > 5 mm, or in the presence of fluid in the uterine cavity or an irregular endometrium, then:
- Endometrial biopsy
- Vulval or vaginal biopsy if any suspicious lesions are seen on examination
- Cystoscopy and sigmoidoscopy to rule out bladder and bowel malignancy if there is a question as to where the bleeding originates from

Management

Underlying malignancy must be excluded (however remote the risk may seem) before commencing any form of treatment. Management of intermenstrual, postcoital and postmenopausal bleeding is directed to the underlying cause.

Intermenstrual bleeding

- Reassurance for physiological mid-cycle bleeding
- Genitourinary (GU) department referral for treatment of chlamydia, gonorrhoea and trichomoniasis. It is essential that the sexual partner(s) undergoes investigation and treatment. Contact tracing needs to be undertaken and this is outwith the scope of a gynaecology department setting
- Adjustment of any hormonal imbalance by increasing the oestrogen component of the COC
- Polypectomy
- Management of fibroids. See Topic 15.
- Appropriate management of any underlying malignancy

Postcoital bleeding

- Cryocautery to cervical ectropion
- Polypectomy
- GU department referral for treatment of chlamydia, gonorrhoea or trichomoniasis
- Removal of IUCD, trimming of threads or consideration of alternative forms of contraception if the bleeding is thought to be secondary to endometritis

- Appropriate management of any underlying malignancy

Postmenopausal bleeding

- Vaginal atrophy can be successfully treated by the administration of topical oestrogen

- Antibiotics are rarely indicated for vaginitis. Oestrogen replacement is usually sufficient.
- Polypectomy
- Management of underlying malignancy as dictated by the stage and grade.

Further reading

Phadnis SV, Walker PG. Modern management of postcoital and intermenstrual bleeding. Trends in Urology, Gynaecology and Sexual Health 2008; 13:24–27.

Bakour SH, et al. Management of women with postmenopausal bleeding: evidence-based review. The Obstetrician & Gynaecologist 2012; 14:243–249.

Annan JJ, Aquilina J, Ball E. The management of endometrial polyps in the 21st century. The Obstetrician & Gynaecologist 2012; 14:33–38.

Related topics of interest

Menopause and hormone replacement therapy

Overview

The menopause is defined as the last menstrual period of a woman's life. This single event characterises a number of significant changes, collectively known as the climacteric, or menopausal syndrome. The changes are primarily due to oestrogen deprivation consequent upon ovarian failure.

Hormone replacement therapy (HRT) is the generic term given to oestrogen therapy for pre-, peri- and postmenopausal women suffering from disturbances of oestrogen deficiency. In those with an intact uterus, it must be combined with a progestogen to prevent unopposed oestrogen-related endometrial hyperplasia and malignancy. It is not contraceptive.

Clinical features

Vasomotor instability   Hot flushes and night sweats are seen in 50–75%, and may last for 5 years in 25%.

Genital atrophy   This is seen in the vulva, vagina, cervix, uterus, ovaries, bladder, urethra, and supporting ligaments, leading to infection, dyspareunia, apareunia, frequency, dysuria and urgency.

Skin and hair   The skin thins and is prone to superficial laceration and bruising. The axillary and pubic hair are slowly lost and the head hair thins. There may be an increase in facial hair.

Psychological   Anxiety, forgetfulness, low self-esteem, loss of confidence, difficulty in concentration.

Osteoporosis   This is caused by an increase in bone resorption and relative loss of trabecular bone. It may be due to an increased skeletal sensitivity to the actions of bone resorbing hormones. It results in a significant rise in the incidence of femoral neck, vertebral body and wrist fractures, with consequent associated losses of mobility, rises in hospitalisation costs and fracture-related deaths.

Cardiovascular   Plasma cholesterol, triglycerides and very low-density lipoproteins (VLDL) will all rise and high-density lipoproteins (HDL) fall. There is an associated increase in ischaemic heart disease in postmenopausal women in parallel with these changes.

Diagnosis

The diagnosis is relatively simple when symptoms are clear-cut. It may be aided by plasma follicle-stimulating hormone (high) and oestradiol (low) levels. Ensure that psychological symptoms are not caused by other life events. Phaeochromocytoma, carcinoid syndrome and thyroid disease may mimic the climacteric.

Management

Treatment significantly reduces the risks of fractures, genital atrophy and psychological symptoms. Mortality from fractures and ischaemic heart disease can be avoided.

Non-hormonal   Publicity after the Women's Health Initiative Study and the Million Women Study has led to women stopping HRT. Due to concerns with safety of HRT treatment, increasingly patients are tending to prefer non-hormonal treatment. Selective norepinephrine reuptake inhibitors (SNRIs) have been shown to be beneficial in the treatment of vasomotor symptoms. There is convincing evidence to suggest that low dose venlafaxine used once at night is effective in the treatment of vasomotor symptoms.

Bisphosphonates have been suggested for the prevention and treatment of osteoporosis. The question of how long to prescribe a bisphosphonate has not been fully clarified yet, because of concerns about 'frozen bone', with complete turning off of bone remodelling with long term use of bisphosphonates and also development of osteonecrosis of the jaw. Five years of treatment with a 2-year 'holiday' has been proposed for alendronate, but there is a lack of evidence to guide treatment for other bisphosphonate drugs.

KY jelly and bioadhesive moisturisers (Replens) have been suggested for treatment of dyspareunia.

Complementary therapy, including phytoestrogens, herbal remedies, acupuncture, reflexology, homeopathy, diet and supplements may be of benefit. Efficacy data are limited and clinical trials often underpowered. Herbal remedies such as St John's wort, Agnus castus and Black Cohosh can have interactions with conventional medications. For example, St John's wort is known to interact with digoxin and selective serotonin reuptake inhibitors.

Oestrogens   These can be given orally, transdermally, vaginally or as a subcutaneous implant.

- **Oral administration** has the disadvantage that hepatic metabolism causes a significant inactivation of much of the oestrogen (the 'first-pass effect'); it may cause an increase in renin substrate production (especially dangerous in hypertensive patients); and it may cause an increase in thromboembolic disease in those with a positive history
- **Subcutaneous** (implants) and **transdermal** (patches) oestrogen produces plasma oestrogen profiles most closely mimicking those of an ovulatory cycle. Implants have been linked with tachyphylaxis (rapid tolerance to a drug dosage) in supraphysiological concentrations and they may be linked with prolonged endometrial stimulation. The addition of subcutaneous or transdermal testosterone may relieve psychosexual problems such as loss of libido

Progestogens   These have been used in women who are unable to take oestrogens (e.g. personal history of oestrogen-sensitive breast cancer). Studies have shown benefit of progestogens over placebo in the control of vasomotor symptoms. However, data from the Women's Health Initiative (WHI) suggested that women on combined HRT were more likely to develop breast cancer than women on oestrogen only preparations. The high dose of progestogen used can also increase risk of venous thromboembolism.

Benefits of HRT

- HRT helps relieve vasomotor symptoms and symptoms of atrophy. There is clear evidence that HRT improves the quality of life in postmenopausal women
- HRT is associated with a reduced incidence of osteoporosis-induced fractures of the wrist, vertebral bodies and hip
- A reduced incidence of heart disease, colorectal cancer and Alzheimer's disease is also a benefit

Risks of HRT

- There is an increased risk of endometrial hyperplasia and malignancy in woman with an intact uterus taking unopposed HRT. This risk is ablated if progestogens are added to their regimen
- There is an increased risk of benign and malignant breast disease in women on HRT regimens for > 10 years after the age of 50 years. This was the finding of the largest studies on HRT (WHI and Million Women studies). However, more recent studies have shown that the recorded risks of breast cancer are statistically small and appear to be linked with the duration of therapy. The only real contraindication to HRT at present is personal or family history of breast cancer
- HRT increases the risk of developing thromboembolic disease and stroke especially when used in older patients (> 60 years of age).

Preparations

The choice of oestrogen is dependent upon the indications, risks, convenience and patient compliance. Vaginitis in postmenopausal women will initially respond to topical oestrogen, but continuation of such a regimen for longer than 12 months may result in unopposed endometrial stimulation due to absorbed oestrogen. The oestrogen utilised include ethinyloestradiol, mestranol, oestradiol, oestriol and conjugated oestrogens. For the postmenopausal women with an intact uterus (> 12 months of postmenopausal amenorrhoea) continuous combined oestrogen and progestogen preparations are available. These result in a thin atrophic endometrium leading to a 'non-bleed HRT' for the majority. Alternatively, there is at least one preparation available as a 3-month long period cycle, again reducing the bleed phase associated with such combined preparations. The gonadomimetic preparation, tibolone, combines oestrogenic and progestogenic activity with weak androgenic activity, is 'non-bleed' and can also be given continuously to the woman with an intact uterus without cyclical progestogens. Oestogen only preparations are also suitable in patients with Mirena coil in situ.

Duration of treatment

Based on the current evidence, starting HRT at the early onset of the menopause and carrying on for a few years, carries little risk in healthy women. Taking medication also confers some benefit to bone strength and a small reduction in the risk of colonic cancer. A recent Danish study has concluded that after 10 years of follow-up, women receiving HRT early after menopause had a significantly reduced risk of mortality, heart failure and myocardial infarction, with no apparent increase in risk of cancer, stroke or thrombosis.

Women with a premature menopause are usually advised to have HRT until the average age of the natural menopause. Women with untreated premature menopause are at increased risk of developing osteoporosis, cardiovascular disease, dementia and cognitive decline. There is no evidence that HRT until the age of natural menopause increase risks in this group of patients. Women should be advised to use the lowest dose which gives symptom relief, and to continue after the natural age of the menopause for a limited period of time.

Further reading

Tong IL. Nonpharmacological treatment of postmenopausal symptoms. The Obstetrician & Gynaecologist 2013; 15:19–25.

Marsden J. Hormone replacement therapy and breast disease. The Obstetrician & Gynaecologist 2010; 12:155–163.

Cumming GP, Mauelshagen AE, Parrish MH. Postmenopausal sexual dysfunction. The Obstetrician & Gynaecologist 2010; 12:1–6.

Related topics of interest

Menstrual cycle physiology

Overview

The menstrual cycle is a coordinated and repeated series of changes in the structure of the endometrium that averages 28 days in length. It is tightly linked to the ovarian cycle of follicular development. The endometrial cycle can be divided into three phases: the menstrual phase or menses, the proliferative phase and the secretory phase. The phases are under regulation of hormones from both the pituitary glands and the ovaries. Menstruation and the secretory phase of the endometrium occur during the follicular phase of the ovarian cycle and the proliferative phase during the ovarian/luteal phase.

There is very little ovarian follicular development in childhood with mature follicular development only possible with hypothalamic–pituitary–ovarian axis maturation at puberty. Once maturation has commenced follicles proceed to either ovulation or atresia, the fate of the majority. At menarche, the first menstrual cycle of puberty, each ovary contains about 500,000 primordial follicles, each consisting of an oocyte, arrested in meiotic prophase, surrounded by granulosa cells and a membrane, the basal lamina, separating the follicle from surrounding stroma. The phases of the ovarian and endometrial cycles and their hormonal regulation are shown in **Figure 11** for an average 28-day cycle.

The endometrial cycle

Day 1–7 menstrual phase (menses)

The menstrual cycle commences with the onset of menstruation, the degeneration

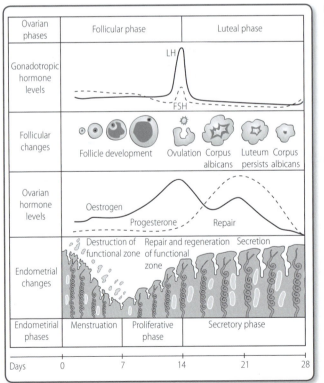

Figure 11 Phases of the female reproductive cycle.

and shedding of the functional zone of the endometrium due to constriction of the spiral arteries reducing blood flow.

Day 7–14 proliferative phase

The deeper basalis layer of the endometrium is not lost during menstruation and after menstruation, the glands of the basalis proliferate across the endometrium and the blood supply is restored giving a new functional zone. This occurs at the same time as the ovarian follicles are enlarging and starting to secrete oestrogen, and oestrogen is required for endometrial proliferation.

Day 15–28 secretory phase

During this phase the endometrial glands respond to the rising oestrogen and progesterone produced by the corpus luteum of the ovarian follicle, by enlarging and increasing the secretion of mucous, peaking at about day 26. The newly formed arteries elongate and spiral through the functional endometrial zone.

The ovarian cycle

Day 1–13 follicular phase

At the start of the follicular phase oestrogen levels are low and follicle-stimulating hormone (FSH) is the dominant hormone released from the anterior pituitary gland. FSH stimulates development of some primordial follicles into multilaminar primary follicles with a central enlarged oocyte surrounded by the zona pellucida and then the stratum granulosum covered by the two theca layers, interna and externa. The thecal cells begin production of the steroid hormone androstenedione which is absorbed by the granulosa cells and converted into oestrogen.

Day 14 ovulation

Granulosa cells coalesce, forming follicular fluid and an antrum in the Graafian follicle. The antrum further enlarges and divides the granulosa cells into the membranum granulosum and the cumulus oophorus. Immediately prior to ovulation the follicle consists of an innermost secondary oocyte with the first polar body, surrounded successively by the zona pellucida, the corona radiata and the cumulus oophorus. The increased oestrogen produced by the tertiary or Graafian follicles stimulates luteinising hormone (LH) secretion from the anterior pituitary which surges at day 14. The LH surge induces completion of meiosis I by the oocyte, rupture of follicle wall and ovulation. Primordial to antral phase development takes 85 days, resulting in a follicle of 2–5 mm in diameter, with subsequent growth being 1–3 mm/day, so that at the time of the LH surge and ovulation a dominant follicle measures 20 ± 3 mm. Each dominant follicle is usually surrounded by 2–3 non-dominant ones measuring < 16 mm, and they are not generally released at ovulation.

Day 15–28 luteal phase

The LH surge promotes progesterone secretion and after ovulation the granulosa and theca cells of the ovary form the gonadotrophic and luteotrophic corpus luteum. Progesterone rises until day 20 (hence the rationale behind day 21 serum progesterones to test for ovulation in the average 28-day cycle with ovulation on day 14).

As progesterone rises, oestrogen decreases and LH continues to maintain the structure and secretory function of the corpus luteum which functions to promote secretion of the endometrial glands in preparation for pregnancy. At about day 26 if no pregnancy occurs, the corpus luteum becomes non-functional and degenerates to form a corpus albicans, oestrogen and progesterone levels fall, FSH levels rise and the cycle starts over again.

Further reading

Rees CMP, Barlow DH. Ovulation and the endometrial cycle. In: Turnbull Sir AC, Chamberlain GC (Eds). Obstetrics. Edinburgh: Churchill Livingstone, 1989: 25–47.

Espey LL, Ben Halim IA. Characteristics and control of the normal menstrual cycle. Obstet Gynecol Clin North Am 1990; 17:275–298.

Ann N. The menstrual cycle: basic biology. Acad Sci 2008; 1135:10–18.

Related topics of interest

- Amenorrhoea (p. 4)
- Contraception: reversible methods (p. 26)
- Premenstrual syndrome (p. 124)

Minimal access surgery

Gynaecologists were amongst the first to embrace the principles of endoscopic surgery and used it widely for diagnostic evaluation. They were then slower than colleagues in other disciplines to widely embrace the therapeutic uses.

Hysteroscopy

The first attempt to visualise the inside of the uterine cavity was by Pantaleoni in 1869, but it was not until recently with the improvements in fibreoptics and instrumentation has hysteroscopy become widely used. Prior to performing hysteroscopic surgery it is essential to gain experience in diagnostic hysteroscopy.

- It is recommended that diagnostic hysteroscopies are performed as outpatient procedures
- Women can be advised to take standard doses of non-steroidal anti-inflammatory agents about an hour before their appointment. There is no benefit in administering opiates beforehand
- Cervical preparation is not required
- Miniature hysteroscopes with a diameter under 3 mm (2.7 mm) are recommended
- Uterine distension with saline appears to be associated with a better view, shorter procedure time and reduced incidence of vasovagal episodes when compared to carbon dioxide
- Vaginoscopy reduces pain and should be the standard method for outpatient hysteroscopy
- Routine cervical dilatation should be avoided
- If a tenaculum is needed then topical local anaesthesia is recommended. Intracervical and paracervical blocks are useful when dilatation is anticipated and larger (5 mm) hysteroscopes are used
- Some simple procedures can be performed at the same time as diagnostic hysteroscopy including directional biopsies, removal of endometrial polyps and retrieval of lost intrauterine contraceptive devices. It is now the investigation of choice compared to Dilation and Curettage (D&C)
- Hysteroscopic polyp removal is superior to avulsion. Simple snares are available as are devices that use bipolar energy to coagulate the base of the polyps
- Advanced procedures are frequently performed under general anaesthesia. They include division of uterine septae (laparoscopy is useful initially to exclude bicornuate uteri, and to assess tubal patency), endometrial resection and division of adhesions (Asherman syndrome). The development of hysteroscopic morcellators is facilitating hysteroscopic myomectomy as an outpatient procedure. Hysteroscopic sterilisation as an outpatient is widely used and has been thoroughly evaluated
- Complications of hysteroscopic surgery include uterine perforation with visceral and vascular damage, fluid overload, infection and haemorrhage. Late complications include treatment failure, haematometra, pregnancy and the possibility of the late presentation of endometrial carcinoma
- Advantages include a short hospital stay, rapid recovery, reduced morbidity and early return to work with reduced cost implications. Outpatient treatment is safe and cost-effective, although some techniques have not been widely adopted due to cost (e.g. sterilisation) although they are significantly better for the patient

Laparoscopy

Professor K Semm at Kiel in Germany was one of the first proponents of laparoscopic surgery in the 1970s. The first report of operative laparoscopy was in 1933 by Fervers, a general surgeon. Gynaecologists adopted laparoscopic techniques to perform sterilisations and the first laparoscopic hysterectomy was performed by Harry Reich in 1989.

Around 250,000 women undergo laparoscopic surgery in the UK each year.

Most are safe, but serious complications occur in about 1 in 1000 cases.

- Laparoscopic surgery is advantageous compared to laparotomy. There are smaller less painful incisions with reduced postoperative analgesic requirements and hospital stay. There is less intraoperative blood loss, adhesion formation, tissue trauma and infection. Faster return to work
- Laparoscopy does have complications with mortality rates of 3.7/100,000 and major complication rates of between 1–12.5/1000. Damage to vessels and viscera, CO_2 embolism and anaesthetic complications are widely reported
- The blind insertion of the Veress needle (closed technique) and trocar are responsible for the majority of vessel and visceral damage. Open laparoscopy (Hasson, 1971) involves a short incision through the skin, fascia and peritoneum prior to the introduction of the trocar under direct vision. This is thought to be safer in terms of reducing vascular injuries and is recommended by the Royal College of Surgeons
- If the closed technique is employed the intra-abdominal pressure should be 20–25 mmHg before the primary port is inserted
- Secondary ports should always be inserted under direct vision after visualisation of the inferior epigastric vessels. Operating pressures of 12–15 mmHg should be maintained after they are inserted
- After inserting the laparoscope, a 360° rotation should be performed to check for adherent bowel
- Palmer's point or the Hasson technique is recommended for primary entry in women who are very thin or morbidly obese

Laparoscopic procedures

Uterus

- Repair of uterine perforation
- Hysterectomy: total, subtotal, laparoscopically assisted vaginal hysterectomy (LAVH), +/– bilateral salpingo-oophorectomy (BSO). With regard to laparoscopic hysterectomy, it should be noted that this operation does not replace vaginal hysterectomy or necessarily make a difficult vaginal hysterectomy easier. Its role may be to convert an abdominal procedure to a vaginal one, or to allow the safe removal of the ovaries at the same time
- Myomectomy
- Cervical cerclage
- Removal of rudimentary uterine horn
- Uterine artery ligation for management of menorrhagia
- Removal of significant adenomyosis

Adnexae

- Adhesiolysis
- Ovarian cyst enucleation
- Tubal surgery: reversal sterilisation, treatment of ectopics
- Ovarian cystectomy, oophorectomy
- Ovarian drilling: polycystic ovary syndrome

Endometriosis

- Endocoagulation
- Excision

Infertility

- In vitro fertilisation (IVF)/gamete
- Intrafallopian transfer (GIFT)/zygote
- Intrafallopian transfer (ZIFT)

Intra-abdominal

- Adhesiolysis
- Management of sepsis – lavage

Cancer

- Laparoscopic lymphadenectomy
- Radical hysterectomy

Prolapse/incontinence

- Laparoscopic sacrocolpopexy (superior to sacrospinous fixation for vault prolapse)
- Laparoscopic hysteropexy
- Laparoscopic colposuspension
- Laparoscopic pelvic floor repair

Pain

- Laparoscopic presacral neurectomy

Single incision laparoscopic surgery (SILS)

SILS is a recent development. It utilises a single port inserted through the umbilicus through which the laparoscope and instruments are introduced. The advantages of laparoscopic surgery prevail with the additional advantage of better cosmesis – just one scar. Operative times may be increased and with the current development of 3 mm instruments the potential better cosmesis may become less of an issue. Although widely adopted in general surgery and urology there is limited data of benefits in gynaecology at present.

Natural orifice transluminal endoscopic surgery (NOTES)

NOTES provides the opportunity for 'scarless' surgery where the laparoscope is inserted through the vagina. This has been employed to remove kidneys and gallbladders but its use has not been evaluated widely in gynaecology.

Robot-assisted surgery

The da Vinci Surgical System robot has been introduced globally and has advantages over ('straight-stick') laparoscopy. These primarily include the 3D view of the operative field, the comfortable setting with the surgeon seated, the complete control of the camera by the surgeon, increased magnification (X 10), and greater degrees of movement. The big disadvantage is the cost and set up time. The robot is providing conventional surgeons with the ability to operate laparoscopically.

Further reading

RCOG Green-top Guideline No. 59. Best Practice in Outpatient Hysteroscopy. London: RCOG, 2011.
RCOG Green-top Guideline 49. Preventing entry-related gynaecological laparoscopic injuries. London: RCOG, 2008.

Hasson HM. A modified instrument and method for laparoscopy. Am J Obstet Gynecol 1971; 110:886–887.
Frappell J. Laparoscopic entry after previous surgery. The Obstetrician & Gynaecologist 2012;14:207–209.

Related topics of interest

Miscarriage

Overview

Miscarriage is defined as the spontaneous loss of a pregnancy at or before 24 weeks of gestation. It occurs in up to 20% of clinical pregnancies. It is most common in the first trimester. Recurrent miscarriage is defined as the loss of three or more consecutive pregnancies and affects up to 1% of couples (See Topic 40).

Clinical features

Women with miscarriage may present with pain and bleeding after a positive pregnancy test. A woman's clinical presentation will aid the choice of investigations and management. A 'missed miscarriage' may occur when a woman is asymptomatic or has minimal symptoms (e.g. brown spotting) and an ultrasonographic diagnosis of miscarriage is made. Women presenting with pain and bleeding in early pregnancy should be managed in an early pregnancy unit (EPU), a dedicated service to improve the efficiency and quality of care they receive.

Aetiology

Increasing maternal and paternal age is associated with increased risk of miscarriage. At the maternal age of 20 years, the risk of miscarriage is 20%, but it rises to 93% above the age of 45 years. Poorly controlled diabetes, smoking, excessive alcohol use and obesity are also linked with miscarriage. The risk of a further miscarriage increases after each consecutive pregnancy loss and is reported as 40% after three losses.

Diagnosis

EPUs should develop and use algorithms for diagnosis and management. It is important to differentiate between ectopic pregnancy, intrauterine pregnancy of uncertain viability and a pregnancy of unknown location.

A woman who presents with heavy vaginal bleeding and pain should be assessed promptly and appropriate resuscitation

Table 13	Sonographic classification of miscarriage
Miscarriages	**Ultrasound findings**
Threatened miscarriage	Intrauterine pregnancy = gestation sac + yolk sac +/– fetal pole and cardiac activity
Inevitable miscarriage	
Incomplete miscarriage	Retained products of conception > 15 mm in diameter (with or without gestation sac)
Complete miscarriage	Empty uterus or retained products of conception < 15 mm in diameter
Missed miscarriage or early fetal demise	Mean gestational sac diameter ≥ 25 mm with no obvious yolk sac or fetal pole with crown–rump length (CRL) ≥ 7 mm and no cardiac activity

undertaken. Clinical examination includes a speculum and pelvic assessment. If the cervical os is open, the miscarriage is inevitable. If products of conception are seen, the miscarriage is either ongoing or complete.

In a majority of women, diagnosis of a miscarriage is made using transvaginal scanning. Ultrasound findings are summarised in **Table 13**. Additional tests include serial serum human chorionic gonadotropin (hCG) levels with a falling serum level indicative of a miscarriage. Serum progesterone levels below 25 nmol/L are associated with non-viable pregnancies.

Management

Patient choice should be paramount in the management of miscarriage, which can be expectant, medical or surgical.

Expectant management

Expectant management involves allowing 'nature to take its course', with no planned medical intervention. Efficacy rates are lower when an intact gestation sac is present. Rates of spontaneous resolution at 2 weeks are 71% for incomplete miscarriage, 53% for an empty sac/blighted ovum and 35% for missed miscarriage. Patient counselling is vital since women with an intact sac may not achieve spontaneous resolution for several weeks.

A Cochrane review of seven trials comparing expectant care with surgical management showed that incomplete miscarriage at 6–8 weeks was more common in the expectant care group (RR 2.56, 95% CI 1.15–5.69). 28% of women eventually required surgical intervention. By comparison, 4% of those who had upfront surgery needed an additional surgical procedure. Rates of infection were more common in the surgery (3%) than the expectant care (1%) group.

Medical management

Medical management of miscarriage generally involves treatment with prostaglandin analogues after antiprogesterone priming. Mifepristone is an antiprogesterone that binds to the progesterone receptor without activating it. This encourages trophoblastic separation, decline in circulating β-hCG and prostaglandin release. Misoprostol is a prostaglandin analogue that is equally effective orally or vaginally. The vaginal route may carry fewer gastrointestinal side effects (nausea, vomiting and diarrhoea). Misoprostol binding to myometrial cells causes strong myometrial contractions leading to expulsion of tissue. Both agents cause cervical ripening with softening and dilation of the cervix.

A variety of protocols are used for the medical management of miscarriage (**Figure 12**). Misoprostol alone can be used in incomplete miscarriage, whilst effective treatment in missed miscarriage requires higher and/or repeated doses of prostaglandin, usually in addition to mifepristone priming. A Cochrane review compared misoprostol with surgical evacuation and found no statistically significant difference in complete miscarriage rates (average RR 0.96, 95% CI 0.92–1.00, eight studies, 1377 women). Surgical intervention was required in 3–16% of women treated with Misoprostol and antibiotics were needed in less than 3%.

Bleeding after medical management can take 3 weeks to subside. Management can be outpatient-based if the unit has protocols in place and the patient has access to emergency advice and admission if required.

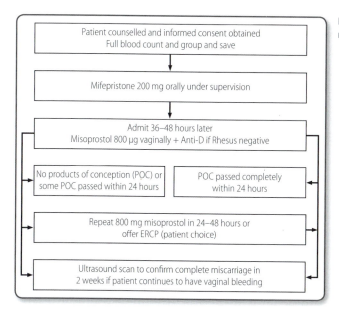

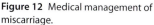

Figure 12 Medical management of miscarriage.

Surgical management

Surgical uterine evacuation [evacuation of retained products of conception (ERPC)] is recommended for persistent, excessive bleeding and haemodynamic compromise, evidence of infected retained products, suspicion of gestational trophoblastic disease or if the patient prefers it.

ERCP is carried out as a day case procedure under general anaesthetic. Preoperative cervical priming with prostaglandins will reduce the risk of uterine and cervical trauma. The patient is placed in lithotomy and an examination under anaesthetic is carried out. The cervix is grasped with vulsella and gently dilated with Hegar dilators (usually 8–10 mm). ERCP should be performed using suction curettage as it results in significantly reduced blood loss. Routine use of a metal curette after suction curettage is not required. Oxytocin can be used to encourage haemostasis and is associated with a significant difference in median blood loss (17.6 mL versus 24.5 mL). In the patient where infection is suspected, it may be prudent to delay surgical intervention for 12 hours to administer intravenous antibiotics first.

Patients should be counselled about serious risks including uterine perforation (5 in 1000 women) and significant cervical trauma (rare). If uterine perforation is suspected, a hysteroscopy and laparoscopy are performed to inspect the uterine and pelvic cavities and assess for visceral damage. The patient is admitted for observation and broad-spectrum intravenous antibiotics given for 24–48 hours. Bleeding that lasts up to 2 weeks is common but rarely is blood transfusion required (1–2 per 1000 women). There is a 4% risk of repeated surgical evacuation and a 3% risk of infection.

Products of conception are examined histologically to exclude ectopic pregnancy and gestational trophoblastic disease. This is particularly important in women with risk factors for these conditions.

Psychological sequelae are commonly associated with pregnancy loss and women should have access to support, follow-up and formal counselling if required. Systems must be in place to ensure that primary care professionals are informed.

Further reading

Sagili H, Divers M. Modern management of miscarriage. The Obstetrician & Gynaecologist 2007; 9:102–108.

RCOG Green-top Guideline No 25. The management of early pregnancy loss. London: ROCOG, 2006.

Cheong Y, Umranikar A. Problems in early pregnancy. In: Luesley DM, Baker, P (Eds). Obstetrics & Gynaecology: An evidence-based text for the MRCOG, 2nd edn. London: Hodder Arnold, 2010:649–667.

Related topics of interest

Ovarian cancer

In the UK, ovarian cancer accounts for more deaths than all the other gynaecological cancers combined. In 2010, 7011 British women were diagnosed with ovarian cancer, and 4295 women died from it. A woman's lifetime risk of developing the disease is estimated as 1 in 54. Most ovarian cancer presents in its advanced stages and the overall 5-year survival rate is just 43%.

Aetiology

The aetiology of ovarian cancer is incompletely understood. The most widely held view is that ovarian cancer results from repeated damage and repair of the ovarian surface epithelium caused by ovulation (the incessant ovulation theory). This is supported by evidence that nulliparous women are at increased risk of ovarian cancer, whilst pregnancy and long term use of the combined contraceptive pill (which inhibits ovulation) are protective. It has recently been suggested that high grade serous tumours of the ovary may in fact originate in the fallopian tube.

Most ovarian cancers are sporadic but 10% may be hereditary, with *BRCA1* (lifetime risk of ovarian cancer 15–65%) and *BRCA2* mutation carriers (10–20% lifetime risk) most at risk. Other hereditary syndromes, including Lynch [Hereditary Non-Polyposis Colorectal Cancer (HNPCC)] and Peutz–Jeghers also increase risk. Risk factors for sporadic ovarian cancer include:

- Advanced age (80% ovarian cancers diagnosed after menopause)
- Nulliparity
- Infertility
- Endometriosis (30–66% increased risk)
- Hormone replacement therapy (HRT) (5 years combined HRT increases risk by 22%)
- Previous benign ovarian cysts (2–9-fold increased risk)
- Previous breast cancer (4-fold increased risk)
- Family history (one first degree family member with ovarian cancer increases risk by 3–4-fold)
- Previous pelvic radiotherapy for cervical cancer
- Smoking
- Obesity (particularly for premenopausal cancers)
- Tall stature (> 1.7 m tall) (increased risk by 40%)
- Talcum powder (33% increased risk)
- Asbestos exposure (3–5-fold increased risk)

Protective factors include:
- Pregnancy (additional protection for each pregnancy)
- Breastfeeding
- Combined oral contraceptives (linked to duration of use; use for > 15 years halves ovarian cancer risk; also protective for *BRCA1* and *BRCA2* mutation carriers)
- Tubal ligation (34% risk reduction)
- Hysterectomy
- Physical activity
- Risk reducing prophylactic bilateral salpingo-oophorectomy (BSO) (still at 3–4% risk of primary peritoneal carcinoma; BSO also reduces risk of breast cancer by 50%)

Clinical features

Most ovarian cancer presents late with advanced disease. The common presenting signs and symptoms are shown in **Table 14**. Recent National Institute for Health and Clinical Excellence (NICE) guidance emphasises the importance of investigating

Table 14 Symptoms and signs of ovarian cancer	
Symptoms	Persistent pelvic and abdominal pain Increased abdominal size Bloating Loss of appetite/feeling full quickly Change in bowel habit Back pain Weight loss Fatigue
Signs	Pelvic or abdominal mass Abdominal distension Ascites Cachexia

vague and non-specific abdominal symptoms in primary care to expedite diagnosis.

There is no established screening programme for ovarian cancer. Studies investigating the use of tumour marker Ca-125 and pelvic ultrasound scans have not demonstrated a survival benefit for general population or high risk population screening. The UKCTOCS study, a large random controlled trial (RCT) of ovarian cancer screening involving more than 200,000 postmenopausal women, will report in 2015. An effective screening test requires a minimum positive predictive value (PPV) of 10% (i.e. 10 laparotomies for every case of ovarian cancer diagnosed).

Diagnosis

A clinical high index of suspicion is vital.

Serum tumour markers

- Ca-125 (raised in 90% advanced epithelial ovarian cancer and 50% early stage disease) **(Table 15)**
- Alpha fetoprotein (AFP) and human chorionic gonadotropin (hCG) (for women < 40 years, raised in germ cell tumours)
- Carcinoembryonic antigen (CEA) and Ca19-9 (to exclude bowel and pancreatic tumours, respectively)

Imaging (Figure 13)

- Pelvic ultrasound [transvaginal ultrasound scan (USS)] to identify and characterise the ovarian cyst (multilocularity, bilateral lesions, solid areas, presence of ascites and evidence of metastasis are suspicious features)
- CT of the thorax, abdomen and pelvis [for staging **(Table 16)**, to exclude metastatic disease, to determine operability and most likely site for biopsy if indicated]. Advanced disease shows a typical distribution on scan, with adnexal masses, ascites, omental disease and peritoneal thickening frequently seen
- Magnetic resonance imaging (MRI) of the pelvis (to define tissue planes, establish proximity to rectosigmoid colon and small bowel, to plan surgery and determine risk of need for bowel resection and colorectal surgical input at laparotomy)

Risk of malignancy index (RMI)

- Simple formula that combines menopausal status, CA-125 level and USS features to determine whether the ovarian cyst is at low, intermediate or high risk of malignancy, in order to determine management (including specialist referral) (See Topic 32.)

Tissue diagnosis

- Where the patient is deemed inoperable or a preference for neoadjuvant chemotherapy is made, an USS or CT-guided biopsy (usually of an omental cake) is necessary to establish the diagnosis and guide choice of chemotherapeutic agents
- A 'staging' laparoscopy may be an alternative in complex cases, to obtain biopsies and determine operability
- Occasionally, where a biopsy is not possible, a sample of ascitic fluid may be sent for cytology to confirm the diagnosis. Rarely, chemotherapy may be commenced with a positive cytology result

Management

Central multidisciplinary team (MDT) meeting

All suspected ovarian cancer diagnoses are discussed at the gynaecological oncology central MDT meeting. Clinical, imaging and histological features are reviewed with a view to planning further management, including who is the most appropriate clinician to initially manage their care.

Patient support

Women with ovarian cancer are supported by:
- Gynaecological oncology clinical nurse specialists
- Information about the cancer, the type of treatment and prognosis
- Education on self-help strategies
- Support groups

Table 15 Classification of ovarian cancers

	Type	Prevalence	Clinical features	Prognosis
Epithelial ovarian	Serous tumours	>50% ovarian tumours Age range: 30–50 years Associated with BRCA mutations	High grade (aggressive) or low grade (indolent) tumours Raised Ca-125 in 90% advanced and 50% early stage tumours	Overall 5-year survival rate: • Low grade serous 56% • High grade serous 34%
	Mucinous tumours	5–10% ovarian tumours Age range: 40–70 years	Associated with mucinous ascites Pseudomyxoma peritonei is a primary appendiceal neoplasm that may present with ovarian metastases	Overall 10-year survival rate: 66%
	Clear cell	6% ovarian tumours Age range: 40–80 years	Associated with endometriosis	Overall 5-year survival rate: 57%
	Endometrioid	8% ovarian tumours Age range: postmenopausal	40% have concurrent endometrial cancer	Overall 5-year survival rate: 70%
	Transitional	Very rare Age range: postmenopausal	Can be very large tumours (10–30 cm)	Not known
Sex cord-stromal	Granulosa stromal cell	2% ovarian tumours Mean age: 50–55 years Also seen in young girls and children	Slow growing tumour Produces oestrogen Presents with irregular or heavy vaginal bleeding Raised inhibin	Overall 5-year survival rate: 92%
	Gynandroblastoma	Exceedingly rare	Mixture of Sertoli and granulosa cells Produces oestrogen and testosterone Combination of feminising and masculinising effects May present with abnormal bleeding, hirsutism and deep voice	Not known
	Sertoli stromal cell	Mean age: 30 years	Produces testosterone Leads to defeminisation and then progressive masculinisation Presents in early stages with anovulation, oligomenorrhoea or amenorrhoea Later stages are associated with hirsutism, voice deepening, clitoromegaly, temporal hair recession and an increase in musculature	Slow growing tumour with good prognosis
	Steroid cell	0.1% ovarian tumours Age range: 20–40 years	Raised androstenedione, α-hydroxyprogesterone, and testosterone levels	Unknown

Contd...

Contd...

Ovarian germ cell	Choriocarcinoma	Rare tumour Age range: gestational type: < 40 years non-gestational type: > 40 years	Aggressive tumour Placental trophoblastic cells tumour Gestational type is metastasis from uterine choriocarcinoma and presents following a pregnancy Non-gestational type is a primary ovarian tumour Presents with irregular bleeding, abdominal pain, nausea and vomiting. Young girls may present with precocious puberty Raised hCG	Overall 15-year survival rate: 94% (gestational type) Exquisitely sensitive to chemotherapy
	Dysgerminoma	1% ovarian tumours Age range: young women (5% in prepubertal girls)	Raised AFP, hCG, Ca-125, inhibin A and B	Overall 10-year survival rate: 92%
	Embryonal	Rare 3% germ cell tumours Median age: 15 years	Sexual precocity and abnormal uterine bleeding Raised hCG, AFP	Not known
	Immature teratoma	1% ovarian tumours Age range: 50% occur between 10–20 years of age	Palpable mass	Overall 5-year survival rate: 90%
	Yolk sac tumour	Rare 10% germ cell tumours Age range: 10–20 years	Abdominal pain with a rapidly growing mass Raised AFP	Overall 5-year survival rate: 94%
	Mixed germ cell	Age range: 15–30 years		Overall 7-year survival rate: 83%
Metastatic tumour	Krukenberg	1% ovarian tumours Age range: any	Metastatic spread from breast or gastrointestinal tumours Mucin-secreting signet-ring cells are pathognomic	

Early stage ovarian cancer

Staging for presumed early stage ovarian cancer includes:

- A midline laparotomy (to facilitate access to omentum and upper abdominal organs, and allow removal of adnexal masses without spillage of cyst contents; an initial subumbilical incision can be extended if necessary)
- Peritoneal washings
- Inspection and palpation of the pelvic and abdominal organs
- Total abdominal hysterectomy and bilateral salpingo-oophorectomy
- Infracolic omentectomy
- Peritoneal biopsies

- Retroperitoneal lymph node assessment (ipsilateral pelvic and para-aortic lymph node sampling)

Disease confined to the ovary (stage Ia) does not require adjuvant chemotherapy. Adjuvant chemotherapy should be considered where disease has spread beyond the ovary (stage Ic); incomplete surgical staging has been performed; or where there are histological features of high risk disease (high grade serous or clear cell tumours). Pelvic and para-aortic lymph node sampling is preferred to systematic lymphadenectomy to reduce surgical morbidity for the majority of patients where the lymph nodes will be negative (bleeding, ureteric injury, nerve injury and lymphocyst formation).

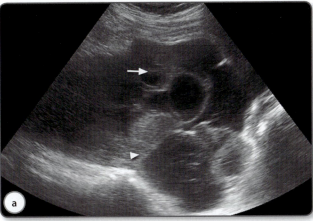

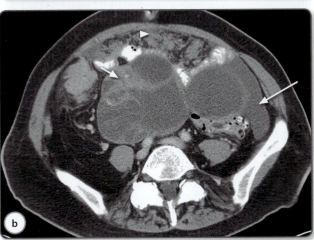

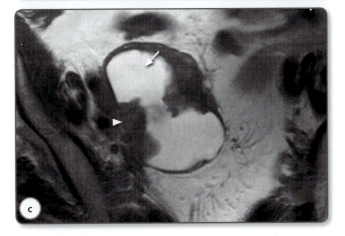

Figure 13 (a) USS showing a multicystic pelvic mass with hypoechoic (arrow) and solid echogenic areas (arrowhead). (b) CT scan showing ovarian cancer, seen as a multicystic mass with solid enhancing areas (short arrow). Omental thickening (arrowhead) and ascites (long arrow) are present. (c) MRI shows ovarian cancer with greater accuracy: the solid areas (arrowhead) are more easily differentiated from cystic elements (arrow).

Advanced disease

The treatment options for advanced disease (stages II–IV) are:

- Primary debulking surgery and adjuvant chemotherapy
- Neoadjuvant chemotherapy with carboplatin or paclitaxel followed (after three cycles) by interval debulking surgery (IDS)

A recent well-conducted RCT showed that neoadjuvant chemotherapy followed by IDS was 'not inferior' to upfront surgery with adjuvant chemotherapy, and the former is generally preferred where surgical debulking is unlikely to be complete, based on preoperative CT scans.

The aim of surgery for advanced ovarian cancer is to completely debulk all macroscopically visible disease. Complete cytoreduction is associated with improved overall 5-year survival rates. Complete cytoreduction rates are higher when the surgery is performed by a gynaecological oncologist rather than a general gynaecologist. Bowel involvement may lead to joint cases with the colorectal surgeons. Extensive upper abdominal disease requiring splenectomy, excision of disease around the porta hepatitis/diaphragm or cholecystectomy is likely to require hepatobiliary surgical input.

Where preoperative imaging indicates inoperable disease, neoadjuvant chemotherapy may be administered to shrink the cancer. After three cycles, disease response is assessed by CT scan and Ca-125 assessment. IDS is recommended for cancers that are operable. This is followed by a further three cycles of chemotherapy. If IDS is not performed, an assessment will be made after six cycles by imaging. Surgery now (delayed

Table 16 International Federation of Gynecology and Obstetrics (FIGO) staging of ovarian cancer	
Stage 1	**Tumour limited to the ovaries**
1a	Tumour limited to one ovary with an intact capsule and no tumour on ovarian surface No malignant cells in ascites or peritoneal washings
1b	Tumour limited to both ovaries with intact capsules and no tumour on ovarian surfaces No malignant cells in ascites or peritoneal washings
1c	Tumour limited to one or both ovaries +/– ruptured capsule, tumour on ovarian surface, malignant cells in ascites or peritoneal washings
Stage 2	**Tumour involves one or both ovaries with pelvic extension**
2a	Extension and/or implants on the uterus and/or tube(s) No malignant cells in ascites or peritoneal washings
2b	Extension to other pelvic tissues No malignant cells in ascites or peritoneal washings
2c	Pelvic extension with malignant cells in ascites or peritoneal washings
Stage 3	**Tumour involves one or both ovaries** **Microscopically confirmed peritoneal metastasis outside of pelvis**
3a	Microscopic peritoneal metastasis beyond the pelvis
3b	Macroscopic peritoneal metastasis beyond the pelvis ≤ 2 cm
3c	Macroscopic peritoneal metastasis beyond the pelvis > 2 cm +/– regional lymph node metastasis
Stage 4	**Distance metastasis**
	Liver parenchyma Pleural effusion with positive cytology

primary debulking surgery) is not evidence-based but is widely practiced in selected cases.

Follow-up

The aim of follow-up is to detect recurrence and manage treatment-related morbidity. Women are seen frequently (every 3–4 months) in the first 2 years, when rates of recurrence are highest. Thereafter, they are typically seen every 6 months (or more frequently if symptomatic) for a total duration of 5 years.

Recurrent disease

Treatment of recurrent disease is individualised according to the site(s) of recurrence and previous response to chemotherapy. Secondary cytoreductive surgery may be performed for isolated pelvic recurrences. There is limited evidence for this and it is only appropriate for carefully selected cases. Women who responded to platinum-based chemotherapy (platinum sensitive) first time round may receive further carboplatin for recurrent disease. Those who did not (platinum resistant) are offered second line chemotherapy (see Chemotherapy).

Borderline ovarian cysts

Borderline ovarian cysts comprise a distinct group of ovarian tumours that show characteristic pathological, clinical and prognostic features. They have high proliferative activity compared with benign tumours but do not show stromal invasion. Compared to ovarian cancer, they affect younger women and have an excellent prognosis, with 5-year survival rates ranging from 95% for stage I to 50–86% for stage III. Ten-year survival rates are 80–90% overall due a tendency for late recurrence.

Serous borderline ovarian tumours are the most common histological subtype (50%) and are bilateral in 30% of cases. Extra-ovarian disease (implants) is commonly encountered, which can be invasive or non-invasive. Mucinous borderline ovarian tumours are associated with pseudomyxoma peritonei in 10% of cases.

Preoperative diagnosis can be difficult as borderline tumours masquerade as benign or malignant disease on imaging, and tumour markers are not reliably raised.

The management of borderline ovarian tumours depends on the stage of disease as well as the age of the patient and her desire for future fertility. In most postmenopausal women, a laparotomy and full surgical staging is appropriate. In premenopausal women with early stage disease, fertility-saving surgery is a reasonable approach (unilateral salpingo-oophorectomy, omental biopsy and peritoneal washings). Where disease has spread beyond the ovary, full or limited surgical resection is advised depending on the patient's wishes and according to the histological features of the tumour, with completion surgery recommended for serous borderline tumours with invasive implants and DNA aneuploidy.

Further reading

Vergote I, Trope CG, Amant F, et al. Neoadjuvant chemotherapy or primary surgery in stage IIIc or IV ovarian cancer. N Engl J Med 2010; 363:943–953.
National Collaborating Centre for Cancer. NICE clinical guideline no.122. Ovarian cancer: The recognition and initial management of ovarian cancer. London: NICE, 2011.
Bagade P, Edmondson R, Nayar A. Management of borderline ovarian tumours. The Obstetrician & Gynaecologist 2012; 14:115–120.

Related topics of interest

Ovarian cysts

Overview

Ovarian cysts may be benign or malignant. The majority of cysts in premenopausal women are benign. 10% of cysts initially thought to be ovarian are paratubal cysts or hydrosalpinges. The management of malignant ovarian cysts is described in Topic 31.

Clinical features

Ovarian cysts may present with pelvic pain or they may be discovered incidentally in asymptomatic women undergoing investigation for unrelated indications. Ovarian cysts are common in women with endometriosis (endometriomas), and these patients usually present with chronic pelvic pain, dyspareunia or dysmenorrhoea. Ovarian cancer presents with non-specific abdominal (bloating, pain, altered bowel habit, nausea and vomiting) or constitutional symptoms (loss of appetite, weight loss).

A large ovarian cyst may be palpable per abdomen. Smaller cysts are detected on pelvic examination in a slim patient.

Aetiology

Ovarian cysts are common and are caused by different processes. Normal physiological processes may cause functional cysts including follicular or corpus luteal cysts.

Diagnosis

Imaging

The diagnosis of an ovarian cyst is made by pelvic ultrasound scan. A transvaginal scan offers greater sensitivity than the transabdominal method. The ultrasound scan report will contain a description of the cyst such as its size and nature.

Tumour markers

Women with a simple cyst of greater than 50 mm, a complex cyst and/or clinical features of ovarian cancer should have their tumour markers measured. Serum cancer antigen 125 (Ca-125) is raised in ovarian epithelial cancer. In women under 40, serum alpha fetoprotein (AFP) and human chorionic gonadotrophin (hCG) should also be measured because they are raised in germ cell tumours.

Risk of malignancy index (RMI)

RMI is used to identify ovarian cysts with a high risk of being malignant. It is calculated by using the formula: U × M × Ca-125. U is an ultrasound score. A value of 1 is given for one or no ultrasound features. A value of 3 is given for two or more features. The ultrasound features scored are multilocularity, bilateral lesions and solid areas, presence of ascites and evidence of metastasis. M is the menopausal status with a score of 1 for premenopausal and 3 for postmenopausal. The result of the Ca-125 blood test in IU/L is multiplied by the menopausal and ultrasound scores. A RMI of less than 25 indicates low risk of malignancy (<3%). A RMI of 25–250 indicates a moderate risk (20%) and more than 250 indicates a high risk of malignancy (75%).

Further imaging

In premenopausal women, magnetic resonance imaging (MRI) is preferable to computerised tomography (CT) to give further information on the type of ovarian cyst.

In postmenopausal women with a high risk of malignancy, CT scan of the abdomen and pelvis must be performed in all cases. It will further evaluate the likelihood of malignancy and disease extent.

Management

The management of ovarian cysts is dependent on menopausal status, the type of cyst and the presence of symptoms.

The principles of management are 3-fold:
- To promote conservative management of benign cysts where appropriate
- To promote laparoscopic removal of benign cysts where possible, to reduce postoperative morbidity

- Appropriate referral to a gynaecological oncologist for women at risk of ovarian cancer

Cysts in the premenopausal period

Asymptomatic simple ovarian cysts

- Ovarian cyst < 50 mm
  Follow-up is not necessary
- Ovarian cyst 50–70 mm
  An annual surveillance with pelvic ultrasound scan is required
- Ovarian cyst > 70 mm
  MRI should be considered to further define the nature of the cyst (Table 17)

- Persistent ovarian cysts > 50 mm
  Calculate the RMI. If the RMI is more than 250, refer to the gynaecological oncology team. If the RMI is less than 250, local surgical management should be offered

Symptomatic ovarian cysts

Regular simple analgesia is recommended. If the cyst continues to be symptomatic then offer surgical treatment:

- Cystectomy is preferable to cyst aspiration since it is associated with a reduced risk of recurrence. A laparoscopic approach confers less postoperative morbidity, faster recovery,

Table 17 Classification of ovarian cysts		
Type	Characteristics	Management
Functional cyst • Follicular • Corpus luteal	Very common Thin wall with fluid only Small cyst measuring 1–5 cm	Conservative treatment
Endometrioma 'chocolate cyst'	Originates from endometrial tissue growing within the ovary Multilocular with thick brown fluid (dark blood)	Laparoscopic ovarian cystectomy or laparoscopic drainage and ablation
Serous cystadenoma	60% of benign tumours Originates from ovarian surface epithelium Unilocular, thin walled cyst with thin clear fluid Rarely multilocular Measures 5–15 cm, 15% bilateral	Ovarian cystectomy or oophorectomy, by laparoscopic or open approach
Mucinous cystadenoma	20% of benign tumours Originates from ovarian surface epithelium Multilocular with thick mucous fluid May grow to 30 cm, 10% bilateral	Ovarian cystectomy or oophorectomy, by laparoscopic or open approach
Mature teratoma 'dermoid cyst'	Common germ cell tumour Thick capsule, contains body tissues such as fat, hair, bone and cartilage May grow to 15 cm or more 10% bilateral	Ovarian cystectomy or oophorectomy, by laparoscopic or open approach
Fibroma	1% of ovarian tumours Composed of mainly fibrous tissue	Ovarian cystectomy or oophorectomy, by laparoscopic or open approach
Thecoma	0.5–1% of ovarian tumours Solid and cystic components 80% present in postmenopausal women Produces oestrogen and uterine bleeding 20% have concurrent endometrial cancer	Ovarian cystectomy or oophorectomy, by laparoscopic or open approach
Borderline ovarian tumours	See ovarian cancer	Laparotomy and full surgical staging or limited surgical staging if fertility-sparing surgery is required
Malignant tumours	See ovarian cancer	Laparotomy and full surgical staging (ovarian cancer)

a shorter hospital stay and is more cost-effective

- Surgery should be performed in a unit with suitable equipment and by an experienced laparoscopic surgeon
- A tissue retrieval bag should be used to avoid spillage of cyst fluid into the abdomen. Spillage can lead to chemical peritonitis. Should the presumed benign cyst be malignant, spillage would result in upstaging of the disease
- The cyst should ideally be removed through the umbilical port which leads to a faster retrieval time and less postoperative pain. Extension of lateral port sites should be avoided since this may cause an incisional hernia
- Laparotomy is advised for large dermoid cysts or other large cysts with solid areas. Women should be informed that an oophorectomy may be required

Cysts in the postmenopausal period

The RMI should be calculated:

- RMI of less than 25
  - Ovarian cysts that are simple and less than 50 mm may be managed conservatively with scans every 4 months. If the cyst resolves or becomes smaller the woman may be discharged. Laparoscopic surgery should be performed for larger cysts or cysts that persist. Bilateral salpingo-oophorectomy is generally preferable to unilateral salpingo-oophorectomy or cystectomy
- RMI of 25–250
  - Laparoscopy or laparotomy in a cancer unit is indicated
- RMI of more than 250
  - Laparotomy in a cancer centre is required

Ovarian cysts in pregnancy

Expectant management may be employed for asymptomatic cysts because of the low risk of acute complications and malignancy. Surgery is appropriate for symptomatic cysts, cysts measuring more than 5–10 cm and those of high suspicion of malignancy. If surgery is required, this should ideally be performed after 15 weeks of gestation, preferably by a laparoscopic approach.

Ovarian cyst accidents

Ruptured or haemorrhagic ovarian cysts

Ruptured ovarian cysts or haemorrhagic cysts present with acute onset lower abdominal pain, which increases with movement. This may be accompanied by nausea and vomiting. The signs include low grade pyrexia, tachycardia, focal or generalised abdominal tenderness and adnexal tenderness. The treatment is initially with analgesia. If the pain has not subsided after 48 hours, a diagnostic laparoscopy should be performed. In those whose pain resolves spontaneously, an ultrasound scan is recommended at 6 weeks to confirm cyst resolution.

Ovarian torsion

Ovarian torsion presents with acute onset of pain, nausea and vomiting. Occasionally, the pain is intermittent and has persisted over days or weeks. On examination, the woman is systemically unwell with tachycardia, tachypnoea and high grade pyrexia. If ischaemia or necrosis has occurred, there will also be hypotension and low blood oxygen saturations. There is generalised abdominal distension, peritonism and adnexal tenderness. The definitive treatment is laparoscopic detorsion. Ovarian fixation may be considered to prevent recurrence, since the risk of recurrent torsion is 10%. Torsion is more common during pregnancy and in the presence of ovarian cysts of 5 cm or more. Surgical management of these cases may involve cystectomy.

Further reading

RCOG Green-top Guideline No. 34. Ovarian cysts in postmenopausal women. London: ROCOG, 2010.

RCOG Green-top Guideline No. 62. Management of suspected ovarian masses in the premenopausal women. London: ROCOG, 2010.

Damigos E, Johns J, Ross J. An update on the diagnosis and management of ovarian torsion. The Obstetrician & Gynaecologist 2010; 14:229–236.

Related topics of interest

- Endometriosis (p. 38)
- Minimal access surgery (p. 91)
- Ovarian cancer (p. 97)

Paediatric gynaecology

Precocious puberty

Precocious puberty is the appearance of physical and hormonal signs of puberty before 8 years in girls and before 9 years in boys.

Premature pubarche and premature thelarche

Premature pubarche and premature thelarche are common, benign, normal variant conditions that can resemble precocious puberty but are non-progressive or very slowly progressive. Premature thelarche is isolated breast development, usually in girls younger than 3 years; premature pubarche is isolated pubic hair in children younger than 7 years. A thorough history, physical examination and growth curve review can help distinguish these normal variants from true sexual precocity.

Precocious puberty

If premature puberty is suspected, the clinician must differentiate between central precocious puberty (CPP) and precocious pseudopuberty. Central precocious puberty is gonadotropin-dependent and refers to early maturation of the entire hypothalamic-pituitary-gonadal (HPG) axis. CPP is idiopathic in 90% of cases. Other causes include inhibition of hypothalamic-pituitary inhibitory system secondary to brain tumours, intracranial infections or trauma.

Precocious pseudopuberty is much less common and is gonadotropin-independent. Causes include gonadal tumours, adrenal tumours, congenital adrenal hyperplasia or exogenous hormonal exposure.

Most patients suspected of precocious puberty are otherwise healthy children whose pubertal maturation begins at the early end of the normal distribution curve.

Diagnosis of precocious puberty

- Oestradiol levels are unreliable
- Adrenal androgen levels [e.g. dehydroepiandrosterone (DHEA), dehydroepiandrosterone sulphate (DHEAS)] are elevated in girls with premature pubarche
- gonadotrophin-releasing hormone (GnRH) stimulation test is gold standard: luteinising hormone (LH) and follicle-stimulating hormone (FSH) levels 30–60 minutes after stimulation with 100 μg GnRH

Treatment of precocious puberty

LH and FSH levels are reduced after 2 weeks of treatment with GnRH agonists through negative feedback. Lupron-Depot comes in 1-month (7.5 mg) or 3-month preparations (11.25 mg).

Follow-up after 4–6 months ensures that progression of puberty has been arrested.

The duration of therapy is individualised according to age and predicted adult height. Most treatment is discontinued at 10–11 years of age.

Prepubertal vaginal discharge

Vaginal discharge is the most common reason for referral of a prepubertal girl to a gynaecologist. Incidence is unknown and age of referral is usually 3–10 years. The most common cause is vulvovaginitis due to non-specific bacterial infection. Other causes include tumours, precocious puberty and sexual abuse.

Gynaecological examination of the prepubertal girl

This must be done with sensitivity and gentleness. If the girl is very young the examination can be done with her on her mother's lap. Gentle separation and retraction of the labia should allow visualisation of the external genitalia, introitus and hymen. Discharge can pool in the posterior fourchette and a swab can be taken from this area. Standard swabs used in adults for high vaginal swabs may be too large, in which case a small, wire, cotton-tipped swab should be used. If visualisation is difficult, placing the child in the knee–chest position can sometimes allow a better view. More detailed examination is likely to require a general anaesthetic.

The neonate and infant

A mucous discharge, sometimes bloody, may come from the oedematous introitus as a result of increased cervical discharge and vaginal transudate caused by the transfer of maternal oestrogen to the fetus.

'Nappy rash', irritation and redness of vulva and buttocks, is an ammoniacal dermatitis caused by hot, wet nappies. Frequent nappy changes, regular skin washing and drying in warm air will help the majority. Sensitive skins will be helped by barrier creams such as dimethicone or zinc oxide cream.

The young girl

Until the oestrogen surge, 1 year before menarche, the vagina is thin with no glycogen and no lactobacilli. It has a neutral pH of 7.2. In addition labia are underdeveloped with no fat pads or pubic hair and in close approximation to the anus. Thus, there is risk of faecal contamination which can lead to infection.

Vulvovaginitis

Non-specific with mixed bacterial flora

Most common and is associated with poor personal hygiene. Vaginal cultures will be reported as mixed bacterial flora or non-specific skin flora. Regular bathing, thorough drying and the use of loose cotton underwear will generally treat it.

Vaginitis leading to secondary vulvitis

This is uncommon and difficult to investigate. It may be the result of a congenital anomaly causing a vaginal discharge, e.g. ectopic ureter. The child may complain of burning on micturition, soreness or discharge; the mother may notice stained underwear.

Infective causes

Group A β-haemolytic streptococcus

The most common infective agent found in prepubertal vaginal discharge. It may be related to an upper respiratory tract infection transmitted from the throat to the vulva by fingers. The onset can be acute and relapse can occur in a third of individuals. Group A streptococci are sensitive to penicillin.

Haemophilus influenzae

This is the second most common cause of vulvovaginitis. Recurrent infections are common. Most strains are sensitive to penicillin.

Gardnerella vaginalis

This usually originates in the bowel. Treat with local instillation of lactic acid 5%, with an eye dropper so as not to interfere with the hymenal ring.

Gonorrhoea

Below the age of 12 years, this is rare and implies sexual contact. If it is found, it warrants admission. Search for other sexually transmitted diseases. The contacts are usually family members. Treat with benzylpenicillin and probenecid.

Chlamydia

This is more common than gonorrhoea and the same rules apply. Do not treat with tetracyclines because of the dental effects.

Threadworms (Enterobius vermicularis)

The worm is common, often carrying coliforms with it. Diagnose by the 'Sellotape' method or vaginal smear microscopy. Treat with mebendazole in those over 2 years of age.

Candidiasis

This is uncommon in young children and if found, a medical reason should be sought, e.g. diabetes or antibiotics. Treat the very young with gentian violet 0.5–1.0% applied with an eye dropper. Nystatin suspension into the vagina with an antifungal on the perineum can be used in the older child.

Trichomoniasis

This is also uncommon and usually results from sexual contact. Treat with metronidazole.

Amoebiasis

This is common and is treated with metronidazole.

Viruses

Condyloma acuminata and herpes simplex can be seen. Condylomata are best treated with cryocautery, as podophyllin causes skin ulceration. Herpes simplex is rare in infants (apart from those whose mothers are excretors), and if found, it implies sexual contact.

Systemic infections

Some systemic infections such as varicella, measles, rubella, diphtheria and shigella can cause vulvovaginitis. Resolution is usually complete.

Vulval dermatitis

Irritant dermatitis has been reported with use of soap or bubble bath, playing in a sandpit, as well as prolonged contact with urine and faeces. Avoidance of the irritative agent should lead to resolution of symptoms.

Foreign body

This is a common source of infection, vaginal discharge and/or bleeding. Rectal examination may detect the object and may facilitate 'milking' the object down to the introitus where it can be removed with a pair of nasal forceps. An examination under anaesthetic (EUA) may be necessary. The most common foreign body is small pieces of tissue paper but other items that have been removed include coins, beads and small toys (e.g. Barbie doll shoe).

Ulcer

A round ulcer with a granular base, from which no organism can be cultured, and which when biopsied shows only granulation tissue, is known as a Lipschutz ulcer. It may occur at any age. Good hygiene is the best treatment, and they usually disappear spontaneously.

Other forms of ulcerating vulval conditions, such as Behcet's syndrome, Crohn's disease and herpes, are quite uncommon and require the appropriate immunological, histological and virological investigations.

Labial adhesions

These are relatively common, non-infective in origin and best treated with gentle outward pressure with the thumbs on the labia, followed by a little Vaseline for a few days. Oestrogen treatment is not indicated for this.

Urethral prolapse

This is seen in 4–6 year olds. The prominent urethra plus tight underclothing and poor hygiene will result in a red, friable, bleeding urethral meatus. Diagnosis is confirmed by passing a catheter. An EUA and excision is the best treatment.

Sarcoma

Sarcoma botryoides is a highly malignant lesion, most common under 2 years of age, but it can be seen in older children. It presents with bleeding from a polyp or haemorrhagic mass in the lower vagina. Advanced cases will also have a palpable mass per abdomen. Rhabdomyoblasts are present. Management will include an EUA and cystoscopy and rectal examination, with chemotherapy being the initial treatment of choice. Surgery, in the form of a Wertheim's hysterectomy with a total vaginectomy, is indicated if tumour regression is incomplete after chemotherapy. Radiotherapy is sometimes used. These regimens result in a better prognosis than historically reported.

Child abuse and safeguarding

Child sexual abuse is forcing or enticing a child to take part in sexual activities, including prostitution, whether or not the child is aware of what is happening. The activities may involve physical contact, including penetrative or non-penetrative acts. They may include non-contact activities, such as involving children in looking at, or in the production of, sexual online images, watching sexual activities, or encouraging children to behave in sexually inappropriate ways.

The care of complainants of sexual assault requires a multi-agency team. Health services, the police, social services and the legal system are all involved. Relevant medical professionals include: forensic physicians, paediatricians, gynaecologists, general practitioners and child and adolescent mental health services (CAMHS) amongst others.

The presentation of the child varies according to age and can range from sexualised behaviour noticed at school to vaginal bleeding. The paediatric forensic examination consists of: obtaining a thorough history; 'top-to-toe' examination; written, graphical and photographic documentation; collecting forensic samples; sexually transmitted infection (STI) screening; arranging aftercare; writing a report; and the insurance that child protection procedures are properly observed.

Further reading

Stricker T, Navratil F, Sennhauser FH. Vulvovaginitis in prepubertal girls. Arch Dis Child 2003; 88:324–326.

Garden AS, Topping J. Paediatric and Adolescent Gynaecology for the MRCOG and Beyond. RCOG Press: London, 2001.

Tirumuru SS, Arya P, Latthe P, et al. Understanding precocious puberty in girls. The Obstetrician & Gynaecologist 2012; 14:121–129.

Related topics of interest

- Abnormality of the genital tract (p. 1)
- Amenorrhoea (p. 4)
- Forensic gynaecology (p. 52)

Pelvic inflammatory disease

Overview

Pelvic inflammatory disease (PID) is an ascending infection of the upper female genital tract. The exact incidence is unknown as establishing an infective cause in women with pelvic pain is difficult. Additionally, the absence of confirmed infection in the lower genital tract does not exclude PID.

Clinical features

Symptoms of acute PID include severe lower abdominal pain which is worse on movement, abnormal vaginal bleeding (intermenstrual, postcoital), offensive vaginal discharge and malaise. The patient may also complain of dyspareunia. Women with acute PID may present with pyrexia. In more severe cases, they may be tachycardic, hypotensive and septic. Abdominal examination will usually elicit tenderness in the lower abdomen with rebound and guarding. Vaginal examination may be uncomfortable and cervical motion tenderness (cervical excitation) can be a feature. It may be possible to palpate an inflammatory adnexal mass. Mucopurulent or blood-stained discharge may be seen.

Women with chronic PID may complain of generalised malaise and fatigue. Chronic lower abdominal pain is a common complaint and this may be characterised as constant with exacerbations, typically during menstruation. There may be an intermittent offensive vaginal discharge. There may be generalised lower abdominal tenderness accompanied by pelvic discomfort and cervical excitation on pelvic examination. Pelvic examination may also reveal the presence of a bulky tender uterus and/or a tender adnexal mass of tubo-ovarian origin.

Aetiology

Risk factors for PID include early sexual debut (< 25 years old), multiple sexual partners, unprotected sexual intercourse and a history of sexually transmitted infections (STIs).

STIs such as *Chlamydia trachomatis* and *Neisseria gonorrhoeae* have been implicated in a third of cases. Acute PID has been observed in 2–5% of women testing positive for chlamydia prior to receiving treatment. Other causative agents include *Mycoplasma genitalium*, *Gardnerella vaginalis* and anaerobes frequently found in the vagina. Mixed infections are common.

Women with intrauterine contraceptive devices (IUCDs) have an increased risk of PID in the first 3 weeks following insertion. Pelvic actinomyces is increasingly rare with the use of modern copper IUCDs and hormonal coils. Pelvic tuberculosis is a rare cause of chronic PID and may occur in immigrants from the developing world.

Diagnosis

PID is a clinical diagnosis and bacteriological investigations may be negative. It is appropriate to have a low threshold to commence empirical treatment because of the lack of definitive clinical diagnostic criteria. Additionally, delaying treatment, particularly in chlamydial infections, increases both the severity of the infection and the potential long-term sequelae. Appropriate investigations include:

- A urinary hCG to exclude pregnancy
- Full blood count (positive findings of leucocytosis and anaemia, the latter in chronic PID)
- Erythrocyte sedimentation rate (ESR) and C-reactive protein (CRP) tend to be raised
- Microbiological investigations should include a high vaginal swab, a nucleic acid amplification test (NAAT) either from the endocervix or a self-taken vaginal swab for chlamydia and gonorrhoea, and serology for HIV. Women at risk may also be offered testing for syphilis. Primary care physicians may wish to refer patients to a genitourinary medicine (GUM) service for these investigations
- Transvaginal ultrasound can identify inflamed or dilated tubes or a tubo-

ovarian mass. Free fluid is commonly seen in the Pouch of Douglas (POD)

- Laparoscopy can be helpful both in confirming suspected cases, obtaining fluid for culture, assessing complicated or unresolved infection, draining an inflammatory mass or assessing chronic PID prior to a definitive procedure. The presence of perihepatic adhesions suggests the Fitz-Hugh–Curtis syndrome (chlamydia).

Management

Empirical treatment should be started based on local pathogens and antibiotic policy. The patient history should include current or recent treatments.

Table 18 illustrates appropriate outpatient and inpatient antibiotic regimens. Broad spectrum antibiotic therapy is usually required. It is appropriate to avoid ofloxacin in women who are at high risk of gonococcal PID, as there is increasing quinolone resistance to gonococcus. Patients who are managed in the outpatient setting should be reviewed in 72 hours to ensure adequate compliance and response to treatment.

In addition to treatment, patients should be aware of the long term implications of the condition and the need for partner treatment to prevent reinfection. Patients should be advised that the earlier treatment is given, the lower the risk of future fertility problems and that repeat episodes of PID are associated with significantly greater risks of infertility. Opportunistic sexual health education particularly regarding the importance of barrier contraception should be provided.

Admission to hospital is required if a surgical emergency (appendicitis, ectopic pregnancy, torted ovarian cyst) cannot be excluded or if patients are clinically unwell. Admission is also appropriate if the patient is pregnant or there is a lack of response or intolerance to oral therapy.

An IUCD may need to be removed, particularly if symptoms are ongoing after 72 hours. It is important to take into account the risk of pregnancy in women who have had intercourse in the preceding 7 days. Emergency oral contraception may be used in these situations. A woman at risk for further episodes of PID requesting an intrauterine device (IUD) for contraception should be offered the Levonorgestrol intrauterine system (LNG-IUS), which is associated with lower infection rates.

Surgical treatment to drain a pelvic abscess may be required. Ultrasound-guided drainage should be considered first. Laparoscopic division of adhesions and

Table 18 Evidence-based antibiotic regimens for acute pelvic inflammatory disease
Outpatient Regimens
• Intramuscular (IM) ceftriaxone 250 mg single dose followed by oral doxycycline 100 mg twice daily + metronidazole 400 mg twice daily for 14 days
• Oral ofloxacin 400 mg twice daily + oral metronidazole 400 mg twice daily for 14 days
• IM ceftriaxone 250 mg, followed by azithromycin 1 g per week for 2 weeks*
• Oral moxifloxacin 400 mg once daily for 14 days**
Inpatient Regimens
• Intravenous (IV) ceftriaxone 2 g daily plus IV doxycycline 100 mg twice daily followed by oral doxycycline 100 mg twice daily plus oral metronidazole 400 mg twice daily for 14 days
• IV clindamycin 900 mg three times daily + IV gentamicin (2 mg/kg loading dose) followed by 1.5 mg/kg three times daily followed by either oral clindamycin 450 mg four times daily or oral doxycycline 100 mg twice daily plus oral metronidazole 400 mg twice daily to complete 14 days*
• IV ofloxacin 400 mg twice daily + IV metronidazole 500 mg three times daily for 14 days*
• IV ciprofloxacin 200 mg twice daily + IV doxycycline 100 mg twice daily + IV metronidazole 500 mg three times daily for 14 days*
*Clinical trial evidence for these regimes is limited, but they may be appropriate in cases of allergy or intolerance ** Moxifloxacin carries increased risks of liver reaction and other serious risks such as prolonged QT interval and should only be used when other antibacterial regimens have failed.

drainage of infected material may expedite recovery and resolution of symptoms. In rare cases of the acute abdomen, a laparotomy may be required. Surgical treatment is guided by intraoperative findings and the patient's desire for fertility. A unilateral or bilateral salpingo-oophorectomy and/or hysterectomy may be required, usually after the acute infection has resolved.

Long term sequelae

Principal complications associated with PID include chronic pelvic pain, ectopic pregnancy and infertility. These complications are more common in women with recurrent episodes of PID; the PID evaluation and clinical health (PEACH) study demonstrated that women with recurrent PID were 80% more likely to suffer from infertility and four times more likely to have chronic pelvic pain.

Chronic pelvic pain affects a quarter of patients with a history of PID. This may be due to adhesions or postinfective hydrosalpinx. Impaired fertility can be secondary to scarring/adhesions. There is also a 15–50% increased risk of ectopic pregnancy in women with a history of PID.

Delays in receiving appropriate treatment in the acute infective phase markedly increase the risk of these long term complications. It is important that facilities for diagnosis and treatment are available in the primary health care setting.

Further reading

British Association for Sexual Health and HIV. UK National Guideline for the Management of Pelvic Inflammatory Disease. Macclesfield: BASHH, 2011.

RCOG. Green-top Guideline No 32. Management of acute pelvic inflammatory disease. London: RCOG, 2008.

Mears A, Bingham J. Pelvic inflammatory disease. The Obstetrician and Gynaecologist 2008; 6:138–144.

Related topics of interest

Perioperative complications in obstetrics and gynaecology

Overview

Perioperative complications can be minimised by thorough preoperative assessment, an experienced surgeon, good assistants, adequate exposure of the surgical field, adequate lighting, good anaesthesia and appropriate postoperative care. Even when all these precautions have been taken, however, perioperative complications can still occur. It is important to recognise complications early to have the best chance of resolving them without long term morbidity. The management of sepsis (Topic 83) and venous thromboembolic disease (Topic 108) is covered elsewhere.

Haemorrhage

Where possible, it is important to anticipate haemorrhage preoperatively. Women with thrombophilias, hepatic disorders or those taking anticoagulants are at increased risk of haemorrhage. Anticoagulants (aspirin, warfarin, clopidogrel) will need to be discontinued preoperatively. Certain operations are considered high risk for haemorrhage, e.g. caesarean sections for placenta praevia, myomectomy and laparotomy for malignant disease. Preoperatively, a full blood count, group and save and/or cross match should be performed.

When haemorrhage occurs, it should be managed expeditiously. Good communication and multidisciplinary team work is vital. Ensure that there is adequate lighting, exposure and assistance. Suction may be useful to identify bleeding points and pressure may control the bleeding. Venous bleeding may be stopped by suturing, the use of haemostatic clips or ligation above and below the vein. Absorbable haemostatic agents such as oxidised regenerated cellulose (Surgicel, Surgicel Fibrillar and Surgicel Snow), topical thrombin (Flosseal) and fibrin glue (Tisseel, Evicel) may also be used to achieve haemostasis. Small arterial bleeders may be controlled by cautery. Visible arterial bleeders may be clamped and ligated. Blood loss should be measured and fluids replaced promptly. An ongoing intraoperative blood loss of 1500 mL and more will require transfusion of red blood cells. Fresh frozen plasma (FFP) contains clotting factors and is indicated when there has been a large red cell transfusion requirement. Platelet transfusion is indicated if the platelet count is less than 50×10^9 /L. In the postoperative period, when the woman is stable, a blood transfusion is considered when the haemoglobin level is less than 80 g/dL.

A return to theatre in the immediate postoperative period is necessary when there is clinical concern that the patient is actively bleeding. Clinical features of ongoing haemorrhage include tachycardia, hypotension, reduced urine output, pallor, abdominal pain and distension, high output from surgical drains, dizziness and collapse. An ultrasound scan will reveal haemoperitoneum or profuse vaginal bleeding may be observed. An early return to theatre will prevent coagulation disturbances (e.g. disseminated intravascular coagulation) and the need for high dependency unit or critical care unit input afterwards.

Ileus and bowel obstruction

Ileus is decreased motor activity of the bowel from non-mechanical causes. Bowel obstruction is caused by a mechanical obstruction which occurs most often in the small bowel (77%). It can lead to ischaemia and strangulation of the bowel. If this is unrecognised, peritonitis, perforation, sepsis or death may occur. Proximal small bowel obstruction presents with upper abdominal or generalised abdominal pain, bilious vomiting and high pitched hyperactive bowel sounds. Sudden onset of a quiet abdomen with fever, leucocytosis or leucopenia is an ominous finding associated with strangulation, or ischaemia from mesenteric arterial or venous thrombosis. Radiographic findings consistent with partial or complete obstruction include air fluid levels in the bowel, birds peak luminal narrowing and the absence of air in the distal lumen. A computed tomography (CT) scan with gastrograffin contrast is often necessary to determine the likely cause and site of obstruction. Partial obstruction may respond to the stimulatory effect of gastrografin on bowel motility.

Paralytic ileus and partial bowel obstruction will resolve in 80% of postoperative patients with medical management. Initial management consists of nasogastric tube insertion, fluid replacement and nutritional support. Partial obstruction should respond within 24–48 hours. If there is no response, laparotomy may be required to prevent ischaemia or perforation. Surgical management consists of resection of the involved segment with primary anastomosis or bypass.

Bowel perforation

Bowel perforation can be caused by accidental injury during surgery. Sometimes it is recognised intraoperatively and repaired at that time. Bowel perforation caused by a thermal injury may not be diagnosed until the woman presents with peritonitis 7–8 days later. Risk factors include previous abdominal surgery, Crohn's disease, pelvic inflammatory disease, endometriosis and pelvic malignancies. Common clinical features are abdominal pain, vomiting, pyrexia, tachycardia, abdominal distension, abdominal tenderness and rigidity. Inflammatory markers are raised and there is intraperitoneal free air on an abdominal X-ray or air under the diaphragm on an erect chest X-ray. Bowel perforation results in faecal peritonitis which carries a 50% mortality rate. Urgent treatment by broad spectrum antibiotics and surgical exploration is required. Wide resection of the bowel may be needed with reanastomosis if possible.

Ureteric injury

Ureteric injuries should be managed by a multidisciplinary team involving the urologist and the radiologist. Ureteric injuries are more likely to be sustained during pelvic gynaecological surgery rather than during an obstetric operation. Large pelvic masses, previous surgery or radiation increase the risk of ureteric injuries. Types of ureteral injuries include transection, ligation and crush injuries. In gynaecological surgery, the first step in preventing ureteric injuries is good visualisation and exposure of the surgical field. Early identification of the ureter is essential to minimise risk of inadvertent laceration or ligation. The peritoneum lateral to the ovarian vessels should be divided and the ureter visualised as it crosses the bifurcation of the common iliac artery. This should be done before placing the clamps on the infundibular pelvic ligaments at oophorectomy or hysterectomy. Ureteric injuries may also be sustained as the ureter runs below the uterine artery. Care must be taken when clamping the uterine pedicles and during insertion of haemostatic sutures.

Unrecognised ureteric injuries manifest in the postoperative period as ureteric obstruction, leaks or fistulas. Ureteric obstruction presents with flank pain, nausea and vomiting. There is loin tenderness and signs of sepsis. Chronic obstruction may lead to renal failure. Bilateral obstruction will lead to anuria. Investigations include full blood count, blood urea, creatinine and electrolyte levels, and intravenous urography to assess the anatomy and function of the urinary tract.

Ureteric leaks present 1–2 weeks after surgery with unilateral abdominal or back pain. They can lead to the formation of pseudocysts (urinomas), abscesses and electrolyte imbalances. The diagnosis is confirmed by contrast enhanced CT with delayed imaging. Small leaks may be managed conservatively, but extensive leaks require ureteric stenting and insertion of a percutaneous urinary drainage catheter.

Ureteric fistulas most commonly involve the vagina (ureterovaginal fistulae). They present with uncontrolled urinary leakage. Most fistulas will manifest within the first 2 weeks after surgery. The diagnosis is confirmed by CT scan. The management of fistulae is described in Topic 16.

Wound complications

Wound complications are more common among obese and diabetic women, those who have had previous radiotherapy and in cases where wound suturing has led to the skin or tissue being under tension.

Wound complications include haematoma, wound dehiscence, infection, delayed and poor wound healing. Haematomas may resolve spontaneously but will require surgical drainage if they increase significantly in size or haemodynamic instability occurs. Wound dehiscence may be allowed to heal by secondary intention. If the rectus sheath has dehisced, it will need to be resutured in theatre. Incisional hernias may develop in the long term. Groin lymphadenectomies may result in the formation of lymphocysts which may require drainage if they become large, painful or infected. Most hospitals have tissue viability nurses who have expertise in wound healing and can advise on appropriate wound care, including the need for special dressings and vacuum-assisted closure (VAC) therapy. Prolonged wound healing issues can usually be managed in the outpatient setting with the help of specialist nurse input.

Further reading

Croissant K, Shafi M. Preoperative and postoperative care in gynaecology. Obstetrics, Gynaecology and Reproductive Medicine 2009; 19:68–74.

Lew W, Weaver F. Clinical use of topical thrombin as a surgical hemostat. Biologics 2008; 2:593–599.

Fanning J, Valea FA. Perioperative bowel management for gynaecologic surgery. Am J Obstet Gynecol 2011; 205:309–914.

Related topics of interest

Polycystic ovarian syndrome

Overview

Polycystic ovarian syndrome (PCOS), first described in 1935 by Stein and Leventhal, is a complex endocrine disorder affecting up to 10% of women of reproductive age. The main pathological abnormality is enlarged ovaries with multiple cystic follicles. It is associated with anovulatory menstrual cycles, oligomenorrhoea or amenorrhoea, and is one of the leading causes of female subfertility. The major endocrine abnormality is excessive androgen secretion and many patients also have abnormal insulin activity. There is great heterogeneity in presentation and several definitions exist but general diagnostic traits are hyperandrogenism, chronic anovulation and polycystic ovaries on scan. Evidence is emerging that women with PCOS are at increased risk of long term health problems such as type II diabetes, cardiovascular disease, endometrial cancer and other cancers.

Clinical features

PCOS is a complex disorder with a variety of signs and symptoms including: anovulatory menstrual cycles, oligomenorrhoea, hirsutism (60%), acne, obesity (60%) and acanthosis nigrans. There have been many attempts to define PCOS and its diagnostic criteria are a topic of considerable ongoing debate. The two main definitions of PCOS are the 1990 National Institutes of Health (NIH) criteria which requires the presence of chronic anovulation plus clinical or biochemical signs of hyperandrogenism, and the 2003 Rotterdam criteria which requires the presence of two or more of chronic anovulation, clinical or biochemical signs of hyperandrogenism, and polycystic ovaries. Patients with PCOS are also at increased risk of a range of adverse health outcomes including hypertension, hyperlipidaemia, obesity and insulin resistance, known collectively as the metabolic syndrome, which in turn predisposes to diabetes and cardiovascular disease. Furthermore, they are at risk of endometrial and other cancers.

Aetiology

The initiating event in PCOS is unclear. It is thought that abnormal gonadotrophin secretion [overproduction of leutinising hormone (LH), relative to follicle-stimulating hormone (FSH)] may induce hyperactivity of ovarian stroma, antral follicular atresia and excess androgen production which is then converted to oestrogen. In support of this hypothesis, 60–80% of women with PCOS have high circulating concentrations of testosterone and other androgens. Furthermore, polycystic ovaries have a thicker theca cell layer than normal ovaries, and in vitro are capable of excessive androgen secretion in response to LH stimulation.

PCOS is associated with hyperinsulinaemia in > 75% of patients which often progresses to type II diabetes, but it is at present unclear whether hyperinsulinaemia is cause or effect of PCOS.

Diagnosis

The diagnosis of PCOS may be made in a patient with clinical signs and symptoms of infertility, irregular periods, hirsutism and obesity. The following tests are helpful in diagnosis:

1. *FSH and LH levels.* A blood test is taken within the first 5 days of the menstrual cycle. A LH:FSH ratio of approximately 3:1 is consistent with PCOS. N.B. This is the reverse of the normal ratio
2. *Testosterone.* Raised in PCOS
3. *Oesterone.* Raised in PCOS (> 300 pmol/L)
4. *Androstenedione.* Raised in PCOS (> 9.8 nmol/L)
5. *Prolactin.* Commonly found raised in 15% of patients

6. *Insulin I.* Classically raised
7. *Ultrasound scan.* The classic picture is of a necklace of 12 or more small follicles all < 5 mm in diameter positioned along the periphery of the ovary. The ovaries may be enlarged, or exhibit an increased amount or density of stroma
8. *Laparoscopy.* Classically enlarged ovaries with a thickened white cover
9. Histological assessment of ovaries

Differential diagnosis

- Congenital adrenal hyperplasia
- Cushing's syndrome
- Hyperprolactinaemia
- Androgen secreting tumours
- Acromegaly
- Hyperthyroidism

Management

Hirsutism and acne   These conditions result from stimulation of the hair follicles and sebaceous glands by excess androgens and are associated with considerable psychological morbidity. Oral contraceptives are widely prescribed for both hursuitism and acne, especially in younger women as they also give contraceptive protection. Cyproterone acetate is an antiandrogenic progestogen, and combined with ethinyloestradiol can be used for up to 6 months to suppress androgens giving effective treatment of hirsutism and some benefit in acne. Gonadotrophin releasing hormone (GnRH) analogues work by normalising androgen levels after 1–2 months of treatment. They are as effective as cyproterone acetate in reducing hirsutism, and when combined with the oral contraceptive pill are more efficacious than the pill alone in improving gonadotrophin secretion and ovulation 6 months after stopping treatment.

Other treatments which have given variable results include the antiandrogen flutamide, the diuretic spironolactone, the steroid dexamethasone and bromocriptine. Cosmetic and hair removal treatments are also routinely used in management of hirsutism, either alone or in combination with systemic therapies.

Anovulation and infertility   Anovulation is the most common reason for infertility in women with PCOS. Lifestyle measures such as weight loss and exercise are always advised in obese patients. The first line pharmacological treatment is clomiphene citrate, a selective oestrogen-receptor modulator that is thought to work by reducing LH levels and increasing FSH levels thereby stimulating ovulation. Although highly successful this treatment is associated with an increased risk of multiple pregnancies and other complications and some women are resistant to clomiphene. In those women with PCOS who are resistant to clomiphene, gonadotrophins are an effective second line treatment at stimulating ovulation. Furthermore, recent studies have shown that metformin is also highly effective at inducing ovulation in clomiphene-resistant PCOS patients.

Surgical treatment for PCOS was traditionally by ovarian wedge resection. This has now been superseded by laparoscopic ovarian drilling using diathermy or laser which is an effective second line treatment for ovulation induction in women with PCOS. Risks with the drilling procedure include damage to other organs, adhesion formation and ovarian atrophy.

Prevention of endometrial carcinoma   Endometrial carcinoma is a potential complication for any woman in the presence of chronic oestrogen stimulation. Regular menstrual cycles are recommended and the use of the combined oral contraceptive pill, cyclical progestogens and metformin are used to induce menstruation. In those women unable or not wanting to take medication, regular ultrasound scans to assess endometrial thickness is advised.

Further reading

Stein IF, Leventhal ML. Amenorrhoea associated with birateral polycystic ovaries. Am J Obstet Gynecol 1935; 29:181–191.

RCOG Green-top Guideline No. 33. Long-term consequences of polycystic ovary syndrome. London: RCOG, 2007.

Zawadzki JK, Dunaif A. Diagnostic criteria for polycystic ovary syndrome: towards a rational approach. In: Dunaif A, Givens JR, Haseltine FP, Merriam GR (eds), Polycystic ovary syndrome. Boston: Blackwell Scientific, 1992;377–384.

Rotterdam ESHRE/ASRM - sponsored PCOS Consensus Workshop Group 2004 revised 2003

Consensus on diagnostic criteria and long term health risks related to polycystic ovary syndrome. Fertil Steril; 81:19–25.

Costello MF, Ledger WL. Evidence-based lifestyle and pharmacological management of infertility in women with polycystic ovary syndrome. Women's Health, 2012; 8:227–290.

Costello M, Ledger WL. Evidence-based management of infertility in women with polycystic ovary syndrome using surgery or assisted reproductive technology. Women's Health 2012; 8:291–300.

Related topics of interest

- Hirsutism (p. 64)
- Amenorrhoea (p. 4)
- Uterine tumours (p. 155)

Pre- and postoperative care and the enhanced recovery programme

Overview

High quality perioperative care minimises intraoperative and postoperative complications. The enhanced recovery programme maintains a high standard of care whilst promoting a faster recovery and safe discharge from hospital.

Preoperative care

Preoperative assessment ensures that the woman is in optimal health prior to her operation. This is an opportunity for the woman to be fully informed about the operation and the postoperative period. The level of risk for each woman is estimated. Coexisting medical conditions are identified. A thorough history is taken and examination performed. Full blood count, group and save are routine investigations. Some women will require additional investigations to complete their assessment. For example, those with chronic obstructive pulmonary disease would require a chest X-ray and pulmonary function tests. Those with previous heart surgery would require an electrocardiogram (ECG), echocardiogram (ECHO) and/or cardiopulmonary exercise test (CPET).

Anaesthetic referral

Women with comorbidities and risk factors are referred for an anaesthetic assessment prior to surgery. Preoperative anaesthetic assessment reduces the rate of cancellation on the day. It also reduces intraoperative complication and mortality rates. The anaesthetist takes into account the operative urgency whilst optimising the woman's condition. The preparation of high risk cases may take weeks to plan and coordinate. An important part of the anaesthetic assessment is determining the level of postoperative care that will be required, such as high dependency unit (HDU) or ward care. In addition to clinical reasons, this also has practical implications since in some hospitals the HDU bed needs to be booked in advance.

Consent

Written consent must be obtained preoperatively. The woman should be informed of the operation itself, its risks and benefits, and alternative treatments. The consent must be given voluntarily. The woman must make the decision herself and not be coerced by her family, friends or health care professionals. The woman giving her consent must have the capacity to make this decision. The written informed consent should ideally be taken by the person performing the operation. Alternatively, written consent may be obtained by a doctor capable of performing the operation.

Postoperative care

In the day surgery setting, women who have had minor procedures such as hysteroscopy will only require a few hours of postoperative care. If no complications occur, they are discharged home. Those who have had major operations such as hysterectomy will require a few days of postoperative care on the gynaecology ward. Women with complex medical problems, poor surgical outcomes or serious complications may require high dependency or intensive care unit nursing.

Fluid management

A fluid balance chart is needed to aid the management of fluids in the postoperative period. The daily requirements of fluid are administered and abnormal losses are replaced. Electrolyte abnormalities are monitored and corrected. Volume depletion and electrolyte abnormalities are not uncommon after surgery. They can be exacerbated with the development of acute illnesses, ileus, diabetic ketoacidosis, vomiting, tachypnoea or fever. Fluid management may be particularly important for women at risk of significant fluid shifts postoperatively (e.g. those who have had litres of ascites drained in theatre) as well as those for whom overfilling would cause harm (e.g. cardiac disease).

Pain management

The objective of pain management is to provide effective pain relief with minimal side effects. It is important to control pain because it is an unpleasant sensation and increases the workload of the heart. It reduces physical activity which may lead to venous stasis and thrombosis. It decreases gut motility which may lead to postoperative ileus and vomiting; and decreases urinary motility leading to urinary retention. Women with pain from abdominal wounds may limit their respiratory effort and resist coughing, leading to increased risk of chest infections. Preoperative siting of an epidural or ultrasound guided transabdominal blocks reduce postoperative pain. Intraoperative administration of local anaesthetic to the wound reduces pain in the immediate postoperative period. Postoperatively, patient controlled analgesia (PCA) with opioids, regular oral analgesia such as diclofenac and paracetamol are effective in controlling pain. PCA is better than intermittent intramuscular opioids but not as effective as epidural opioid analgesia. Local anaesthesia is effective only for a short time.

Management of nausea and vomiting

The treatment of nausea and vomiting is by antiemetics, fluid replacement and correction of electrolyte imbalance. Additional treatment may be required depending on the cause. In the immediate postoperative period, vomiting is often caused by drugs and if caused by anaesthesia should settle within 24 hours. One week after surgery, it may still be drug related but due to opiates rather than anaesthetic agents. Other causes are urinary tract infection, paralytic ileus or bowel obstruction.

Mobilisation

Early postoperative mobilisation is very beneficial and should be encouraged. It reduces the risk of thromboembolism, pulmonary complications and pressure damage. Patients who mobilise early are likely to be discharged from hospital sooner. Effective postoperative pain control enables early mobilisation.

Preventing sepsis

Sepsis is the clinical syndrome that results from a dysregulated inflammatory response to infection. Sepsis carries a high mortality rate (20–40%), so anticipating, preventing, recognising and promptly treating infection is of paramount importance. A meticulous aseptic surgical technique will minimise the risk of wound infection. Intraoperative prophylactic antibiotics should be given for all surgical cases with a high risk of infection and all major cases. Postoperatively, the surgical wound and drains must be kept clean. Early mobilisation reduces the risk of chest infection. Removal of the catheter as soon as possible reduces the risk of urinary tract infection.

Preventing deep vein thrombosis (DVT)

DVT is caused by venous stasis, hypercoagulability and blood vessel wall changes. The identification of risk factors and estimating the level of risk for developing thrombosis is the first step to preventing DVT. Risk factors include pregnancy, obesity, thrombophilia, malignancy, surgery and immobilisation. Intraoperatively, thromboembolic deterrent stockings and/ or intermittent pneumatic compression devices are required. Early postoperative mobilisation and leg exercises involving the calf muscles increase blood flow through the deep veins. In those with a high risk of developing thrombosis, prophylactic doses of subcutaneous heparin (enoxaparin) should be administered postoperatively. Enoxaparin alters the coagulation process and prevents the formation of blood clots.

Enhanced recovery programme

Enhanced recovery encompasses a structured approach to intraoperative and postoperative management with early mobilisation (Table 19). The objectives of the enhanced recovery programme (ERP) are to increase the rate of postoperative recovery and improve

Table 19 The enhanced recovery programme (ERP)

Steps	Interventions	Benefits to women
Preoperative preparation for surgery	Informed consent Involve family and carers in the plan Preoperative assessment Discharge planning High carbohydrate drinks before admission Intake water 2 hours before surgery	Full understanding of the operation Improved patient understanding Optimise medical status Safe and efficient discharge Keeps gut motile Maintains hydration
Reduce the physical stress of the operation	Combined general and regional anaesthesia Additional local anaesthetic or nerve block techniques Minimally invasive surgery Prevent hypothermia Maintain fluid balance Use of modern drugs	Improved postoperative pain relief Improved postoperative pain relief Less trauma to tissue and organs Improves recovery from surgery Identification of fluid depletion Some lead to faster recovery
Improved postoperative care	Effective pain relief Early oral fluids and diet Routine laxatives Prophylaxis for nausea and vomiting Early recognition and treatment of infections	Early mobilisation, deep breathing and appropriate coughing. Reduce the chest infection and venous thromboembolism (VTE) Early recovery of normal bowel function, maintains nutrition status to encourage wound healing Encourage bowel motility, reduce 'wind pain', allow earlier discharge Increased postoperative comfort Faster postoperative recovery
Early mobilisation	Early feeding and normal diet Avoid prolonged use of intravenous infusions, drains and urinary catheters Mobilisation within 24 hours	Reduces the body's stress response Early mobilisation, shorter recovery time and prevention of infections Faster postoperative recovery, prevention of thrombosis and chest infections

patient outcomes. The first step of the ERP is effective preoperative assessment and planning. The second step is reducing the physical stress of the operation, e.g. using minimal access rather than open surgery, epidural analgesia and keeping the woman warm. Introduction of the ERP reduces hospital stay by an average of 28–50%. The ERP is associated with a low rate of complications and readmission rates are less than with conventional care (3% vs. 10%). Patient satisfaction rates are also high (85–95%).

Further reading

Wodlin NB, Nilsson L. The development of fast-track principles in gynaecological surgery. Acta Obstet Gynecol Scand 2013; 92:17–27.

Salkind AR, Rao KC. Antibiotic prophylaxis to prevent surgical site infections. Am Fam Physician 2011; 83:585–590.

Carter J. Fast-track surgery in gynaecology and gynaecologic oncology: a review of a rolling clinical audit. ISRN Surg 2012:368014.

Related topics of interest

Premenstrual syndrome

Overview

Premenstrual syndrome (PMS) is a condition which manifests with distressing physical, behavioural and psychological symptoms, in the absence of organic or underlying psychiatric disease, which regularly recurs during the luteal phase of each menstrual cycle and which disappears or significantly regresses by the end of menstruation.

The degree of symptoms varies from woman to woman. Only 5% of women experience no premenstrual changes, whereas 20–40% will suffer symptoms severe enough to consult their doctor. 5% of these will be severely incapacitated by them.

PMS appears more prevalent in women who are obese, perform less exercise and are of lower academic achievement.

Aetiology

The aetiology of PMS is uncertain, but cyclical ovarian activity and the effect of estradiol and progesterone on the neurotransmitters serotonin and gamma-aminobutyric acid (GABA) appear to be important. Absence of PMS before puberty, in pregnancy and after the menopause supports the theory that cyclical ovarian activity is important.

Diagnosis

The diagnosis is dependent on timing the symptoms in relation to menstruation. Also, the presence of a symptom-free phase of at least 7 days after menstruation helps distinguish PMS from other menstrual problems. When assessing women with PMS, symptoms should be recorded prospectively, over two cycles using a symptom diary. A retrospective recall of symptoms is unreliable. There are many diaries available but the daily record of severity of problems (DRSP) is well established and simple for patients to use.

Clinical features

Typical psychological symptoms include mood swings, irritability, depression and feeling out of control; physical symptoms include breast tenderness, bloating and headaches; behavioural symptoms include reduced visuospatial and cognitive ability, and an increase in accidents.

Differential diagnosis

- Psychiatric disorders
- Psychosexual problems
- Causes of breast symptoms
- Lethargy/tiredness – anaemia/ hypothyroidism
- The menopause

Management

Women with marked underlying psychopathology and PMS should be referred to a psychiatrist. Symptom diaries (daily record of severity of symptoms) should be used to assess the effect of treatment.

When treating women with PMS, referral to a gynaecologist should be considered when simple measures have failed and symptoms are severe.

Ideally, women with severe PMS should be managed by a multidisciplinary team which includes a hospital or community gynaecologist, psychiatrist or psychologist, dietician and counsellor.

When treating women with PMS, an integrated approach is beneficial. This may include complementary medicines which themselves may not be evidence based.

- General advice about exercise, diet and stress reduction should be considered before starting any treatment
- Pyridoxine (vitamin B6) commonly used in doses of 50–300 mg/day. Thought to increase the levels of dopamine and serotonin. However, long term use with doses over 25 mg/day has been associated with reversible peripheral neuropathy
- Among the complementary therapies, best data exist for vitamin D/calcium, magnesium, Agnus Castus and evening primrose oil. When prescribing complementary therapy (e.g. St. John's wort), interactions with other medications should be considered

- There is increasing evidence to show that selective serotonin reuptake inhibitors (SSRI) such as fluoxetine significantly reduce symptoms. SSRIs are therefore first line pharmacological agents for use in patients with severe PMS. When treating women with PMS, luteal phase or continuous dosing of SSRI is recommended. SSRI should be withdrawn gradually following treatment of women with PMS
- There is evidence to show that oral contraceptive pills with newer progestogens (e.g. Yasmin) when used continuously rather than cyclically is helpful in treatment of PMS
- Oestrogens are used in order to suppress ovulation on the basis that PMS is cyclical and that removal of the natural menstrual cycle will abolish PMS. This can be given as implants, the combined pill and oestrogen dermal patches; obviously regular courses of progesterones or a Mirena coil are essential to prevent endometrial hyperplasia. It has been found that this is one of the few methods of treatment which is better than placebo for all symptoms monitored

- Danazol has been used on a similar basis to oestrogen implants, in which it suppresses ovulation. The problem is that the doses required to suppress ovulation are associated with irreversible androgenic side effects, and therefore should not be used
- Gonadotrophin-releasing hormone (GnHR) analogues have been used successfully in PMS, but continual usage cannot be recommended due to the unwanted effects of hot flushes, vaginal atrophy and osteoporosis. GnRH analogues with add-back hormone replacement therapy (HRT) reduce the clinically relevant oestrogen responsive symptoms. This should not be used as first line treatment in patients with severe PMS. Lack of responsiveness to GnRH analogues questions the diagnosis

As a last resort, it is theoretically possible to cure intractable symptoms by performing a hysterectomy along with a bilateral salpingo-oophorectomy. This will cure the PMS, but at some cost in terms of physical and psychological morbidity, mortality and need for continuous HRT.

Further reading

Endicott J, Harrison W. Daily record of severity of problems (DRSP): reliability and validity. Arch Womens Ment Health 2006; 9:41–49.

Dimmock PW, O'Brien PM. Efficacy of selective serotonin-reuptake inhibitors in premenstrual syndrome: a systematic review. Lancet 2000; 356:1131–1136.

Vigod SN, Ross LE, Steiner M. Understanding and treating premenstrual dysphoric disorder: an update for the women's health practitioner. Obstetrics and Gynecology Clinics of North America 2009; 36:907–924.

Related topics of interest

Radiotherapy

Ionising radiation causes injury to the genetic apparatus of a dividing cell leading to death of the cell at subsequent mitosis. This occurs directly by damage to the DNA or indirectly subsequent to the creation of free radicals which bind with and damage DNA. The differential effect of ionising radiation on normal and cancer cells relies on the ability of healthy cells to be able to repair them whereas tumour cells have a lesser ability to recover.

The aim of radiotherapy is to deliver a lethal dose to the tumour while minimising the damage to adjacent tissues.

Physics

The dose of ionising radiation is that energy absorbed by a unit mass of tissue, the SI unit being the gray, which is equivalent to 1 J/kg.

- Ionising radiation in gynaecological malignancy is delivered in two ways: via beam sources (external) and brachytherapy sources (internal)
- Beam sources deliver radiation in the form of photons or γ-rays. High-energy sources are preferred because they deliver the maximum dose at greater depth, which is essential for pelvic treatment. It is essential to know the dose delivered at a specific depth of tissue, and also the dose delivered to surrounding tissue, from knowledge of the isodose curve at a given depth
- Brachytherapy sources are radionuclides placed in body cavities within or near to the treatment site. The commonly used source is caesium-137. The total dose required at each insertion is carefully calculated, and this determines the time the source is left in situ

Radiobiology

Ionising radiation affects genetic material but not the metabolic function of a cell.

- Effects on tissues will depend on the rate of mitosis of the constituent cells

- Tumour cells have a rapid mitotic rate and consequently should be relatively radiosensitive. This is not true for all tumours for reasons which are incompletely understood. Hypoxic cells are relatively radioresistant, and the proportion of such cells in a given tumour will influence the response to treatment

Toxicity

- Normal cells show an early effect from radiation, with death in rapidly dividing cells such as intestinal epithelium and bone marrow
- Acute toxicity can lead to fatigue, diarrhoea, cystitis, skin reactions, nausea and myelosuppression
- Later effects relate to a failure of the tissue owing to lack of replacement cells consequent upon depletion of the stem cell population
- Features of late toxicity following pelvic radiotherapy include early menopause and infertility, bowel and bladder fistulae and strictures, vaginal stenosis, sacral insufficiency fractures and lymphoedema

Planning

Each patient is carefully assessed, with particular regard to the size and spread of the tumour, its relation to vital organs and the size of the patient.

- The area to be irradiated may also include probable sites of metastatic spread, e.g. the pelvic side walls, where the pelvic lymph nodes are situated
- For external beam treatment, the dose requirement and area to be treated are calculated from a series of X-rays taken with the patient on a simulator with identical movements to the external beam treatment machine. Conformal and intensity-modulated radiotherapy utilise CT images to plan and shape radiation fields to fit the tumour and in the case of intensity

modulated radiotherapy adjust the dose of radiation whilst avoiding critical structures and thus minimising toxicity

- Planning of brachytherapy treatment involves insertion of containers, moulds or needles with dummy sources, into the relevant site with the patient anaesthetised. The position and orientation of the sources may be checked by X-rays or CT scans of the treatment site, followed by afterloading of the radioactive source, manually or via an afterloading machine.

Radiotherapy in gynaecology

Radiotherapy is utilised for primary treatment, adjuvant treatment, treatment of recurrent cancer and palliative therapy.

Radical primary radiotherapy with curative intent

- Radiotherapy is the primary form of treatment for patients with locally advanced cancer of the cervix. The results are generally similar to surgery in early-stage disease, but the latter treatment is generally preferred because of side effects of irradiation. Radiotherapy is usually given in combination with weekly single agent cisplatin-based chemotherapy, as this has been shown to improve survival rates (by 10% overall) and reduce the risk of recurrence (13% improvement in progression-free survival) compared to radiotherapy alone
- Radical radiotherapy is also considered in patients with medically inoperable cancers of the endometrium
- Cancer of the vagina is commonly treated with radiotherapy. However, surgery may be preferred for early stage disease.

Adjuvant radiotherapy

- Adjuvant radiotherapy is used to treat microscopic disease of the surgical bed and the draining lymph nodes. It is used in the postsurgery setting when treatment is given with curative intent.
- Adjuvant radiotherapy is advised in cancers of the cervix and vulva where there have been positive or close excision margins and/or evidence of regional nodal metastases
- Adjuvant radiotherapy is used postoperatively in women with high-intermediate risk endometrial cancer, as it has been shown to reduce the risk of local recurrence (but with no effect on overall survival). Vaginal brachytherapy is preferred to external beam or combination radiotherapy as it has a lower toxicity profile with equivalent locoregional recurrence rates. High risk and stage III endometrial cancer is generally treated with adjuvant chemotherapy, which may be combined with radiotherapy to reduce locoregional recurrence rates

Palliative radiotherapy

- Recurrent pelvic cancer, especially of the cervix, may be amenable to radiotherapy, depending on the original treatment and the feasibility of exenterative surgery. Vaginal recurrence of an endometrial primary may be successfully treated by local insertion of iridium wires (brachytherapy). Importantly, radiotherapy can never be given to the same area twice (due to the likelihood of severe complications), so primary or adjuvant treatment with radiotherapy would preclude the use of radiotherapy in the recurrence setting
- Palliative radiotherapy may be given to relieve pain or obstruction of blood and lymph vessels of the lower limb by tumour. It may also be given to relieve symptoms at distant sites

Further reading

van der Velden J, Fons G, Lawrie TA. Primary groin irradiation versus primary groin surgery for early vulvar cancer. Cochrane Database Syst Rev, 2011; (5) CD002224.

Coles C. Radiotherapy for gynaecological cancers. In: Shafi MI, Earl HM, Tan LT, (Eds). Gynaecological Oncology, 2nd edn. Cambridge University Press 2009: 79–90

Kong A, Johnson N, Kitchener HC, et al. Adjuvant radiotherapy for stage I endometrial cancer: an updated Cochrane systematic review and meta-analysis. J Natl Cancer Inst 2012; (11)7;104(21):1625–1634.

Related topics of interest

Recurrent miscarriage

Overview

Recurrent miscarriage is defined as the loss of three or more consecutive pregnancies and affects up to 1% of couples. Of note, the US definition of recurrent pregnancy loss is defined as two or more failed clinical pregnancies.

Aetiology

Parental (maternal and paternal) age and an increasing number of previous miscarriages are two independent risk factors for further miscarriage. It is recognised that advanced maternal age is associated with a decline in number and quality of oocytes. The age-related risk of miscarriage increases from 11% in 20–24 years old women to 93% in the ≥ 45 years old age group. Each successive pregnancy loss increases the risk of a further miscarriage with a risk of 40% after three consecutive pregnancy losses. Other environmental risk factors include maternal cigarette smoking, caffeine consumption (>3 cups of coffee/day) and heavy alcohol consumption. More recently, maternal obesity (body mass index ≥ 30 kg/m^2) has been demonstrated to significantly increase the risk of miscarriage in couples with unexplained recurrent miscarriage (OR: 1.793; 95% Cl 1.06–2.38).

Maternal endocrine disorders have been linked to miscarriage; however, the prevalence of diabetes mellitus and thyroid dysfunction in women who suffer recurrent miscarriage is similar to that reported in the general population. Although well-controlled diabetes and thyroid disease is unlikely to have an adverse effect, poorly controlled maternal diabetes is linked with foetal malformation and miscarriage. Polycystic ovary syndrome (PCOS) and its related insulin resistance and hyperandrogenaemia are also associated with an increased risk of miscarriage.

Between 2–5% of couples suffering from recurrent miscarriage may have a genetic cause, where one partner has a balanced chromosomal anomaly. Carriers of a balanced translocation are usually phenotypically normal, but their pregnancies are at increased risk of miscarriage or may result in a live birth with congenital mental or physical abnormalities. Spontaneous chromosomal abnormalities, especially trisomy, cause 30–57% of miscarriages and this risk increases with maternal age.

Congenital uterine anomalies (e.g. uterus didelphys, bicornuate uterus) can also contribute to miscarriage. The reported prevalence in the recurrent miscarriage population varies between 1.8–37.6% and is more likely for women with recurrent second-trimester miscarriages.

Cervical incompetence is another recognised cause of second-trimester miscarriage which is diagnosed following a history of second-trimester miscarriage preceded by spontaneous rupture of membranes or painless cervical dilation.

Antiphospholipid syndrome (APS) is associated with adverse pregnancy outcomes, including recurrent miscarriage. There are a variety of antibodies associated with this syndrome, the most relevant and validated being lupus anticoagulant, anticardiolipin and anti-β_2 glycoprotein-I antibodies. These antibodies have a variety of effects on the trophoblast, including the inhibition of trophoblastic function and differentiation leading to thrombosis of the uteroplacental vasculature, induction of syncytiotrophoblast apoptosis and initiation of maternal inflammatory pathways on the syncytiotrophoblast surface. Inherited thrombophilias (e.g. activated protein C and abnormalities in antithrombin III and prothrombin) have been associated with early miscarriage, but have stronger associations with late pregnancy loss.

Severe infections that cause bacteraemia or viraemia can cause sporadic miscarriage. Proven bacterial vaginosis (BV) in the first trimester of pregnancy has been reported as a risk factor for second-trimester miscarriage and preterm delivery. The treatment of BV in the second trimester of pregnancy has been demonstrated to significantly reduce the incidence of second-trimester miscarriage and preterm birth in a randomised controlled trial. There is insufficient evidence to associate immune factors, e.g. human leucocyte antigen incompatibility, or the absence of maternal leucocytotoxic antibodies with recurrent miscarriage.

Diagnosis

Investigations for recurrent miscarriage should be performed at a specialist clinic. All women with recurrent first-trimester miscarriage and all women with one or more second-trimester miscarriage should be screened before a subsequent pregnancy for antiphospholipid antibodies. The laboratory and clinical criteria required to make a diagnosis of antiphospholipid syndrome are detailed in **Table 20**. Cardiolipin is the dominant antigen used in most serologic tests for syphilis, thus patients may have a false-positive result for syphilis. Other associated clinical features recognised as antiphospholipid-associated clinical features but not included in the criteria include cardiac valve disease, livedo reticularis, thrombocytopenia, nephropathy and neurologic manifestations. Women with second-trimester miscarriage should be screened for inherited thrombophilias including factor V Leiden, prothrombin gene mutation and protein S deficiency.

Products of conception from the third and subsequent miscarriages should be sent away for cytogenetic analysis. If there are abnormalities, parents should have peripheral blood karyotyping. The clinician should consider the possibility of maternal tissue contaminating the products of conception and in the event that cytogenetic analysis reveals a 46 XX karyotype, differentiation between foetal genetic material and maternal contamination can be made using reflex DNA extraction and analysis of maternal blood by means of microsatellite analysis. Diagnosis of uterine anomalies can be made by pelvic ultrasound. Other procedures that may aid diagnosis include hysteroscopy and laparoscopy.

Management

A positive diagnosis of antiphospholipid syndrome should prompt treatment with low dose aspirin and low molecular weight heparin according to the individual patient's risk. A meta-analysis comparing aspirin and unfractionated heparin compared with aspirin alone demonstrated a significant reduction of miscarriage rate by 54% with both drugs (RR: 0.46, 95% Cl 0.29–0.71). Heparin does not cross the placenta, thus does not carry a teratogenic risk. This treatment is started after an ultrasound scan confirms fetal viability (usually at 6 weeks). It is important to recognise that these pregnancies remain at high risk of complications including pre-eclampsia, preterm delivery and fetal growth restriction.

Genetic counselling is important when a structural chromosomal anomaly is identified. Couples with genetic abnormalities may require assisted

Table 20 Diagnosis of antiphospholipid syndrome	
Laboratory tests (≥ 1 criteria on ≥ 2 occasions at least 12 weeks apart)	• Anticardiolipin antibodies (IgG/IgM in medium/high titre > 40 g/L/mL/L or > 99th percentile) • Anti-β_2 glycoprotein-I antibodies (IgG/IgM > 99th percentile) • Lupus anticoagulant
Clinical criterion (at least one) **	• ≥ 1 clinical episodes of venous, arterial or small vessel thrombosis (e.g. deep vein thrombosis, pulmonary embolus, stroke). In any tissue/organ • ≥ 1 late-term spontaneous abortions (< 10 weeks) • ≥ 1 premature births of a morphologically healthy neonate because of severe pre-eclampsia/clampsia or placental insufficiency (< 34 weeks) • ≥ 3 unexplained spontaneous, consecutive abortions (< 10 weeks)
[Adapted from Miyakis S, et al. International consensus statement on an update of the classification criteria for definite antiphospholipid syndrome (APS). J Thromb Haemost 2006; 4(2):295–306.]	

conception with preimplantation genetic diagnosis (PGD) and in vitro fertilisation (IVF). Patients with proven fertility have a higher (55–74%) chance of achieving a healthy live birth in future untreated pregnancies following a natural conception than is currently achieved after PGD/IVF (31–35%). Amniocentesis or chorionic villus samplings (CVS) are also options to detect genetic abnormalities in the fetus.

There is a lack of evidence to assess the effect of corrections of uterine septate defects. Non-randomised data has suggested a beneficial effect (n = 366, average live birth rate 83.2%). Open surgery is in itself associated with postoperative infertility and carries the risk of uterine scar rupture during pregnancy. These complications can be reduced using a transcervical hysteroscopic approach.

Cervical cerclage can be offered to selected patients with a singleton pregnancy and a history of one second-trimester miscarriage attributed to cervical incompetence if the cervical length before 24 weeks is 25 mm or less.

There is insufficient evidence to advocate the use of progesterone supplementation to prevent miscarriage in women with recurrent miscarriage. A randomised controlled trial (PROMISE) is currently recruiting patients to inform this intervention. A Cochrane systematic review suggests that the use of progestogens is effective in the treatment of threatened miscarriage (RR: 0.53, 95% Cl 0.35–0.79).

Other interventions like human chorionic gonadotrophin supplementation, suppression of luteinising hormone levels in PCOS, metformin supplementation (PCOS) and immunotherapies (paternal cell immunisation, third-party donor leucocytes, intravenous immunoglobulin) have not been proven to improve live birth rates.

In 50–75% of couples with recurrent miscarriage, no apparent causative factor is identified. These patients should be reassured that their chance for a future successful pregnancy can exceed 50–60%, depending on maternal age and parity. Although the value of psychological support has not been tested in a randomised controlled trial, data from non-randomised studies have demonstrated that providence support from a dedicated early pregnancy unit has a beneficial effect. The data also suggests that empirical treatment of women with unexplained recurrent miscarriage is unnecessary.

Further reading

RCOG Green-top Guideline No. 17. The investigation and treatment of couples with recurrent first-trimester and second-trimester miscarriage. London: RCOG, 2011.

American Society of Reproductive Medicine. Evaluation and treatment of recurrent pregnancy loss: a committee opinion. Fertil Steril 2012; 98:1103–1111.

Utting D, Bewley S. Family planning and age-related reproductive risk. The Obstetrician & Gynaecologist 2011; 13:35–41.

Related topics of interest

Sexual function

Overview

Normal sexual experience is dependent upon intact pelvic organs with functioning vascular and neurological mechanisms. All changes because of sexual arousal are irrevocably linked with cognitive processes.

Anatomy and physiology

Masters and Johnson's classification (1966) divides human sexual response into four phases:

- Excitement
- Plateau
- Orgasm
- Resolution

This classification does not take into account libido or desire, which is a vital part of any sexual dynamics. Each phase is incremental upon the preceding, and each is necessary for the subsequent phase to occur. Each phase has genital and systemic components, e.g. changes in colour and size of the labia and vagina and penis, increase in pulse, respiratory rate and blood pressure. The corticosensory experience of orgasm represents the peak of the pleasurable sensation of sexual activity, followed by a generalised state of relaxation and well-being.

The sexual response model has undergone many changes since this original classification and important differences have been identified between male and female sexual responses. For example, emotional intimacy is the single most important factor determining a woman's initial state of arousal, while genital events predominate for men.

Neurotransmitters play an important role in sexual responsiveness, with dopamine and norepinephrine involved in the 'excitement' phase and serotonin playing an inhibitory role, vital for satiety and the refractory phase. The balance between excitatory and inhibitory neurotransmitter activity is crucial for a normal sexual response. Oestrogen, progesterone and androgens influence the motivational state towards or against sexual activity. Testosterone increases sexual desire, arousal and receptivity to sexual activity.

Female sexual dysfunction

Female sexual dysfunction affects as many as 12% of women over the age of 18 years. Dysfunction implies disturbances in sexual function that are accompanied by psychological distress. Female sexual dysfunction comprises several disorders, including dyspareunia/apareunia, vaginismus and orgasmic dysfunction (**Table 21**) but most common are the arousal disorders.

Many never present with their problems. Kinsey found that at least 10% of women in their thirties are anorgasmic. Orgasmic dysfunction does not necessarily mean sexual dysfunction, and a normal physiological sexual experience does not preclude sexual dysfunction. It is believed that gynaecological clinic attendees have higher than average sexual dysfunction, with female attendees more likely to complain of loss of enjoyment,

Table 21 Female sexual dysfunction	
Disorders	**Primary symptoms**
Sexual arousal disorder	Lack of sexual arousal or desire
Persistent genital arousal disorder	Intrusive and unwanted genital arousal
Women's orgasmic disorder	Lack of orgasm despite high sexual arousal
Dyspareunia	Persistent or recurrent pain on penetration
Vaginismus	Involuntary spasm of the vagina that prevents penetration
Sexual aversion disorder	Anxiety or disgust regarding sexual activity

whereas male attendees complain of loss of genital function. In at least one-third of couples, in which one partner in a relationship complains of sexual dysfunction, the other partner will be found to also have a problem.

Aetiology

Consider physiological causes (diabetes, endocrine disorders, cardiovascular disease, major chronic physical illness, multiple sclerosis), previous surgery, especially for gynaecological cancer, and posthysterectomy syndrome. Cancer treatments, including chemotherapy and pelvic radiotherapy can cause premature menopause, and radical radiotherapy for cervical cancer causes vaginal shortening and stenosis. Psychological causes are common (depression and anxiety). Drugs may be implicated [antidepressants, especially selective serotonin reuptake inhibitors (SSRIs), antiandrogens and oral contraceptives], particularly alcohol. Dyspareunia and apareunia after childbirth are relatively common, and all gynaecologists are familiar with having to re-repair the perineum, vulva and vagina after an episiotomy which has healed incorrectly.

Diagnosis

A frank and detailed sexual history and then a careful physical examination are required. Check for normal secondary sexual characteristics and possible causes, e.g. infection and poorly sutured episiotomy scars. Vulval pain disorders and vaginismus have pathognomonic physical signs. 20% of women have a retroverted uterus which can be a cause of deep dyspareunia. Chronic pelvic infection and endometriosis may cause deep dyspareunia.

Management

Treatment will depend on the underlying cause. Organic physical causes should be treated in line with current recommendations.

Vaginal atrophy causes dryness, itching, irritation, dyspareunia and vaginal bleeding during sexual intercourse. Local or systemic hormone replacement therapy preparations are effective treatments. Tibolone, with oestrogenic, progestogenic and androgenic effects, improves libido as well.

Exogenous testosterone treatment by patch (300 µg/day), gel, implant or pessary has been shown to improve sexual function in postmenopausal women with arousal disorders.

Non-hormonal treatments include:

- **Flibanserin** (50/100 mg nocte), a selective neurotransmitter modulator, which decreases serotonin and increases dopamine and norepinephrine to rebalance these systems in women with arousal disorders. It has been shown to improve sexual function in clinical trials
- **Phosphodiesterase type-5 inhibitors** (PDE5i, e.g. Viagra) enhance genital vasocongestion and may be useful for the treatment of women with neurodegenerative disease leading to female sexual dysfunction. Their wider use in arousal disorders has not been convincingly demonstrated to date.
- **Melanocyte-stimulating hormone analogues** (e.g. bremelanotide) have shown early promise in the treatment of arousal disorders but further studies are needed

None of these non-hormonal treatments has yet achieved regulatory approval.

Psychological support includes basic counselling, cognitive behaviour therapy, sensate focus and couple therapy. Sensate focus is a modern behaviour based technique, which initially 'bans' sexual intercourse. Time, empathy, communication and confidentiality are of the essence in the relationship between a couple, and between the couple and the therapist.

Assessment of 'success' is difficult. It is believed that 65% will report at least an improvement after intensive sexual counselling, but many studies have shown a high relapse rate.

Male sexual dysfunction

This includes:

- Erectile dysfunction
- Premature ejaculation
- Dyspareunia
- Other ejaculatory dysfunction

Erectile dysfunction has an organic cause in up to 50% of cases. Damage to the nervi erigentes will delay or prevent erection, and severe damage to the nerves following prostate or colorectal surgery may not be reversible. On the other hand, medical disorders such as cardiovascular diseases and diabetes, which simply decrease blood flow to the penis, may be medically reversible. Drug-induced erectile dysfunction (e.g. antihypertensives, antipsychotics, alcohol) should be excluded. Psychological causes can be helped by counselling and support. About 60% of men with erectile dysfunction will respond to treatment with PDE5 inhibitors (such as Viagra).

Further reading

Masters WH, Johnson VE. Human sexual response. Toronto; New York: Bantam Books, 1966.

Fooladi E, Davis SR. An update on the pharmacological management of female sexual dysfunction. Expert Opin Pharmacother 2012; 13:2131–2142.

Maclaren K, Panay N. Managing low sexual desire in women. Women's Health 2011;7:571–583.

Nappi R, Polatti F. The use of estrogen therapy in women's sexual functioning. J Sex Med 2009; 6:603–616.

Related topics of interest

Sexually transmitted infection

The term sexually transmitted infection (STI) applies to conditions which are transmitted by genital, anogenital or orogenital contact. These may be bacterial, viral, spirochetal or protozoan. Coinfection with more than one STI is common. A routine screen for STIs in an asymptomatic patient would include testing for chlamydia, gonorrhoea, syphilis and human immunodeficiency virus (HIV). Testing for hepatitis B is reserved for higher risk groups.

Patients presenting with symptoms suggestive of an STI, or requesting testing for STIs, should have a sexual history taken (a detailed account of sexual contacts), usually for the preceding 12 months. If a positive diagnosis is made the process of partner notification [(PN), also known as contact tracing] is initiated, so that contacts can be tested and treated, and onward transmission and reinfection is prevented. The main exceptions to this are infection with herpes or human papillomavirus (HPV), where PN is not beneficial.

Treatment regimes for all STIs are regularly reviewed by the British Association for Sexual Health and HIV (BASHH). Up to date guidance documents can be found on the BASHH website (see further reading).

Blood borne viruses

Certain groups have been identified as being at greater risk of acquiring blood borne virus infection (HIV, hepatitis B and C): men who have sex with men, people from high prevalence countries, sex workers, intravenous drug users, and sexual partners of these groups. In a genitourinary medicine (GUM) setting a risk assessment for blood borne viruses is performed routinely.

HIV

Uptake of HIV testing in the UK has increased over the last decade, with adoption of 'opt-out' strategies in GUM clinics and antenatally. This means that these individuals are offered and recommended an HIV test as part of routine care. Despite these measures late

diagnosis of HIV is still common (47% in 2011), and is associated with increased mortality and morbidity. It is estimated that 24% of HIV in the UK is still undiagnosed. The most common route of transmission for HIV in the UK is now sexual. In 2011, the number of new heterosexually acquired infections (half of these probably acquired in the UK) nearly equalled those acquired by men who have sex with men. Vertical transmission from mother to child and intravenous drug abuse are now uncommon routes of transmission.

Hepatitis B and C

Hepatitis B can be transmitted sexually or through blood products. Hepatitis C is primarily transmitted through blood products, but can occasionally be transmitted sexually, particularly between HIV positive men. In GUM settings hepatitis B and C testing is currently only offered to at-risk groups. However, recent National Institute for Clinical Excellence (NICE) guidance (2013) encourages awareness raising and lowered thresholds for testing. Hepatitis B vaccination is offered to those considered at higher risk.

Syphilis

The reported incidence of syphilis has been increasing since the late 1980s. This increase has been seen amongst men who have sex with men as well as those having sex abroad and overseas visitors/migrants.

- The causative organism is a spirochete (*Treponema pallidum*). Other spirochetes are a cause of the skin conditions yaws and pinta which can make interpreting serology difficult
- Primary syphilis can cause a genital ulcer or chancre at the site of acquisition, with regional lymphadenopathy
- Untreated this can lead to secondary or systemic syphilis commonly presenting with the following: generalised rash (often affecting the palms and soles), lymphadenopathy, malaise, mucosal (snail track) ulceration and condylomata lata. It can also affect any other system in the body

- Latent syphilis is the name given to *Treponema pallidum* diagnosed on serological testing with no signs or symptoms
- Symptomatic late syphilis may affect the nervous system (tabes dorsalis, meningovascular or dementia) or cardiovascular system (aortitis). There may be progressive destructive lesions or gummata
- Congenital syphilis is caused by the spirochete crossing the placenta during pregnancy, resulting in widespread infection in some affected babies. It is rare in the UK
- Confirmatory diagnosis is through serological tests; the venereal disease research laboratory (VDRL) and rapid plasma reagin (RPR) are non-specific tests, whereas treponema pallidum hemagglutination assay (TPHA) and enzyme immunoassays (EIA) are specific tests. Interpretation of syphilis serology is complex and should be discussed with a genitourinary medicine physician
- First line treatment is intramuscular benzathine penicillin. Second line is usually oral doxycycline

Gonorrhoea

Although still not a common infection, diagnosis of gonorrhoea is rising in the UK. This can be partly explained by increased sensitivity of available tests.

- The gram-negative diplococcus (*Neisseria gonorrhoeae*) is highly infectious and can affect the lower genital tract, oropharynx, rectum and eye, as well as causing disseminated and joint infection. The most common symptom is urogenital discharge. It can ascend leading to pelvic inflammatory disease. It is also a cause of Bartholin's abscess, ophthalmia neonatorum and seronegative arthropathy
- Diagnosis, which is most often by nucleic acid amplification test (NAAT), should be confirmed by culture of the organism from the affected site(s), which allows antibiotic sensitivity tests to be undertaken
- Emerging antibiotic resistance remains a problem when treating gonococcal

infections. The treatment of choice today is intramuscular ceftriaxone 500 mg, given with oral azithromycin 1 g, for which resistance is beginning to emerge. Recommended treatment regimes for gonorrhoea have changed several times in the last few years: up to date dosage regimes should be checked in BASHH guidance (see further reading).Test of cure is recommended in all cases

Chlamydia

Chlamydia trachomatis is the most common bacterial STI, with sexually active young people at highest risk. The causative organism is an obligate intracellular parasite containing both DNA and RNA, having characteristics of both bacteria and viruses. Urogenital infection is usually caused by the subtypes DK. However, lymphogranuloma venereum (LGV) strains (L1, L2 and L3), although still rare, are increasingly being reported in men who have sex with men. In 2006, the national chlamydia screening programme was launched in the UK with the aim to screen up to 35% of the population of those under 25. Looking at the impact of this programme, Health Protection Agency (HPA) modelling suggests that the substantial increase in the number of diagnoses made in England between 2000 and 2010/2011 has probably decreased the prevalence of chlamydia among sexually active under 25 years old, relative to 2000.

- Chlamydial infection is frequently asymptomatic in women: vaginal discharge, dysuria, postcoital bleeding and mild pelvic discomfort may indicate infection. The organism is often found in conjunction with gonococcal infection. If left untreated 10–40% of women will develop pelvic inflammatory disease. Other complications include conjunctivitis, neonatal infection, perihepatitis (Fitz-Hugh–Curtis syndrome) and sexually acquired reactive arthritis
- The diagnostic accuracy of chlamydial testing has improved dramatically with the advent of nucleic acid amplification (NAAT) tests. These can detect chlamydia infection in urine, endocervical or

self-taken vaginal swabs, and can also be used for detection of pharyngeal and rectal chlamydia infection
- The drug of first choice is azithromycin 1 g stat, while doxycycline or erythromycin are alternatives

Genital herpes

Herpes simplex virus (HSV) is a DNA virus with two main subtypes: HSV-1 and 2. Both can affect the genital area. HSV-1 acquisition on the genitals can occur during orogenital contact.
- A primary episode can cause tingling and burning in the affected area prior to the appearance of painful vesicles/ulcers in the genital area (**Figure 14**). Dysuria is a commonly associated symptom. Secondary bacterial or fungal infection can occur delaying the healing process
- After acquisition the virus migrates via sensory nerves to the sacral root ganglia, where it remains latent until reactivation occurs
- Sufferers have reported reactivation to occur during systemic illness, immuno-suppression, fatigue, stress, menstruation and during pregnancy
- Recurrent episodes are well-localised, short-lived and produce fewer symptoms
- Diagnosis is usually on clinical grounds but should be confirmed by polymerase

chain reaction (PCR) or culture and serotyping
- Treatment is with aciclovir, valaciclovir or famciclovir. Treatment is more effective if commenced as soon as symptoms appear, reducing the severity and duration of the episode
- Primary diagnosis in pregnancy is associated with first-trimester miscarriage. If infection is acquired within 6 weeks of delivery, caesarian section should be offered to prevent neonatal transmission. Treatment is with acyclovir 400 mg three times daily which should be continued until delivery. Pregnant women with prior herpetic diagnosis should alert their midwife/general practitioners. For these women, suppression treatment with acyclovir may be considered from 36 weeks' gestation.

Genital Warts

Anogenital warts are caused by the HPV, of which there are many types. Types 6 and 11 are commonly associated with genital warts. Other types are associated with cervical intraepithelial neoplasia (CIN), vulval intraepithelial neoplasia (VIN), cervical cancer and vulval cancer, the most common of these being types 16 and 18. HPV vaccine is now being offered to schoolgirls in the UK, effective against types 6, 11, 16 and 18.
- Genital warts can be pleomorphic and are associated with itching
- Warts may enlarge during pregnancy or immunosuppression
- Diagnosis is on clinical grounds with a low threshold for biopsy of atypical lesions
- Treatment is commonly with podophyllotoxin applied to the affected area (contraindicated in pregnancy), topical imiquimod (not recommended in pregnancy) or cryotherapy
- Warts which fail to respond to medical treatment may need surgical removal
- Recurrence of warts is common

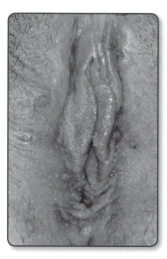

Figure 14 Multiple labial ulcers typical of genital herpes. Courtesy of Dr Emma Crosbie.

Trichomonas vaginalis

This is a flagellated protozoan. Infection can be asymptomatic but women can present

with vaginal discharge, itching, offensive odour and dysuria.
- Diagnosis is usually made by typical appearance on microscopy. Culture is sometimes employed as it is more sensitive and specific
- First line treatment is with metronidazole

Further reading

British Association of Sexual Health and HIV, Clinical Guidelines. Macclesfield: BASHH, 2012.
Pattman R. Oxford Handbook of Genitourinary Medicine, HIV and Sexual Health, 2nd edn. Oxford University Press 2010.

Mayor MT, Roett MA, Uduhiri KA. Diagnosis and management of gonococcal infections. Am Fam Physician 2012; 86:931–938.

Related topics of interest

- Human papillomavirus vaccination (p. 67)
- Pelvic inflammatory disease (p. 112)
- Vaginal discharge (p. 160)

Subfertility: aetiology and diagnosis

Overview

Between 10% and 15% of couples suffer from an involuntary delay in achieving a pregnancy. Subfertility may be classified as primary (no previous pregnancies) or secondary (previous pregnancies). In the general population, more than 80% of women will conceive within the first 12 months, and over 90% by the end of 2 years. The probability of conceiving each month, known as fecundity, reduces significantly with advancing female age. There is a sharp decline in fecundity after the age of 35 years, with the chance of conception being very low after 40 years of age.

Couples presenting with subfertility should be seen together as diagnostic measures and treatment choices will affect both partners. Ideally, they should be seen in a dedicated clinic with access to suitable information and counselling services if they wish. Subfertility causes significant psychological stress.

Aetiology

Causes of subfertility:
- Anovulation: 25%
- Tubal factor: 20%
- Uterine or peritoneal disorders: 10%
- Male factor: 30%
- Unexplained: 25%

Many couples will present with both male and female factors. A full history is essential to exclude other causes, such as coital difficulty.

Diagnosis
History

It is important to assess both partners. Both must be asked about their previous medical, surgical, medication and family history, about any sexually transmitted disease and coital history. The female partner should be asked about her menstrual pattern, whether she has any previous gynaecological history (e.g. cervical surgery) and whether she has had previous pregnancies. The male partner should be asked about previous pregnancies and testicular surgery. Information must also be noted of anything that could impact during a pregnancy, e.g. if the female partner has diabetes, as the subfertility clinic must also optimise preconception advice. Information regarding smoking, alcohol and recreational drug use must be obtained as this may impact on the chance of conception and may have consequences for the welfare of children conceived. The female partner should be advised to ensure she is up to date with cervical screening and that she should take 0.4 mg folic acid daily (she is taking antiepileptic medication 5 mg daily, is diabetic or has a history of previous spina bifida).

Examination

The female partner should be examined to check her body mass index (BMI) which should be between 19 and 29 to maximise her chances of pregnancy. A pelvic examination should be performed to exclude pathology. The male partner need not be examined, unless there is a significant abnormality found after semen analysis.

Investigations – initial

Female – all
Rubella titre
- Confirm immunity prior to treatment

Mid-luteal phase progesterone
- It is likely that women with regular menstrual cycles are ovulating
- Measurement of progesterone 7 days before expected menses will confirm ovulation if a level > 16 pmol/L is measured

Follicle-stimulating hormone (FSH)/ luteinising hormone (LH)/oestradiol
- Day 2–5 of cycle
- FSH 4–7 IU/L

- LH 3–6 IU/L (should be lower than FSH)
- Oestradiol < 180 pmol/L
- FSH > 10 IU/L suggests a reduction in ovarian reserve. This is seen as women age and is associated with a lower chance of conception
- LH levels higher than FSH levels are frequently seen in women with polycystic ovarian syndrome (PCOS)

Transvaginal ultrasound scan
- Antral follicle count
- Ovarian morphology, e.g. features of PCOS
- Uterine anomaly
- Presence of fibroids/polyps
- Chlamydia screen (urine)

Anti-Müllerian hormone (AMH) (although this investigation is still not available in all hospitals)
- Indicative of ovarian reserve
- Relatively new investigation and absolute value ranges are still not agreed. Current data would support:
  - < 5 pmol/L – indicative of reduced reserve
  - > 25 pmol/L – indicative of increased reserve, possible PCOS

Female – specific
Prolactin
- Do not measure routinely
- Only measure if amenorrhoea, profound oligomenorrhoea or galactorrhoea

Testosterone and sex hormone binding globulin (SHBG)
- Only measure if clinically indicated – suspicion of hyperandrogenaemia and/or PCOS

Karyotype
- If clinical suspicion of chromosomal rearrangement

Male – all
Semen analysis
- Day 3–4 abstinence from ejaculation
- World Health Organization (WHO) criteria 2010 – normal values (5th and 95th confidence intervals)
  - Volume > 1.5 mL (1.4–1.7 mL)
  - Concentration 15×10^6/mL ($12–16 \times 10^6$)
  - Progressive motility 32% (31–34%)
  - Morphology 4% (3–4%)

If a semen sample shows a reduction in any of the above parameters, it should be repeated after 3 months to exclude a temporary disruption to spermatogenesis, e.g. from intercurrent illness.

Male – specific
If azoospermia (absence of any sperm in the ejaculate) is diagnosed, further investigations must be carried out to try to elucidate the cause. However, in two-thirds of cases, no cause will be found. Azoospermia may be because of hypothalamo-pituitary axis failure, testicular failure or to an obstructive cause in the genital tract.
- **Karyotype** Chromosomal rearrangements, e.g. Klinefelter's syndrome, balanced translocations are seen much more frequently in men with azoospermia and may be associated with testicular failure
- FSH and LH levels should be measured to exclude a hypothalamo/pituitary cause. Low levels of gonadotrophins are associated with hypothalamo/pituitary disorder whilst high levels are associated with testicular failure
- **Screen for cystic fibrosis** Congenital absence of the vas deferens (CBAVD) is a cause of obstructive azoospermia and is frequently associated with a cystic fibrosis mutation

If profound oligospermia is diagnosed ($< 2 \times 10^6$/mL) a karyotype should be arranged as there is an increased incidence of karyotypic abnormality.

Further assessment
Tubal Assessment
Before arranging tubal patency testing, it is important to consider how the results of testing will alter patient management. If a severe male factor is found, the couple should be referred for assisted conception treatment and this will not be affected by whether or not the female partner has patent tubes. However, if for example, a couple are to embark on drug treatment to induce ovulation, it is essential to confirm tubal patency beforehand. If tubal patency testing is thought necessary, the

method chosen will depend on whether or not the woman is considered to be low or high risk for a tubal factor.

- Low risk – no previous history of abdominal surgery/pelvic infection, perform either
  - Hysterosalpingogram (HSG)
    - Injection of radio-opaque dye through the cervical canal
    - X-ray to confirm spill of dye
  - Hysterosalpingography (HyCoSy)
    - Injection of echogenic contrast through the cervical canal
    - Transvaginal scan to confirm spill from tubes
- High risk – previous abdominal surgery/ pelvic infection
  - Previous history will raise suspicion of tubal disease
  - Laparoscopy and dye test
  - Consent for adhesiolysis during the procedure if clinically indicated
  - Consent for tubal division/ salpingectomy if patient considering in vitro fertilisation treatment and in-operable hydrosalpinges are found at the time of laparoscopy
- Very high risk – extensive previous abdominal surgery – e.g. Crohn's disease
  - Do not assess tubal patency, as even if tubal patency was suggested by HSG, there would still be suspicion of poor tubal function. Laparoscopy often contraindicated
    - Treat as if tubal factor diagnosed
- Hysteroscopy
  - If ultrasound scan suggests the presence of a uterine anomaly
  - May need to undertake with laparoscopy – if there is uncertainty about abnormality seen, e.g. large septum or bicornuate uterus
  - To exclude polyps suggested on scan
  - If there is a suspicion of Asherman's syndrome
- 3D ultrasound scanning/ magnetic resonance imaging (MRI) scanning
  - This may be carried out instead of a hysteroscopy and laparoscopy in the first instance if available
  - If there is a suggestion of uterine anomaly
  - Safer than hysteroscopy and laparoscopy
  - Will help decision making with respect to surgical intervention, e.g. large septum or bicornuate uterus
- Ovarian reserve testing
  - Term given to collection of results indicating the reserve of oocytes that a woman has left
  - Ovarian reserve declines steeply with age, particularly after the age of 35 years
  - AMH, antral follicle count and basal FSH levels can be used in combination to assess reserve

Further reading

Anderson RA, Nelson SM, Wallace WH. Measuring anti-Müllerian hormone for the assessment of ovarian reserve: when and for whom is it indicated? Maturitas 2012; 71:28–33.

Karavolos S, Stewart J, Evbuomwan I, et al. Assessment of the infertile male. The Obstetrician and Gynaecologist 2013; 15:1–9.

Saunders RD, Shwayder JM, Nakajima ST. Current methods of tubal patency assessment. Fertil Steril 2011; 95:2171–2179.

Related topics of interest

Subfertility: medical and surgical management

Overview

When caring for a couple with subfertility, it is important to decide both when and how to treat to increase their chance of conception. These decisions must be made after considering how long the couple has been trying to conceive, the age of the female partner, the ovarian reserve of the female partner and the results of additional investigations. It is important to advise couples to optimise their chance of conception by having sexual intercourse every 2–3 days and to tell them about the detrimental effect of smoking and high alcohol intake.

In Topic 43, the causes of subfertility were discussed. This topic will detail the options open to couples dependent on their diagnosis. Should these treatments be unsuccessful, the couple should be considered for assisted conception treatment. It is important to remember that most couples presenting with subfertility have only a reduced chance of conception and many conceive spontaneously either before or after fertility treatment.

Anovulation

The World Health Organization (WHO) has defined three types of anovulatory disorder
1. WHO I – *Hypo*gonadotrophic *hypo*-oestrogenic
2. WHO II – *Normo*gonadotrophic *normo*-oestrogenic
3. WHO III – *Hyper*gonadotrophic *hypo*-oestrogenic

WHO I

Presentation

Amenorrhoea. May present with low body mass index (BMI).

Investigations

Low follicle-stimulating hormone (FSH), low luteinising hormone (LH), low oestradiol.

Check serum prolactin to exclude a prolactinoma. Ultrasound scan may show 'multicystic' ovaries.

Causes

Hypothalamic dysfunction (congenital/acquired), low body fat (anorexia/excessive exercise), pituitary disease (congenital/acquired, e.g. tumour, radiotherapy), hyperprolactinaemia.

Treatment

Treat underlying cause if found, e.g. anorexia. Women must be encouraged to increase their weight and reduce exercise if these are factors. If semen analysis is normal and there are bilaterally patent tubes, consider ovulation induction with human menopausal gonadotropin (hMG) or a combination of FSH plus LH. There is a need for close monitoring by ultrasound scan as there may be multiple follicular developments. There is a risk of multiple pregnancy of 10–20% after close monitoring.

Patients with hyperprolactinaemia should be treated with a dopamine agonist such as bromocriptine. Bromocriptine is highly effective in reducing levels of prolactin leading to the resumption of ovulatory cycles; however, it is associated with unpleasant side effects such as hypotension. Newer dopamine agonists (e.g. cabergoline) are associated with fewer side effects, but there are limited long term safety data following their use and manufacturers recommend discontinuation before pregnancy. Therefore, bromocriptine should be the drug of choice for first line treatment.

If there is also a tubal problem or a reduction in semen parameters, the patient should be treated with in vitro fertilisation (IVF) +/– intracytoplasmic sperm injection (ICSI).

WHO II

Presentation

The woman may present with oligomenorrhoea or amenorrhoea.

Additionally, she may complain of hirsutism and/or acne and may have a raised BMI. Approximately 85% of women with anovulatory cycles fall within this group. Polycystic ovarian syndrome (PCOS) is diagnosed according to the Rotterdam European Society of Human Reproduction and Embryology (ESHRE)/American Society for Reproductive Medicine (ASRM) consensus of 2003 by the finding of at least two of the following three features:

1. Oligo/anovulation
2. Raised androgens (clinical features/biochemistry)
3. Polycystic ovarian syndrome (PCOS) features on ultrasound scan

Investigations

Gonadotrophins within 'normal' range, although may see reversal of FSH/LH ratio with raised LH levels. May see raised serum testosterone, low sex hormone binding globulin with consequent raised free androgen index (FAI). Anti-Müllerian hormone (AMH) levels will be raised. Typical PCOS appearance on ultrasound scan (ovarian enlargement > 10 cc, peripherally arranged follicles, dense stroma, high antral follicle count-appearances may be limited to only one ovary).

Causes

PCOS, but may also be seen without PCOS in women with a raised BMI.

Treatment

Advise patient to lose weight to attain a BMI of < 30. Losing weight may re-establish ovulatory cycles. Treatment should not be started for women with a raised BMI as there is a significantly lower chance of a successful outcome. If semen analysis is normal, tubal patency has been confirmed and BMI is < 30, consider oral ovulation induction agents. If the woman is amenorrhoeic, it is important to induce a withdrawal bleed using an oral progestogen, such as norethisterone for 7–10 days, before starting ovulation induction agents.

Clomiphene citrate (an antioestrogen that blocks negative feedback of oestradiol to pituitary, and results in increased FSH secretion encouraging folliculogenesis).

Initially offer 50 mg on day 2–6 of cycle (or following induced bleed). If there is no response then increase dose to 100 mg. In exceptional circumstances try 150 mg. Women should be advised of the risk of a multiple pregnancy. Monitoring with ultrasound scan should be undertaken in the first cycle to reduce the risk of hyperstimulation and high order pregnancies, although it is rare to have higher order multiple pregnancies than twins. If ovulatory cycles establish, treatment should be continued for a maximum of six cycles.

Metformin may be used either alone or in combination with clomiphene citrate. Metformin is an insulin sensitiser and treatment results in lower levels of insulin which in turn reduce the production of androgens.

In women resistant to clomiphene, treatment with the aromatase inhibitor letrozole can be considered. Letrozole reduces the production of oestrogen by granulosa cells, which in turn reduces the negative feedback of oestradiol to the pituitary. The pituitary responds by producing more FSH to encourage folliculogenesis. Ovulation rates with Letrozole are similar to clomiphene although there is a suggestion of a lower risk of multiple pregnancies with Letrozole. Long term follow up studies are not available, and therefore clomiphene citrate remains the first line treatment choice. If ovulation does not occur after oral ovulation induction agents, the patient can be considered for either:

1. *Ovulation induction with gonadotrophins.* This treatment involves daily injections of FSH or hMG. It is essential to monitor the patient closely by ultrasound to ensure that no more than three follicles develop. If there is excessive response, the treatment must be stopped. After the development of a preovulatory follicle, ovulation is induced using an injection of hCG to mimic the LH surge. The couple are advised to have intercourse. Ovulation induction should be carried out for six cycles if a pregnancy does not occur. The patients must be advised of the risk of multiple pregnancies – approximately 20%

2. *Ovarian drilling.* The patient undergoes a laparoscopy and six to eight diathermy 'stabs' are made in one or both ovaries. The diathermy is thought to interfere with the intraovarian hormonal environment possibly by reducing AMH levels to allow spontaneous ovulation to occur. If ovulatory cycles resume, this is usually for a limited period of approximately 12 months

WHO III

Presentation

Amenorrhoea, may complain of hot flushes.

Investigations

Low oestradiol, raised FSH, raised LH, low AMH. In women under the age of 30 years, it is important to check thyroid function, karyotype and carrier status for Fragile X.

Causes

Genetic, immunological, frequently no cause is found.

Treatment

Recommend hormone replacement therapy to control symptoms, and for osteoprotection. If the woman wishes to conceive, she would need to undergo treatment using donated oocytes.

Tubal disease

Tubal surgery should be limited to those women with mild tubal disease and who are young. Women with isolated cornual block may be treated with hysteroscopic tubal cannulation. Although rarely available within the National Health Service (NHS), reversal of sterilisation can effectively restore tubal function, especially in young women. Women over 35 years of age or with moderate/severe tubal disease should be referred for assisted conception treatment rather than tubal surgery. If hydrosalpinges are found at laparoscopy, they should be removed or divided in preparation for IVF treatment as there is good evidence of a significant reduction in pregnancy rates with IVF in the presence of hydrosalpinges.

Endometriosis

Endometriosis is associated with subfertility. Medical treatment of endometriosis does not increase the chance of conception. Laparoscopic ablation of endometriosis is associated with an increased chance of conception and should be offered. Following a consensus, the European Society of Human Reproduction and Embryology agreed that an ovarian endometrioma should be removed if it is more than 4 cm in diameter. However, endometriomata should not be removed if they are bilateral or there is evidence of a reduced ovarian reserve. There remains ongoing debate about the best treatment for endometriosis for subfertility.

Male factor

Couples with male factor subfertility should be referred for assisted conception treatment. Rarely, a cause for azoospermia (no sperm in ejaculate) may be found, such as obstruction or hypogonadotrophic hypogonadism. In these cases, medical and surgical treatments are of value. In other cases, there is no evidence to support the use of medical agents or surgical intervention to improve semen quality.

Unexplained subfertility

Where the female partner is under 36 years, couples should be encouraged to attempt spontaneous conception for 2 years, if no cause of subfertility has been found. After 2 years, couples should be referred for IVF treatment. In women over 36 years of age or women with reduced ovarian reserve, it may be appropriate to refer for IVF treatment earlier. There is no place for empirical treatment with clomiphene citrate.

Fibroids, polyps and uterine anomaly

Uterine abnormalities including fibroids and polyps are found in 10–15% of women with subfertility.

Fibroids are associated with subfertility and poor pregnancy outcome. The decision as to whether to remove fibroids must be made after considering the patient's history as well as the size and position of fibroids. Submucosal fibroids significantly reduce the chance of embryo implantation and should be resected hysteroscopically if possible. For patients with a history of subfertility, large intramural and subserosal fibroids of > 7 cm in diameter should probably be removed via laparotomy or laparoscopy. It may be appropriate to remove smaller fibroids depending upon the history. However, there is very little evidence about the effect of fibroids on the chance of conception and the beneficial effect of removal.

Polyps > 1 cm in diameter are associated with an increased risk of miscarriage and should be removed hysteroscopically.

Uterine anomalies must be assessed on an individual basis. It is essential to accurately diagnose any uterine anomaly to decide whether surgical intervention is necessary. Additionally, women with a uterine anomaly are at increased risk of premature delivery, and therefore all efforts must be made to reduce the risk of a multiple pregnancy. When a uterine anomaly is suggested from scan, a hysteroscopy should be carried out to confirm the diagnosis. Although there is little evidence, it may be beneficial to remove a uterine septum in patients presenting with subfertility.

If Asherman's syndrome is suspected, a hysteroscopy and division of adhesions should be carried out. It is of benefit to insert an intrauterine contraceptive device (IUD) after surgery for 6 months to prevent further scarring. After 6 months, the IUD should be removed and the patient told to attempt to conceive.

Further reading

NICE Clinical Guidance No. 156. Assessment and treatment for people with fertility problems. London: NICE, 2013.

Fernandez H, Morin-Surruca M, Torre A, et al. Ovarian drilling for surgical treatment of polycystic ovarian syndrome: a comprehensive review. Reprod Biomed Online 2011; 22:556–568.

Bhattacharya S, Harrild K, Mollison J, et al. Clomiphene citrate or unstimulated intrauterine insemination compared with expectant management for unexplained subfertility: pragmatic randomised controlled trial. BMJ 2008; 337:a716.

Related topics of interest

Termination of pregnancy

Overview

Termination of pregnancy (TOP) or induced abortion is a topic that is both emotive and controversial. Both pro-choice (for) and pro-life (anti) groups are fixed and vehement in their views. Despite advances in contraceptive options for women and consistent use of effective methods of contraception, TOP for unwanted pregnancy remains a part of everyday gynaecological practice in the UK. In 2011, 189,931 TOPs were carried out in England and Wales.

Legal issues

TOP in England, Scotland and Wales but not Northern Ireland is governed by the Abortion Act, 1967. TOP is illegal under most circumstances in Northern Ireland. A legally induced abortion must be:

- Carried out in a hospital or specialist licensed clinic
- Justified under one or more of the approved statutory grounds (**Table 22**) according to two registered medical practitioners

Table 22 Statutory grounds for termination of pregnancy	
Statutory grounds	
A	The continuance of the pregnancy would involve risk to the life of the pregnant woman greater than if the pregnancy was terminated
B	The termination is necessary to prevent grave permanent injury to the physical and mental health of the pregnant woman
C	The pregnancy has not exceeded its 24th week and the continuance of the pregnancy would involve risk, greater than if the pregnancy was terminated, of injury to the physical or mental health of the pregnant woman
D	The pregnancy has not exceeded its 24th week and the continuance of the pregnancy would involve risk, greater than if the pregnancy was terminated, of injury to the physical and mental health of any existing child (children) of the family of the pregnant woman
E	There is substantial risk that if the child was born it would suffer from such physical or mental abnormalities as to be seriously handicapped

There is a gestation limit of 24 weeks for TOPs under statutory grounds C and D, but statutory grounds A, B and E are without gestation limits. The law also states that a doctor can decline to certify a woman for a TOP if they have a moral objection to abortion, but must recommend another doctor who is willing to help.

A woman contemplating TOP should be provided with accurate information about different methods of abortion available, so that she can make a fully informed choice and give informed consent.

Girls under the age of 16 years can consent to TOP if the clinician assesses them to be Gillick competent (able to fully understand the proposed medical procedure and its implications). It is essential to consider child protection issues when treating these girls and consider whether it is appropriate to involve social services.

Methods of TOP

TOP procedures are either surgical or medical. Women should be offered adequate analgesia [non-steroidal anti-inflammatory drugs (NSAIDs), opiates]. Surgical procedures are performed up to 20 weeks' gestation.

Surgical methods

- In the UK, vacuum aspiration is preferred to sharp curettage as it is associated with shorter operating times and reduced blood loss. This method is appropriate up to 14 weeks' gestation. Manual vacuum aspiration (MVA) uses a handheld syringe, which allows this procedure to be performed in an outpatient clinic under local anaesthetic. Difficulties have been encountered when MVA is carried out after 9 weeks' gestation
- Vacuum aspiration under 7 weeks carries a greater risk of failure, and it is usual practice to wait until 7 weeks if the woman presents beforehand. It is important to inspect the aspirated tissue for products of conception
- For pregnancies above 14 weeks' gestation, surgical abortion by dilation and evacuation

(D&E) can be carried out, but there are increased risks of bleeding and uterine perforation

- Cervical preparation with vaginal misoprostol is recommended before surgical TOP and may be of particular benefit when there is an increased risk of cervical injury or uterine perforation (age < 17 years, advanced gestational age, cervical anomalies, previous surgery)

Medical methods

- Regimens of oral mifepristone (antiprogesterone) followed by misoprostol (prostaglandin analogue) can be used safely and effectively for TOP at any gestation. **Table 23** illustrates recommended regimens. Women who wish to complete the TOP at home following misoprostol may do so provided there is access to 24-hour advice and assistance and appropriate follow up arrangements are in place.

Complications

Women should be adequately counselled regarding risks associated with both medical and surgical TOP. Estimated complication rates are 1 per 1000 TOPs. Women undergoing medical TOP at less than 14 weeks' gestation report more pain and gastrointestinal symptoms during the procedure, and more bleeding after the first 2 weeks compared to those undergoing surgical TOP. Severe bleeding requiring blood transfusion is lower with early TOPs, occurring in less than 1 per 1000, but rising to about 4 per 1000 at gestations greater than 20 weeks.

Surgical TOP carries the risk of uterine perforation of 1–4 per 1000 and this risk is increased at higher gestations. Cervical trauma is also a risk with surgical TOP and can be reduced by cervical priming with prostaglandins.

Both surgical and medical TOPs carry a small risk of failure (less than 1 in 1000), necessitating a further procedure. There is also a small risk of retained products of conception requiring intervention.

Infection, which is usually caused by pre-existing microbes, can occur in both medical and surgical TOP. Opportunistic screening for chlamydia and gonorrhoea will allow for appropriate treatment. Some units advocate prophylactic antibiotic use (e.g. 1 g PR metronidazole).

Women should be reassured that there are no proven associations between TOP and subsequent ectopic pregnancy, placenta praevia or infertility. The risk of placenta praevia may have been increased with sharp curettage abortions, but the increased risk has not been observed in vacuum aspiration. Women should be counselled about the range of emotional responses they may experience following a TOP, including grief and regret.

Table 23 Recommended regimens for medical TOP	
Pregnancy gestation	Recommended medical TOP protocol
≤ 63 days	Mifepristone 200 mg PO 24–48 hours later Misoprostol 800 µg PV/Buccal/Sublingual*
9–13 weeks	Mifepristone 200 mg PO 36–48 hours later Misoprostol 800 mg PV followed by four further doses of misoprostol 400 µg PV at 3 hourly intervals PV/PO
13–24 weeks	Mifepristone 200 mg PO 36–48 hours Misoprostol 800 µg PV followed by four further doses misoprostol 400 µg PO/PV 3 hourly If treatment fails to induce an abortion, mifepristone can be repeated 3 hours after the last dose of misoprostol, and 12 hours later misoprostol may be recommended

* vaginal administration of misoprostol may reduce gastrointestinal side effects but does not affect efficacy
Adapted from RCOG Evidence-based Clinical Guideline No. 7, 2011.

Care after abortion

Women who are Rhesus negative should be given Anti-D IgG within 72 hours following TOP regardless of the method and gestation. There is no need for routine follow-up; however, women undergoing medical TOP where a successful abortion has not been confirmed should be offered follow-up to exclude an ongoing pregnancy.

Women should be counselled regarding contraceptive choices and the TOP service should be able to provide all methods of contraception including long-acting methods.

The chosen method of contraception should be started immediately.

Further reading

Royal College of Obstetricians and Gynaecologist. Evidence-based Clinical Guideline No. 7. The Care of Women Requesting Induced Abortion. London: RCOG, 2011.

Aston G, Bewley. Abortion and domestic violence. The Obstetrician & Gynaecologist 2009; 11:163–168.

Von Hertzen H, Piaggio G, Wojdyla D. et al. For the WHO Research Group on Post-ovulatory Methods of Fertility Regulation. Two mifepristone doses and two intervals of misoprostol administration for termination of early pregnancy: a randomised factorial controlled equivalence trial. BJOG 2009; 116:381–389.

Related topics of interest

Urinary incontinence and voiding difficulties

Overview

Urinary incontinence is defined as involuntary leakage of urine. Most cases are caused by stress incontinence or overactive bladder (OAB). Mixed incontinence implies that both stress incontinence and overactive bladder contribute to the patient's symptoms. A symptomatic diagnosis should be made in the first instance and conservative treatments commenced by community based continence practitioners. If conservative treatments fail the woman should be referred to secondary care for a urodynamic diagnosis and discussion of management.

Clinical features

The clinical features of leakage depend on the underlying cause. Stress incontinence is associated with leakage on exercise, movement, cough and essentially any action which results in a rise in intra-abdominal pressure. The main symptom of overactive bladder is urgency to void. This may be associated with frequency of micturition and nocturia. The urgency may or may not be associated with urinary leakage. It is therefore further classified in to OAB wet and OAB dry. Constant unprovoked leakage is suggestive of a fistula, overflow or a congenital abnormality. Postmicturition dribbling is suggestive of a urethral diverticulum.

Aetiology

The aetiology is very much dependent on the type of incontinence. For example:
- Urodynamic stress incontinence – childbirth
- Detrusor overactivity – idiopathic, diabetes, bladder stone or tumour, infection, obstruction, postradiation therapy, neurologic injury
- Overflow incontinence – pelvic mass, severe constipation, obstruction, postchildbirth (following over distension injury)

Also:
- Fistulae – surgical, childbirth, radiation, diverticular disease
- Congenital anomalies – aberrant ureter, epispadias
- Cognitive impairment, e.g. dementia, acute confusional state
- Miscellaneous – urethral diverticulum

This is not an exhaustive list.

Stress urinary incontinence (SUI)

SUI is defined as involuntary loss of urine when the intravesical pressure exceeds the maximum urethral pressure, in the absence of detrusor activity. The term stress incontinence is used to describe a symptom, a sign and is a diagnosis. This can cause confusion.

The symptom of stress incontinence is leakage provoked by activity such as cough, sneeze, running or walking. The sign of stress incontinence is the visualisation of leakage from the urethral meatus with cough or Valsalva. It is important to note that if a patient is examined after recently voiding, the sign of stress incontinence may not be elicited because the bladder is empty. The diagnosis of stress incontinence can really only be confirmed at urodynamics and is called urodynamic stress incontinence (the term genuine stress incontinence is no longer used).

Treatment

First line treatment is lifestyle advice about weight loss, stopping smoking and doing pelvic floor exercises. This may be followed by supervised pelvic floor physiotherapy. Continence devices such as rings or urethral plugs may be considered. If these fail, urodynamics are used to confirm the diagnosis of SUI prior to considering surgery.

The most common procedure for the treatment of SUI in the UK is the mid urethral sling (MUS), inserted by either retropubic [transvaginal tape (TVT)] or transobturator [trans obturator tape (TOT)] approach. The tape is made of polypropylene type 1 mesh. There is level 1 evidence for both procedures; however, care should be taken about the type of commercial tape used because they are not all the same, and do not all have the same level of published evidence. The cure rate following primary MUS is 80–90%. Common complications following MUS are OAB, voiding difficulties and mesh exposure in the vagina. Less common are delayed perforation of the bladder or urethra.

Other procedures which are used include colposuspension and fascial slings. Both have cure rates similar to MUS. In some cases, there is an indication for periurethral injections of bulking agents; however, the cure rate with fillers is much lower than MUS.

Recently, single incision slings have been developed. Whilst likely to be useful in the management of SUI, these do not yet have enough evidence to use outside the setting of a research trial.

OAB

OAB is diagnosed by symptoms. These include urgency +/– urge incontinence, frequency and nocturia. Note pain is not a symptom of OAB. The aetiology of OAB is poorly understood and most cases are idiopathic. It is effectively a diagnosis of exclusion. Infection, haematuria and diabetes should be excluded first.
Conservative treatments for OAB include:
Lifestyle advice   On fluid management (both volume and type) as well as weight loss. Bladder retraining should be considered.
Pharmacotherapy   There a several long and short-acting anticholinergic drugs available in oral and transdermal preparations. The National Institute for Health and Clinical Excellence (NICE) recommends the use of short-acting oxybutinin as first line pharmacotherapy. Recently, a new class of drugs has been developed which may offer hope for the treatment of OAB, called β_3-agonists.

If these conservative treatments do not work then more invasive treatments are available. Urodynamics should be performed first. The presence of involuntary detrusor contractions associated with urgency or leakage confirms the diagnosis of detrusor overactivity. Second line treatments include injection of botulinus toxin (Botox) in the bladder wall, sacral nerve stimulation or posterior tibial nerve stimulation. For intractable, severe cases, one may still consider a clam cystoplasty or urinary diversion.

Overflow incontinence

This uncommon condition is because of voiding difficulties which are either caused by urethral obstruction or detrusor underactivity. It is defined as an involuntary loss of urine when the intravesical pressure exceeds the maximum urethral pressure because of an elevation of intravesical pressure associated with bladder distension. It presents as continual dribbling or voiding small volumes in conjunction with stress incontinence. It is often diagnosed by the large palpable bladder, or on ultrasound. The differential diagnosis includes an upper motor neuron lesion, regional anaesthesia, drugs, surgery, a pelvic mass, including a retroverted gravid uterus in the second trimester, or genital inflammation. The treatment is tailored to the cause.

Occult incontinence

Women who have severe vault or anterior vaginal wall prolapse are at risk of developing urinary incontinence once their prolapse is corrected. It is thought that the 'kinking' of the urethra caused by the prolapse prevents stress incontinence. In some women, once the prolapse is reduced with a pessary or surgery, stress incontinence may be unmasked. Many people have tried to develop methods to predict who will develop SUI following prolapse surgery, e.g. a urodynamic study with a ring pessary, but currently all methods have predictive values no better than chance.

Voiding difficulties

Most commonly these are the result of an underactive detrusor, which is difficult to treat. Clean intermittent self-catheterisation is convenient and easily taught to the majority, and has a very low infection rate. Sacral nerve stimulation is useful in some cases. Another cause of voiding difficulties is prolapse. It is, however, difficult to predict whether correcting the prolapse will improve the voiding difficulty. Urethral stricture can also cause voiding difficulties but true strictures are uncommon in women. Urodynamics should be used to distinguish between an underactive detrusor and urethral stricture.

Further reading

Hussain U, Kearny R. Surgical management of stress urinary incontinence. Obstetrics, Gynaecology & Reproductive Medicine 2013; 23:108–113.
NICE Clinical Guideline No. 40. The management of urinary incontinence in women. London: NICE, 2007.

Abboudi H, Fynes MM, Doumouchtsis SK. Contemporary therapy for the overactive bladder. The Obstetrician & Gynaecologist 2011; 13:98–106.

Related topics of interest

- Fistulae in obstetrics and gynaecology (p. 50)
- Genital prolapse (p. 55)
- Urodynamics (p. 152)

Urodynamics

Overview

Urodynamics is the term that encompasses a number of tests used in the investigation of women with lower urinary tract symptoms (LUTS). The bladder's dual roles of storage and expulsion of urine is measured objectively. Urodynamic investigations should not be performed blindly, but rather are carried out to answer a specific question and inform management. This is termed the 'urodynamic question'.

Up to 50% of women may be affected with a continence or voiding problem at some time in their life. In the past, urodynamics were used in the initial assessment of women with urinary symptoms because the bladder was considered an 'unreliable witness'. Less emphasis was placed on the patients' symptoms and more on the outcome of urodynamics, an objective test. Currently, urogynaecologists recommend that conservative treatments for simple bladder problems are undertaken prior to urodynamics and this is reflected in National Institute for Health and Clinical Excellence (NICE) guideline CG40.

Terminology used for LUTS should comply with the joint International Association of Urogynaecology and International Continence Society standards and urodynamics should be performed in accordance with standards published by the International Continence Society.

Urodynamic tests

Non-invasive tests

Urinary dipstick   This test can be used to screen for infection and/or haematuria which if found should be investigated as a priority. Occasionally, the pathophysiology of frequency and urgency is transitional cell carcinoma of the bladder. Always exclude menstruation as a cause of haematuria prior to any other investigations.

Bladder diary   All patients presenting for urodynamic evaluation should have completed a urinary diary, preferably for 3 days, recording time, volume and type of intake and the time and volume of urine output. They should also record related symptoms of urgency, incontinence and pain.

Pad tests   These can be used to evaluate the amount of urine lost. Patients are given pre-weighed pads which they wear for usually 24 hours. The pads are then reweighed to determine the amount of urine lost. Pyridium (phenazopyridine) stains urine bright yellow. It is occasionally given prior to a pad test to establish if the loss is urine or vaginal discharge.

Free flow studies   The patient, with a comfortably full bladder, voids in private through a flow meter. The flow rate graph should be a smooth bell shape curve. The Liverpool nomogram should be used to evaluate the flow and volume. Low or intermittent flow rates may be due to outlet obstruction or poor detrusor contractility that needs further evaluation using pressure flow studies. The residual volume should be recorded either by catheterisation or with ultrasound [bladder volume (mL) = depth (cm) × height (cm) × width (cm) × 0.7].

Invasive tests

There is little morbidity associated with urodynamics, apart from a low risk of urinary tract infection and occasional discomfort. Infection must be excluded and eradicated before proceeding to urodynamic investigation.

Cystometry   This is the test which most people associate with urodynamics. Cystometry measures the intravesical pressure, from which the detrusor pressure can be calculated by subtracting the intra-abdominal pressure. The pressures are measured during the different phases of the bladder cycle, namely storage and voiding. The detrusor pressure (P_{det}) can be calculated:

$$P_{det} = P_{ves} - P_{abd}$$

P_{ves} = Intravesical pressure,

P_{abd} = Intra-abdominal pressure

Intra-abdominal pressure is approximated from a pressure catheter placed in the rectum, vagina or a stoma. The intravesical pressure is measured by a pressure catheter transducer placed in the bladder. During the test the bladder is filled with sterile water via a filling catheter, usually at 100 mL per minute; however, the filling rate may be slower in specific clinical conditions, e.g. neurological disease or severe detrusor over activity (DOA). **Figure 15** shows a typical urodynamic trace.

Cystometry first assesses the bladder storage phase, wherein DOA, abnormal bladder sensations, reduced or increased capacity and poor compliance may be elicited. Once filling is completed, provocation tests are undertaken. These include coughing, listening to running water and exercises such as star jumps. These provocation tests are designed to replicate the triggers known to cause the bladder symptoms in the specific patient, thereby answering their urodynamic question. The most common provocation tests are designed to elicit stress urinary incontinence. Sometimes it is not feasible to replicate the provocation factor, e.g. urinary leak caused by orgasm.

The voiding phase assesses detrusor contractility as well as pelvic floor and urethral function. Normal women void with a combination of a low pressure detrusor contraction (i.e. pressure < 15 cm H_2O) and simultaneous relaxation of the pelvic floor.

It is vitally important that urodynamics are only performed by fully trained staff, who understand the calibration and quality control procedures required to ensure the results are valid.

Video cystourethrography   This employs radiological screening during cystometric assessment, so that in addition to the normal cystometry parameters, the anatomy and function of the lower urinary tract may be seen dynamically. This is an expensive form of investigation and gives a radiation dose equivalent to a single chest film. In most units, this test is reserved for patients with complex neurological conditions or complex previous surgery. It will allow the dynamic assessment of, e.g. bladder diverticulae and vesicoureteric reflux.

Ambulatory urodynamics   Ambulatory monitoring is used solely as a second line investigation where standard urodynamics have failed to provide an explanation of symptoms. There are a number of controversial issues around ambulatory monitoring, and therefore it should only be performed at tertiary centres. The patient wears a lightweight recording device which

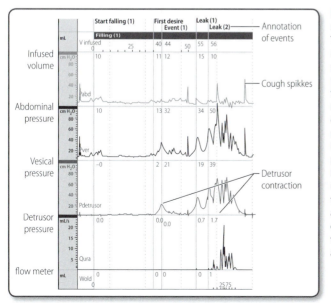

Figure 15 Urodynamic trace showing detrusor overactivity. The trace has five lines which record infused volume, abdominal pressure, vesical pressure, detrusor pressure (subtraction of abdominal from vesical pressure) and flow rate (i.e. leakage). A detrusor contraction is labelled. The pressure rise is seen on both the detrusor line and the vesical line but is not present on the abdominal line. During the detrusor contraction, urinary leakage is demonstrated by the flow meter. Cough spikes are also shown. During urodynamics coughs are regularly performed to test the subtraction of the vesical and abdominal lines.

measures bladder and abdominal pressure measurement by natural filling. It has a hand-operated device to record important events during the test including cough, urgency and leakage.

Urethral function studies   There are different techniques for measuring urethral function. Urethral pressure profilometry and leak point pressure measurement are the most common ones in current use. They can help inform the management of women with complex incontinence or following failed surgery for stress incontinence, but their use is controversial.

Electromyography (EMG)   This is a complicated test and primarily measures the electrical activity around the urethral sphincter. It is used in tertiary centres to investigate detrusor sphincter dyssynergia, Fowler's syndrome, neuropathy and myopathy.

Urodynamic report

Following urodynamics, a systematic and detailed report should be written by the person performing the test. The test results should be analysed in the context of the urodynamic question and the patient's experience. International Urogynecological Association (IUGA) and International Continence Society (ICS) have published definitions of urinary symptoms and urodynamic diagnoses. Two of the most common definitions are urodynamic stress incontinence (USI) 'the involuntary leakage of urine during increased abdominal pressure, in the absence of a detrusor contraction' and detrusor overactivity 'an urodynamic observation characterised by involuntary detrusor contractions during the filling phase which may be spontaneous or provoked'.

Further reading

Haylen BT, de Ridder D, Freeman RM, et al. An International Urogynecological Association (IUGA)/International Continence Society (ICS) joint report on the terminology for female pelvic floor dysfunction. International Urogynecol Journal 2010; 21:5–26.

Schäfer W, Abrams P, Liao L, et al. Good urodynamic practices: uroflowmetry, filling cystometry, and pressure-flow studies. Neurourol Urodyn 2002; 21:261–274.

Swithinbank L, Webster L. Basic understanding of urodynamics. Obstetrics, Gynaecology and Reproductive Medicine 2012; 22:315–320

Related topics of interest

- Urinary incontinence and voiding difficulties (p. 149)
- Genital prolapse (p. 55)
- Fistulae in obstetrics and gynaecology (p. 50)

Uterine tumours

The uterus is composed of two main tissues, the myometrium, which forms the smooth muscle wall of the uterus, and the endometrium, which lines the internal cavity of the uterus and consists of glandular structures within a stromal matrix. Benign and malignant tumours of the uterus can originate in either of these components but tumours of the myometrium tend to be benign, whereas those of the endometrium are more often malignant.

Benign tumours

Benign tumours of the myometrium, leiomyomata (fibroids), are the commonest benign tumours encountered in gynaecological practice and are discussed in Topic 15.

Benign tumours of the endometrium, endometrial polyps, are localised masses of endometrial tissue that project into the lumen of the uterus. They may be single or multiple and may be asymptomatic or cause abnormal vaginal bleeding (intermenstrual, menorrhagia or postmenopausal). Although usually benign, polyps can occasionally contain malignancy at a rate of 0.5–5%. Polyps are usually removed surgically during hysteroscopy for investigation of abnormal bleeding.

Precancerous lesions of the endometrium

Endometrial hyperplasia is overgrowth of the glandular component of the endometrium. Many epidemiological and molecular studies have provided evidence of a relationship between endometrial hyperplasia and endometrial cancer, whereby there is a continuum of proliferative glandular changes from simple hyperplasia to complex hyperplasia with atypical, malignant appearing cells, and culminating, in some cases, in endometrial carcinoma. Endometrial hyperplasia is associated with prolonged oestrogen exposure of the endometrium and simple hyperplasia often regresses with removal of oestrogen stimulant. The rate of malignant progression for simple hyperplasia is approximately 1% if without atypia and 8% with atypia. Complex hyperplasia with atypia may coexist with an endometrial carcinoma or if left untreated may progress to carcinoma in 25–50% of women, and hence hysterectomy is often the treatment of choice. For women who are at high risk of surgical morbidity (e.g. those who are morbidly obese) and those who wish to retain their fertility, treatment with high dose oral progestogens (e.g. megestrol acetate) or the intrauterine system [equal efficacy rates but fewer systemic progestogenic side effects, e.g. weight gain and venous thromboembolism (VTE)] may be appropriate, alongside careful surveillance and follow-up.

Malignant tumours

Malignant tumours of the myometrium

Leiomyosarcomas are rare tumours arising from the myometrium. They have a peak incidence at age 40–60 years, often recur after removal and frequently metastasise. They may arise in a pre-existing fibroid (0.2–1%) but more commonly arise de novo in the myometrium. The vast majority of uterine leiomyosarcomas are sporadic, but it has been suggested that patients with germline mutations in fumarate hydratase are at increased risk. Previous radiotherapy for pelvic malignancy is also a risk factor. These poor prognostic tumours are not usually confined to the uterus at time of presentation and are relatively chemo and radiotherapy-resistant.

Malignant tumours of the endometrium

The majority of malignant tumours of the body of the uterus are endometrial carcinomas. They are the most common invasive gynaecological cancer of developed countries, with nearly 8000 new cases in England and Wales annually. Over the past 20 years there has been a sharp rise in the incidence (40%) and death rate from endometrial cancer (20%), despite improvements in overall survival. This may reflect an ageing population, increased use of tamoxifen for the treatment of breast cancer, uterine-sparing treatments for heavy menstrual bleeding and the obesity epidemic.

Endometrial carcinoma is rare in premenopausal women, the maximum incidence being age 55–65 years. Development of endometrial cancer is predominantly related to excess oestrogen exposure. Risk factors include obesity, diabetes, hypertension, polycystic ovarian syndrome, unopposed oestrogen therapy, tamoxifen treatment, early menarche, late menopause and nulliparity. It often presents with abnormal or postmenopausal vaginal bleeding, and most women with endometrial cancer are diagnosed at an early stage with uterine-confined tumours.

The majority of endometrial carcinomas are thought to be sporadic but there some genetic syndromes associated with the disease, the most common being hereditary non-polyposis colorectal cancer syndrome (HNPCC) also known as Lynch syndrome, an autosomal dominant cancer-susceptibility syndrome associated with mutations in DNA mismatch repair genes. Endometrial cancer associated with HNPCC tends to occur in young women with an estimated lifetime risk of endometrial cancer of 40–60%.

A diagnosis of endometrial cancer can be suspected from increased endometrial thickness on vaginal ultrasound (cut off of 4 mm is considered normal in a postmenopausal woman), and formally determined by histological assessment from endometrial biopsies or curettings from pipelle or hysteroscopy specimens.

There are two major types of endometrial carcinomas: type 1 account for 80% of cases, are of well-differentiated histology and resemble proliferative endometrial glands, hence are referred to as endometrioid carcinomas. They are related to oestrogen exposure and can arise from the atypical hyperplasia intermediate. In contrast, type 2 carcinomas follow a separate pathway. They usually arise in atrophic glands and their incidence peaks a decade later than type 1 carcinomas. They are usually poorly differentiated tumours and the most common subtype is serous carcinoma, which has a greater propensity to spread outside the uterus resulting in a generally poorer prognosis.

Endometrial carcinomas can grow either as discrete polypoid structures or diffusely over the endometrial surface. Spread usually starts with myometrial invasion then progresses to adjacent organs such as cervix, fallopian tubes, ovaries and peritoneal surfaces. Spread via lymphatics to pelvic or para-aortic nodes eventually occurs but blood stream spread to distant sites such as lungs and liver is a relatively rare and late event.

Staging of endometrial cancer is based on the International Federation of Gynecology and Obstetrics (FIGO) surgical staging system, with stage I disease confined to the uterus and the worst, stage IV disease, involving invasion of the bladder, bowel and/ or distant metastases (FIGO staging system for endometrial cancer, 2009) (**Table 24**).

Treatment of early-stage disease has traditionally been by total abdominal hysterectomy and bilateral salpingo-oophorectomy; however, laparoscopic or laparoscopic-assisted surgery is now the standard of care, since it is associated with fewer postoperative complications, a shorter postoperative stay and faster return to normal activities compared with open surgery. Although most endometrial cancer occurs in postmenopausal women, ovary-sparing surgery is often considered in younger women yet to complete their families, although they are at risk of ovarian recurrence so require close follow-up. Adjuvant radiotherapy can be given for stage I disease with deep myometrial involvement, more advanced local disease, high-grade tumour or positive lymph nodes. Vaginal brachytherapy is the treatment of choice to reduce pelvic recurrence as it has lower toxicity rates than external beam treatment, but neither has been shown to improve survival in the adjuvant setting. For stage III–IV disease adjuvant chemotherapy is generally given as it improves survival and reduces recurrence. Recurrent disease can appear in many different forms ranging from isolated vaginal relapse to widespread disease and, therefore, treatment is highly individualised with surgery, radiation, chemotherapy and hormonal therapy as possible treatments.

Table 24 FIGO staging of endometrial cancer	
Description	
Stage I	Tumour confined to the corpus uteri
Ia	No or less than half myometrial invasion
Ib	Invasion equal to or more than half of the myometrium
Stage II	Tumour invades cervical stroma, but does not extend beyond the uterus*
Stage III	Local or regional spread of tumour, or both
IIIa	Tumour invades the serosa of the corpus uteri or adnexae†
IIIb	Vaginal or parametrial involvement†
IIIc	Metastases to pelvic or para-aortic lymph nodes†
IIIc1	Positive pelvic nodes
IIIc2	Positive para-aortic lymph nodes with or without positive pelvic lymph nodes
Stage IV	Tumour invades bladder, or bowel mucosa, or distant metastases, or all three
IVa	Tumour invades the bladder or bowel mucosa, or both
IVb	Distant metastases, including intra-abdominal metastases or inguinal lymph nodes, or both

At all stages, tumour grade can be 1, 2, or 3.
*Endocervical glandular involvement should be considered only as stage I and no longer as stage II. †Positive cytology has to be reported separately without changing the stage.
(Adapted from Pecorelli S. Revised FIGO staging for carcinoma of the vulva, cervix, and endometrium. Int J Gynaecol Obstet 2009; 105:103–104.)

Further reading

Dossus L, et al. Reproductive risk factors and endometrial cancer: the European Prospective Investigation into Cancer and Nutrition. Int J Cancer 2010; 127:442–451.

MacKintosh ML, Crosbie EJ. Obesity-driven endometrial cancer: is weight loss the answer? BJOG 2013; 120:791–794.

Wright JD, Medel N, Sehouli J, et al. Contemporary management of endometrial cancer. Lancet 2012; 379:1352–1360.

Crosbie EJ, Kitchener HC. Recent advances in the treatment of advanced or recurrent endometrial cancer. Expert Reviews in Obstetrics & Gynaecology 2009; 4:521–532.

Related topics of interest

Vaginal cancer

Overview

If cysts of embryological origin are excluded then benign tumours of the vagina are rare. Likewise primary malignant tumours of the vagina have a lower incidence than cervix and corpus uteri, ovary and vulva. 80% of all vaginal tumours are metastatic tumours, predominantly from the cervix and endometrium.

The vagina is the site of origin of sarcoma botryoides in young children and of clear cell carcinoma in young women whose mothers were given exogenous oestrogens in pregnancy.

Squamous carcinoma

Over 90% of primary malignancies of the vagina are squamous carcinoma. They constitute 1–2% of genital malignancies. This may underestimate the true incidence as large extensive lesions may be classified as cervical or vulval in origin.

- Human papillomavirus (HPV) is found in 2/3 of all squamous carcinomas of the vagina (mostly HPV 16)
- The peak incidence is in the sixth and seventh decades, and predisposing factors include: (i) a history of cervical intraepithelial neoplasia (CIN), particularly if hysterectomy has been performed for CIN and the margins are not clear of disease, with cancer at the vault suture line a particularly difficult management problem; (ii) irritation because of procidentia; long term use of a ring pessary for prolapse; chronic infection; previous radiotherapy
- Vaginal intraepithelial neoplasia (VAIN) is a precursor of squamous carcinoma. 10% of VAIN 3 will progress to cancer if untreated. High grade lesions may be treated with laser therapy, topical agents or rarely by surgery or radiotherapy to prevent progression
- The tumour appears as a lump or an ulcerative mass (**Figure 16**), the squamous cells exhibiting varying degrees of differentiation, occasionally with keratin whorls

- Spread is direct to adjacent tissues, by lymphatic permeation or embolisation. The nodal groups involved depend on the site of the tumour, common sites being the posterior upper third, with spread to pelvic nodes, and the anterior lower third, with spread to both inguinal and pelvic nodes

Clinical features

These patients present with abnormal bleeding, occasionally vaginal discharge and rarely with pain. In the later stages, patients may present with urinary retention, haematuria and constipation or tenesmus. Diagnosis may be as an incidental finding at a routine examination.

Treatment

Accurate staging is crucial in the treatment of the disease, and examination under anaesthesia with cystoscopy and sigmoidoscopy, taking appropriate biopsies, is performed.

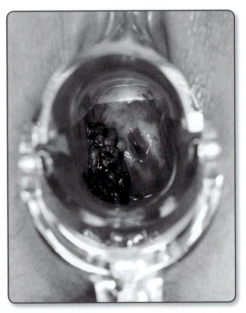

Figure 16 A primary squamous cell carcinoma of the vagina seen during speculum examination of a 48-year-old woman presenting with abnormal vaginal discharge. Photo courtesy of Dr Emma Crosbie.

Table 25 Staging and survival figures for vaginal cancer		
Stage at diagnosis	**Extent of spread**	**5-year survival**
Stage 0	Carcinoma in situ, intraepithelial carcinoma	95%
Stage I	The carcinoma is limited to the vaginal wall	75%
Stage II	The carcinoma has involved the subvaginal tissue but has not extended to the pelvic wall	40%
Stage III	The carcinoma has extended to the pelvic wall	30%
Stage IV	The carcinoma has extended beyond the true pelvis or has involved the mucosa of the bladder or rectum	0–20%
Stage IVa	Spread of the growth to adjacent organs	-
Stage IVb	Spread to distant organs	

Most centres treat all cases with radiotherapy. Better results may be achieved with radical surgery for stage I disease in centres with the necessary expertise. Surgery is reserved in most centres for recurrent or resistant disease. Some patients survive long term after radical surgery, often pelvic exenteration being necessary.

Overall survival depends on stage at diagnosis (**Table 25**)

Rare malignant vaginal tumours

Sarcoma botryoides   An embryonal rhabdomyosarcoma found in the vagina. It is a tumour of childhood, arising at a mean age of 2 years. It presents with bleeding or the appearance of a bloody grape-like mass at the introitus. The treatment of choice is combination chemotherapy, and the number of long term survivors is increasing. Surgery may be necessary as adjunct treatment.

Clear cell adenocarcinoma   An association has been found between the development of clear cell carcinoma of the vagina in young women and intake of diethylstilboestrol by their mothers during pregnancy. Histological features are of typical large cells with clear cytoplasm and 'hobnail' nuclei.
- Over 500 cases have been reported worldwide since the association was first described in Boston, USA, in 1970, by Herbst and Scully
- Local treatment leads to a high incidence of recurrence, therefore radical surgery or radiotherapy is the main treatment modality

Malignant melanoma   This tumour constitutes 1% of vaginal cancers. As with melanoma elsewhere, the prognosis depends on the depth of the lesion, with wide local excision being curative for very superficial lesions, but deeper invasion carrying a very poor prognosis.

Further reading

Creasman T. Vaginal cancers. Current Opinion in Obstetrics & Gynecology 2005; 17:71–76.
Ahmed A, Tan LT, Shafi MI. Cervical and vaginal cancer. In: Shafi MI, Earl HM, Tan LT (Eds). Gynaecological Oncology, 2nd edn. Cambridge University Press 2009; 147–162.

Di Donato V, Bellati F, Fischetti M, et al. Vaginal cancer. Crit Rev Oncol Hematol 2012; 81:286–295.
Herbst AL, Scully RE. Adenocarcinoma of the vagina in adolescence. A report of 7 cases including 6 clear cell carcinomas. Cancer 1970; 4:745–757.

Related topics of interest

Vaginal discharge

Overview

Vaginal discharge is a common presenting complaint in primary and secondary care. There are a variety of physiological and pathological causes. Physiological vaginal secretions are produced by the vulva, Bartholin's and Skene's glands, cervix and endometrium.

Clinical features

The characteristics of the discharge and its accompanying symptoms can often guide the health provider to the likely cause. Bacterial vaginosis (BV) is associated with a thin, fishy-smelling discharge. Candida usually causes a thick, white, cheesy discharge without an offensive odour, and is associated with vulval itch, soreness, superficial dyspareunia and dysuria. The vulva may appear inflamed and there may be fissuring. The discharge of trichomoniasis is offensive and can be accompanied by itching, dysuria and abdominal pain. The vulva, vagina and cervix can all be inflamed and coated with a frothy yellow discharge. The ectocervix is sometimes inflamed and in these cases, described as a 'strawberry cervix'. The woman may also complain of abnormal bleeding.

Aetiology

The normal vaginal pH (3.8–4.4) is maintained by vaginal flora (lactobacilli). The quantity and quality of discharge can vary within the menstrual cycle and with age. Each woman is usually able to recognise what is acceptable or abnormal for her. The acidity of vaginal fluid is maximal at birth and ovulation and minimal during childhood and the menopause. The physiological acidity of the vaginal secretions and the normal flora may have a protective role. Additionally, cervical mucus contains bacteriostatic substances.

Other factors which may influence physiological discharge include hormonal contraception, pregnancy, malignancy, semen and personal hygiene.

Bacterial vaginosis (BV) and vulvovaginal candidiasis (VVC) are the most common pathological causes of vaginal discharge. In BV, the pH of vaginal fluid is elevated and the flora is dominated by anaerobic bacteria. Common culprit organisms include *Gardnerella vaginalis, Prevotella spp., Mycoplasma hominis,* and *Mobiluncus spp.* It remains uncertain if BV is caused merely by an imbalance in vaginal environment or is established as a sexually transmitted infection (STI). BV is associated with a new sexual partner and the presence of other STIs but it can also occur in women who are not sexually active. Other risk factors include frequent vaginal douching, oral sex, black African race and smoking. BV is also associated with pelvic infection after termination of pregnancy, and in pregnancy has been associated with late miscarriage, preterm birth and postpartum endometritis.

VVC is caused by an overgrowth of yeasts, *Candida albicans*, in a majority of cases. In asymptomatic patients, candida does not need to be treated as up to 20% of women will have vulvovaginal colonisation. Immunocompromised women and diabetics are predisposed to candidiasis and antibiotic use can also precipitate this condition.

Other sexually transmitted pathogens include *Trichomonas vaginalis, Chlamydia trachomatis* and *Neisseria gonorrhoea.*

A foreign body (retained tampon or condom), intrauterine devices, allergic responses, genital tract malignancy and fistulae can also cause abnormal discharge. Excessive cervical mucus is seen in up to 10% of women and is often in association with cervical erosion or endocervical polyps.

Postmenopausal women may experience vaginal atrophy secondary to diminished oestrogen levels.

Diagnosis

It is essential to obtain a detailed history, including a sexual and contraceptive history to identify the necessary investigations and management options. Women at low risk of STIs may be treated empirically. Women assessed as being at risk of STIs in primary care may be referred to a genitourinary medicine (GUM) department for specialist management.

Women with persistent vaginal discharge should be examined to exclude serious pathology including gynaecological malignancy. Systemic symptoms including fever and abdominal pain should instigate investigations for pelvic inflammatory disease. When microbiological facilities are available, women should be offered investigations for chlamydia, gonorrhoea, trichomoniasis, bacterial vaginosis, syphilis and HIV. Vaginal pH can be assessed using a narrow-range pH paper with secretions from the lateral sides of the vagina. Women who decline speculum and pelvic examination should be provided with vulvovaginal (self-taken) swabs for chlamydia and gonorrhoea.

Diagnosis of BV can be confirmed using Amsel's criteria, where at least three of the four criteria are present: thin, white, homogenous discharge, clue cells on microscopy of wet mount, vaginal pH > 4.5, or the addition of alkali causes a release of a fishy odour. A Gram stained vaginal smear can also be evaluated with the Hay-Ison criteria which analyses the flora present in the vagina. A high vaginal swab should only be taken in cases of recurrent symptoms, treatment failure, pregnancy or the puerperium, postabortion or recent instrumentation of the uterus.

Management

Syndromic management can be provided based on clinical and sexual history to a patient who is at low risk of STI and has no symptoms indicative of upper reproductive tract infection. Discharge characteristic of *Candida* can be treated with antifungals. Both vaginal and oral azole antifungals have been found to be effective.

An offensive discharge without an itch suggestive of BV should be treated with metronidazole. Oral metronidazole is the recommended first line treatment for BV in the UK. Alternative treatments include vaginal metronidazole and oral clindamycin. Recurrent or ongoing infection should prompt physical and microbiological investigations prior to further empirical treatment.

There is no need to routinely screen or treat partners of women with suspected or proven candidiasis. Routine testing or treatment of male partners in cases of BV is not currently recommended. It may be appropriate to test and treat female partners of women with BV as studies have demonstrated high similarities in the vaginal flora of monogamous women who have sex with women.

Patients who are at higher risk of STI, pregnant and postpartum women, or those who are post gynaecological procedures should be examined and swabs taken prior to treatment. Women who decline speculum examination can be treated empirically after obtaining self-taken swabs.

Positive STIs should be treated in line with local and national guidance and appropriate partner notification undertaken. Trichomonas vaginalis can be treated with oral metronidazole and as it is an STI, treatment of partners is recommended.

Although routine screening is not undertaken for BV in the UK, incidental findings of BV should be treated with metronidazole 400 mg twice daily for 5–7 days. The intravaginal route can also be used. Divided doses of oral metronidazole are thought to be safe in pregnancy but a single 2 g dose is not recommended in pregnant or breastfeeding women.

Women with recurrent BV can be given twice-weekly metronidazole vaginal gel as maintenance treatment. Acidifying vaginal gels may help to reduce relapse rates. Women with recurrent BV on combined hormonal contraception or the copper intrauterine contraceptive device (IUCD) may wish to consider switching to an alternative method of contraception. Women using vaginal treatments should be advised that latex condoms may be damaged and alternative contraceptive precautions should be taken. Women should also be advised to avoid douching and using feminine hygiene products (wipes, washes, etc.) as these may interfere with the physiological microflora of the vagina.

Postmenopausal women with atrophic changes may benefit from intravaginal oestrogen replacement with pessaries and creams. Discharge associated with extensive cervical ectropion may require cryocautery to alleviate symptoms. Women who have persisting symptoms despite treatment of microbiological causes should be referred to a gynaecologist or GUM physician.

Further reading

Faculty of Sexual and Reproductive Healthcare (FSRH), British Association for Sexual Health and HIV (BASHH). Management of vaginal discharge in non-genitourinary medicine settings. London: Faculty of Sexual and Reproductive Healthcare (FSRH), 2012:28.

Mitchell H. ABC of sexually transmitted infections: vaginal discharge—causes, diagnosis and treatment. BMJ 2004; 328:1306–1308.
Spence D, Melville C. Vaginal discharge. BMJ 2007; 335:1147.

Related topics of interest

- Dyspareunia (p. 32)
- Pelvic inflammatory disease (p. 112)
- Sexually transmitted infection (p. 135)

Vulval cancer

Overview

Vulval cancer is one of the rarest gynaecological tumours with approximately 800 new cases in the UK each year. Affecting mostly older women, 90–95% of primary tumours are squamous cell carcinomas. Bartholin's gland adenocarcinomas, Paget's adenocarcinomas, melanomas and basal cell and verrucous carcinomas can also occur.

Clinical features

Elderly women tend to present with advanced disease because of either embarrassment or a failure to appreciate the significance of their symptoms. Diagnosis is sometimes delayed by a lack of familiarity of the clinician with the disease. Common symptoms include vulval discomfort or pruritus, or a vulval mass which may bleed or discharge. Advanced disease can present with a groin mass. Typically a vulval cancer looks like a raised ulcer with rolled edges, but in its early stages can be difficult to distinguish from warty changes (**Figure 17**).

Aetiology

Recognised risk factors for vulval cancer:
- High risk human papillomavirus (HPV) infection
  - 40% of all vulval cancers are associated with HPV infection, commonly HPV 16
- Vulval intraepithelial neoplasia (VIN)
  - Treated VIN has 4–8% lifetime risk of vulval cancer
  - 80–90% of VIN related tumours occur in women under the age of 50 years
  - Untreated VIN may have an 80% progression rate at 10 years
- Lichen sclerosus
  - 3–5% lifetime risk of vulval cancer
  - Tends to affect an older group of women
- Immunosuppression, e.g. transplant patients, heavy smoking and obesity
- Like many cancers, altered expression of proto-oncogene p53 is seen in a significant proportion of vulval cancers
- Risk factors for rare vulval tumours include fair skin and sunlight exposure (malignant melanoma, basal cell carcinoma) and extramammary Paget's disease of the vulva (adenocarcinoma)

Diagnosis

Diagnosis is based on clinical assessment and confirmed with biopsy prior to surgical management. Biopsies should be taken from the edge of the tumour and include some normal skin also. Where excision biopsy is carried out, presurgical photographs may be helpful for planning definitive surgery. In advanced disease a computed tomography (CT) scan or magnetic resonance imaging (MRI) of the groins and pelvis may be helpful

Figure 17 Wide local excision of squamous cell carcinoma (SCC) of the vulva and flap reconstruction. *Continued...*

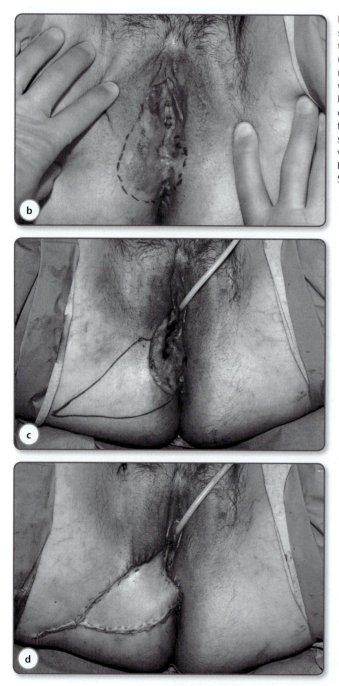

Figure 17 Wide local excision of squamous cell carcinoma (SCC) of the vulva and flap reconstruction. (a and b) Biopsy-proven SCC of right vulva; (c) Lesion is excised with at least 1 cm apparently healthy tissue margin to reduce risk of recurrence; (d) Advancement flap reconstruction to close the skin without tension and restore vulval function and appearance. Photos courtesy of Mr Richard Slade.

to exclude nodal involvement (excellent negative predictive value but false positives occur); however, staging is surgical and retrospective (**Table 26**).

Management

As a rare cancer, vulval cancer should be managed by a multidisciplinary team in

Table 26 Staging and 5–year survival of vulval cancer		
Stage	Extent of disease	5–year survival (%)
I	Tumour confined to vulva	92%
Ia	≤ 2 cm in size, stromal invasion ≤ 1 mm, no nodes	
Ib	> 2 cm in size or stromal invasion > 1 mm, no nodes	
II	Tumour extending to lower 1/3 urethra or vagina, or anus	49%
III	Positive inguinofemoral lymph nodes	32%
IIIa1	1 lymph node metastasis ≥ 5 mm	
IIIa2	1–2 lymph node metastases < 5 mm	
IIIb1	≥ 2 lymph node metastases ≥ 5 mm	
IIIb2	≥ 3 lymph node metastases < 5 mm	
IIIc	Extra-capsular spread	
IV	Tumour invading regional or distant sites	13%
IVa1	Upper urethra/vaginal mucosa, bladder or rectal mucosa, fixed to pelvic bone	
IVa2	Fixed or ulcerated inguinofemoral lymph nodes	
IVb	Distant metastases including pelvic lymph nodes	

a gynaecological cancer centre. The key is individualisation of management.

Preoperative assessment is crucial as patients tend to be elderly with multiple comorbidities, and should include full blood count (FBC), renal function tests, chest X-ray and electrocardiograph (ECG).
Prognostic indicators include:
- Positive inguinofemoral lymph nodes
- Stage and grade of tumour
- Depth of invasion: 1–2 mm = 8% positive lymph nodes, 3–5 mm = 30% positive lymph nodes
- Patient's age and performance status

Excision of primary lesion

The surgical approach is dictated by the size and location of the lesion. Small lateral lesions may be treated by wide local excision with the risk of local recurrence being minimised by ensuring a 1 cm disease free margin, including the deep margin. In most cases where more extensive resection is required a triple incision technique can be utilised to excise the vulval lesion and inguinofemoral lymph nodes. If there is tumour in the skin bridge radical vulvectomy is advocated. Radical surgery may require the use of skin grafts or myocutaneous flaps, with or without plastic surgical input,

to achieve adequate healing and cosmesis (Figure 17).

Groin node dissection

Inguinofemoral lymph node dissection is mandated when depth of invasion is greater than 1 mm (i.e. stage Ib or more). Lesions > 2 cm from the midline are suitable for ipsilateral lymph node dissection; otherwise bilateral lymph node dissection is indicated. However, if ipsilateral lymph nodes prove positive, a contralateral lymph node dissection is indicated.

Attempts to minimise the morbidity of node dissection have been made. Superficial inguinal lymph node dissections have a higher rate of recurrence than inguinofemoral dissections. Work into the identification and removal of the Sentinel node is ongoing, and it is hoped that by identifying and removing the Sentinel node extensive lymph node dissection can be avoided unless this proves positive.

Chemoradiotherapy

Preoperative radiotherapy and 5-fluorouracil may be used for tumour shrinkage, particularly if sphincter preservation is required.

Postoperatively, adjuvant radiotherapy to the vulva and pelvis may be given to women with positive inguinofemoral lymph nodes, as 25% women with positive inguinofemoral nodes have pelvic node involvement. It may also be utilised if surgical margins are close or positive, although re-excision may be considered first. Patients with < 8 mm clear margin have a 57% risk of local recurrence.

Radical radiotherapy and chemotherapy may be used as an alternative to surgery in advanced disease, particularly if there are concerns regarding a patient's fitness for surgery, or if a patient declines surgery.

Recurrent disease

Local recurrence can be resected or treated with radiotherapy with a good chance of prolonged remission. Groin recurrence is often difficult to control and tends to be fatal.

Rarer tumour types

Groin metastases are rare with verrucous or basal cell carcinomas or melanomas, therefore wide local excision is adequate and lymphadenectomy is not indicated. Radiotherapy is contraindicated in verrucous carcinoma as anaplastic transformation has been reported. Malignant melanomas are classified using Breslow's classification.

Treatment related morbidity

Wound breakdown and infection are common problems that can cause prolonged hospitalisation. Lymphoedema is a major cause of long term morbidity as a result of lymphadenectomy. This is minimised by suction drainage of groin wounds, early mobilisation, physiotherapy and support hosiery. Psychological and psychosexual dysfunction is common. Radiotherapy can cause long term bowel and urinary symptoms, vaginal stenosis, and can exacerbate lymphoedema.

Further reading

Crosbie EJ, Slade RJ, Ahmed AS. The management of vulval cancer. Cancer Treatment Reviews 2009; 35:533–539.

Luesley D, et al. Royal College of Obstetricians and Gynaecologists Working Party Report: Management of Vulval Cancer. RCOG: London, 2006.

Acheson N. Sentinel node mapping. The Obstetrician & Gynaecologist 2007; 9:270–275.

Related topics of interest

- Vulval diseases (p. 167)
- Human papillomavirus vaccination (p. 67)
- Radiotherapy (p. 126)

Vulval diseases

Overview

Many conditions affect the vulva, but those most commonly seen are chronic dermatitis, lichen sclerosus and vulval intraepithelial neoplasia (VIN). The treatment and outlook differs significantly, not least because VIN is a precancerous condition that may coexist with malignancy. Diagnostic accuracy is imperative to minimise symptoms and long term risk to the patient, and may be based on clinical assessment or histopathological diagnosis.

Clinical features

Lichen simplex chronicus (chronic vulval dermatitis)

Vulval eczema or dermatitis is a common inflammatory skin condition which causes intractable pruritus. Inflammation often involves the labia majora but can extend to the inner thighs and mons pubis. Erythema and swelling, and latterly skin thickening or lichenification can be seen. Symptoms may be exacerbated by contact with precipitants.

Lichen sclerosus

Lichen sclerosus is an autoimmune dermatosis which can present at any age but is more common in prepubertal girls and postmenopausal women. Its incidence is estimated at 1/1000. It causes severe pruritus which may affect the entire vulva and perianal region. Scratching leads to excoriation and bleeding. Active inflammation of the skin causes erythema and hyperkeratosis, which may appear as thickened white skin patches, often in a figure-of-eight distribution. Skin may be atrophic, have the appearance of parchment, show subepithelial haemorrhages (ecchymoses), and have a tendency to split easily. Ongoing inflammation results in adhesion formation and fusion of the labia minora and clitoris, or skin bridges at the posterior fourchette may be seen (**Figures 18a** and **b**).

Lichen planus

Lichen planus affects skin or mucosal surfaces on any part of the body. It presents with flat, violaceous, purpuric papules and plaques with a fine pale reticular pattern (Wickham striae) (**Figure 18c**). It can be erosive and causes pain more so than pruritus. It affects all ages and is unrelated to menopausal status.

Vulval intraepithelial neoplasia (VIN)

This may present with pruritus, dyspareunia or the presence of an abnormal area on the vulva; however, 20–50% of cases are asymptomatic. Lesions are highly variable and may be leukoplakic, keratotic, ulcerated and erythematous or pigmented (**Figure 18d**). They may turn acetowhite on vulvoscopy. Any area of the anogenital region can be affected.

Aetiology

Lichen simplex chronicus

- Chronic inflammatory changes in the vulval skin because of irritation by external allergens or irritants

Lichen planus and lichen sclerosus

- Probably autoimmune
- More likely to have other autoimmune conditions
  - Thyroid disease, alopecia areata, vitiligo, type I diabetes

Vulval intraepithelial neoplasia

Undifferentiated (usual type)
- Most VIN is undifferentiated
- Often multifocal in younger women
- Associated with human papillomavirus (HPV) infection, predominantly HPV 16, 18 and 33
- Up to 90% are smokers, and more common in immunocompromised women

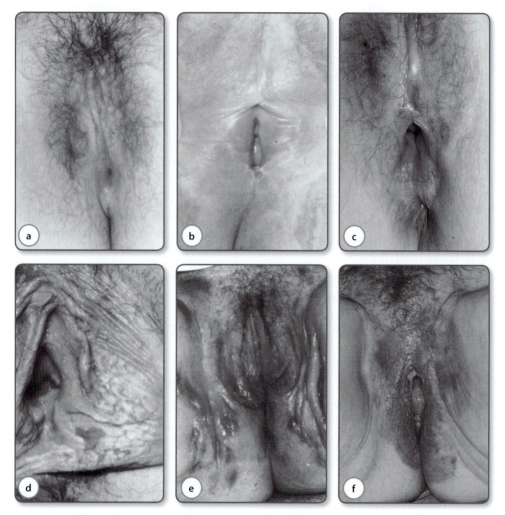

Figure 18 (a) Early vulval lichen sclerosus, showing the typical whitened or leukoplakic appearance of the labia minora; (b) late vulval lichen sclerosus, showing leukoplakia and the loss of vulval architecture; (c) erosive vulval lichen planus; (d) leukoplakic papules of VIN on the left side of the posterior fourchette; (e) extensive vulval Crohn's disease, with oedema, ulceration, abscesses and sinuses; and (f) the erythematous plaques of extramammary Paget's disease of the vulva. Photographs courtesy of Dr Jennifer Yell.

- (Relatively) low risk of developing squamous cell carcinoma

Differentiated
- Lesions are characteristically small, firm, punched-out ulcers or warty papules
- Rare and usually only seen in association with lichen sclerosus, in postmenopausal women
- Excision is mandated as it confers a significant risk of developing squamous cell carcinoma.

Diagnosis

A routine gynae history may not identify all relevant symptoms in relation to vulval complaints. The history must explore symptoms at other sites, faecal or urinary incontinence, medication use and family and personal history of other medical conditions, in particular autoimmune conditions and atopy.

Similarly, the examination should assess extragenital sites, e.g. mouth, nails and scalp, and examination of the vulva should be done with good light and exposure of the area. Skin biopsy may not always be necessary, if clinical examination yields a confident diagnosis. If VIN or cancer is suspected, or if symptoms fail to respond to first line treatment, skin biopsy is indicated.

Management
General advice

General vulval skin care advice is relevant to all of the conditions discussed, and is a fundamental component of treatment:

- Avoid potential irritants that may exacerbate symptoms
  - Soap, perfumed products, synthetic fabrics, preservatives in topical treatments
- Use soap substitutes, e. g. E45 cream
- Emollients/barrier creams protect the skin, especially if incontinent
- Discontinue extraneous over the counter preparations

Routine enquiry should be made about sexual function, and referral to psychosexual counselling services should be available.

Chronic vulval dermatitis

Skin patch testing may be helpful. Serum ferritin should be checked as correction may alleviate symptoms. The mainstay of management is avoidance of allergens, vulval care and emollients and soap substitutes. Antihistamines may be useful, particularly at night.

Lichen sclerosus and lichen planus

Potent topical steroids have high response rates but relapse is common. Clobetasol proprionate 0.05% (Dermovate) ointment or cream is commonly used. It should be applied sparingly to the affected area once daily for 4 weeks, then alternate days for 4 weeks, then twice a week for 4 weeks. Eventually it should be used rarely, if at all. One 30 g tube should last 3 months.

Up to 10% of women will be steroid resistant. Second line treatment such as topical tacrolimus, may be used by dermatologists. Vaginal lichen planus may require hydrocortisone foams.

The lifetime risk of invasive vulval cancer is increased to 2–4%. Women should be advised of symptoms to report, and be encouraged to self-examine. They should be referred back to secondary care if symptom control fails or suspicious changes manifest.

Vulval intraepithelial neoplasia

Treatment of VIN aims to relieve symptoms, exclude invasive disease and reduce the long term risk of developing cancer. Gold standard is local excision, but excision of larger lesions, or repeated excisions for recurrent disease can have serious physical and psychological morbidity. Reconstructive surgery may be required in some cases.

Medical treatments spare the vulval anatomy but have higher rates of treatment failure and recurrence. Topical imiquimod, an immune response-modulating cream licensed for the treatment of genital warts, has been used with success in the treatment of VIN. It can cause local erythema and pain, which can adversely affect compliance. Laser ablation of VIN is useful for multifocal disease or when excision is most likely to have adverse effects, e.g. when disease involves the clitoris.

Women should be seen at least annually for assessment for invasive disease or recurrent VIN. Following surgical excision women have a 4% risk of developing vulval cancer.

Other vulval diseases
Psoriasis

Psoriasis can affect the vulval skin but spares the vaginal mucosa. It often presents as smooth, non-scaly, erythematous discrete lesions. Emollients, soap substitutes, topical steroids and calcipotriene are used; however, coal tar preparations are avoided. Secondary bacterial infection can result and the use of an antibacterial or antifungal containing steroid cream may be helpful.

Vulval Crohn's disease

Crohn's disease is a chronic inflammatory bowel condition which can affect the vulva via direct extension from affected bowel or from 'metastatic' granulomas. It rarely precedes the bowel disease and tends to present as an oedematous, painful, ulcerated vulva, with granulomas, abscesses and sinuses (**Figure 18e**). Metronidazole and oral immunomodulators are the mainstay of treatment. Surgery should be avoided.

Extramammary Paget's disease (EMPD)

This is a rare vulval complaint of postmenopausal women, predominantly presenting with pruritus. It has a characteristic appearance, with raised erythematous plaques covered in a white 'cake-icing' effect (**Figure 18f**). It is intraepithelial (premalignant) in 90% of cases, but an invasive focus of adenocarcinoma can be detected in up to 10%, so careful mapping vulval biopsies are required at presentation to exclude this. In addition, an associated underlying malignancy of the breast, colon or genitourinary tract is seen in up to 30% of patients, necessitating examination and investigation (e.g. mammogram, chest X-ray, colonoscopy, hysteroscopy). Surgical excision will treat symptoms and exclude an underlying invasive adenocarcinoma. Surgery aims to include a 2–3 cm margin of apparently normal skin as microscopic spread can be extensive. Involved surgical margins are common and recurrence is the norm. Extensive EMPD may warrant radical vulvectomy with flap reconstruction.

Further reading

RCOG Green-top Guideline No. 58. The management of vulval skin disorders. London: RCOG, 2011.

Cullis P, Mudzamiri T, Millan D, et al. Vulval intraepithelial neoplasia: making sense of the literature. The Obstetrician & Gynaecologist 2011; 13:73–78.

Shepherd V, Davidson EJ, Davies-Humphreys J. Extramammary Paget's disease. BJOG 2005 112:273–279.

Related topics of interest

Vulval pain syndromes and pruritus vulvae

Vulval pain syndromes

Pain can be inflammatory or neuropathic in origin. Tissue damage causes inflammatory pain, where sensory hypersensitivity with hyperalgesia and allodynia (pain from a stimulus that would not be expected to cause pain) are seen. Neuropathic pain is usually a result of central or peripheral nervous system damage, and manifests as diffuse burning and aching pain.

Vulval pain is an increasingly common condition of developing countries, which affects women of all ages and backgrounds and can have profound effects on their everyday lives. Vulvodynia has been defined by the International Society for the Study of Vulvo-Vaginal Disease (ISSVD) as vulval discomfort, often a burning sensation, in the absence of abnormality of the skin or neurological system.

Clinical features

The ISSVD has proposed the following classification (**Table 27**) of vulval pain syndromes (VPS):
- Generalised vulval dysaesthesia (GVD): Previously known as dysaesthetic

Table 27 ISSVD classification of vulval pain		
Vulval disease	Infection	Candidiasis, herpes
	Inflammation	Lichen sclerosus/planus
	Neoplasia	SCC, Paget's disease
	Neurological	Herpes neuralgia
Vulvodynia	Generalised	Provoked Unprovoked Mixed
	Localised	Provoked Unprovoked Mixed

SCC, squamous cell carcinoma (Adapted from Lynch PJ, et al. 2006 ISSV classification of vulvar dermatoses: pathologic subsets and their correlates. J Reprod Med 2007; 52:3–9.)

vulvodynia, GVD tends to occur in older women who report chronic vulval discomfort which may be worse at the end of the day but is not usually aggravated by intercourse
- Localised vulval dysaesthesia (LVD): Previously described as vulvar vestibulitis, and can affect the vestibule (vestibulodynia – most commonly), clitoris (clitorodynia) or other localised areas. This tends to affect young women who describe superficial dyspareunia with ongoing pain after intercourse, or pain on inserting tampons, cycling or horse riding

VPS tend to follow a relapsing and remitting course. In time most patients will improve or recover completely. A small number of patients have intractable symptoms that do not resolve.

Aetiology

Although the aetiology is unclear VPS are widely regarded as part of the spectrum of complex regional pain disorders. As such they may evolve similarly to reflex dysaesthesia wherein pain persists in the absence of injury. Histologically patients with LVD have shown peripheral nerve hyperplasia in vestibular tissue, but the condition is not related to the presence of inflammation.

Diagnosis

VPS can be under-recognised but should be considered when patients have:
- Chronic or recurrent vulval pain
- Fail to respond to therapeutic measures
- Vulva appears normal
- Tender to touch in the case of LVD, even to light touch with a cotton bud
- Negative investigations, e.g. swabs for *Candida*, biopsy for dermatoses

There are no specific investigations for VPS, and diagnosis is based upon exclusion of other pathology (which may require a vulval biopsy and/or infection screening) and on a full history and thorough examination. An accurate pain history is essential, as well as knowledge of aggravating and relieving factors.

Management

In VPS most specialists adopt a combined medical, psychological and psychosexual approach. Written information and details of support available should be given to the patient at an early stage. Patients may benefit from having a diagnosis, or from being reassured that there is no underlying abnormality and that spontaneous resolution of symptoms is probable.

Topical agents may sometimes help, in the form of emollients, corticosteroids or local anaesthetic agents. They rarely produce long term improvement, however. Tricyclic antidepressants (TCAs) may be of use, as they have anxiolytic and analgesic effects. If amitryptylline is going to work it tends to be at doses of 40–75 mg but higher doses may be required, and after 3–6 months a dose reduction can be trialled. Patients must be counselled that TCAs are not being used as antidepressants, and that they are not dependency inducing drugs. Gabapentin is commonly used in those who have not responded to TCAs. Refractory cases may require the involvement of chronic pain specialists, the use of Botox, alternative therapies and surgery (vestibulectomy).

Almost all patients with VPS will report sexual impairment, predominantly reduced libido or secondary vaginismus and this aspect of the disease must be addressed, via counselling, biofeedback and practical advice.

Pruritis vulvae

Clinical features

Pruritus vulvae is marked and persistent itching of the vulva without any apparent primary cause. The itching does not involve the vagina and does not generally involve the anal area, whereas primary pruritus ani will tend to spread to the vulva. Lichen simplex chronicus (LSC) can develop secondary to persistent excoriation.

Aetiology

Itching sensory pathways are not well delineated. Pain and itch probably both arise in the free networks of nerve fibres without necessity for specialised end organs. Pain and itch are not synonymous, and itch is not sub-threshold pain. The superficial plexus at the dermoepidermal junction is particularly involved in itching. It has been shown that the epidermis itself is not essential. The itch sensation is probably initiated by one or more chemical stimuli, produced either locally or elsewhere by vasodilatation or scratching damage. Prostaglandin E may be involved. Scratching will relieve 'normal' or 'physiological' itching as it causes large nerve fibre impulses to the central nervous system to override impulses from small nerve fibres. In pathological states similar stimuli result in earlier and more prolonged severe itching. Prolonged scratching liberates more irritants because of the trauma to the skin and hence a vicious circle is created.

LSC may initially be triggered by a vulval skin disorder, and is characterised by intractable itching, and scratching during sleep. It is a self-perpetuating secondary condition wherein the only signs are caused by scratching and the vulval skin is otherwise normal.

Diagnosis

In LSC lichenification (thickening) and excoriation of the vulval skin may be seen; however, it is essentially a diagnosis of exclusion.

Management

In managing the problem of chronic vulval itch, night sedation may help to break the cycle of nocturnal itch and scratch. Sedating antihistamines such as hydroxyzine may be used. Local anaesthetics and antihistamines will only further sensitise the area. Hormone replacement therapy (HRT) will help when atrophy is a cause. Any associated depression should be treated seriously and sympathetically. The importance of routine vulval care applies, as in all vulval skin conditions.

Further reading

Nunns D, Murphy R. Assessment and management of vulval pain. BMJ 2012;344:e1723.

Sargeant HA, O'Callaghan FV. The impact of chronic vulval pain on quality of life and psychosocial well-being. Aust NZJ Obstet Gynaecol 2007; 47:235–239.

Stewart KM. Clinical care of vulvar pruritis, with emphasis on one common cause, lichen simplex chronicus. Dermatol Clin 2010; 28:669–680.

Related topics of interest

Amniotic fluid embolism

Overview

Amniotic fluid embolism (AFE) remains a rare and incompletely understood obstetric emergency, in which amniotic fluid, fetal hair or fetal cells enters the maternal circulation through the endocervical veins or the placental bed triggering an allergic-type reaction leading to disseminated intravascular coagulopathy (DIC) and cardiorespiratory collapse. The estimated mortality rate of AFE is between 1 in 8,000 and 1 in 80,000 pregnancies.

In the UK between the years 2006 and 2008, 261 women died as a result of a direct or an indirect association with pregnancy. Of these 13 (5%) were due to AFE giving a mortality rate of 0.57 per 100,000 maternities (CMACE, 2011). Hence AFE remains an important cause of maternal death in the UK although there is some evidence that mortality due to AFE is decreasing, between 2006 and 2008 AFE fell from the second to the fourth leading cause of direct maternal death. Although, previously AFE was regarded to have near universal mortality rate, the latest CMACE report gives a case fatality rate of 16.5%. All cases are reportable to the UK Obstetric Surveillance System (UKOSS), a surveillance system to investigate and review rare disorders in pregnancy and postpartum (UKOSS, 2010). UKOSS identified 60 women over a 4-year period between 2005 and 2009 who presented with AFE. This approach has described a case fatality rate of 20% all within 1 day of onset of symptoms.

Aetiology

The occurrence of AFE is increased in maternal age > 35 years. There also appears to be an association with ethnic minority groups, although this may be because of differences in access of care and language barriers.

It appears that in order for AFE to occur there should be either one of the following:
- Ruptured membranes
- Ruptured cervical or uterine veins
- A pressure gradient from uterus to vein

Hence AFE is associated with any of the following events:
- Abdominal trauma
- Amniocentesis
- Artificial rupture of membranes
- Caesarean section*
- Cervical laceration
- Eclampsia
- Induction of labour
- Placental abruption
- Placenta praevia
- Polyhydramnios
- Uterine rupture
- Spontaneous rupture of membranes

*UKOSS demonstrated that 73% AFE occurred after a cesarean section.

Clinical features

Symptoms have a sudden onset and present as dramatic cardiorespiratory collapse of the patient. All women experience at least one of the cardinal symptoms (*) and a quarter experience four of the following symptoms:

Cardiovascular system:
- *Hypotension – blood pressure may drop suddenly with loss of diastolic component
- Cardiac arrhythmias
- Cardiorespiratory arrest

Respiratory system:
- *Respiratory distress – laboured breathing, tachypnoea
- Pulmonary oedema on clinical examination or chest X-ray

Neurological system:
- Tonic–clonic seizures – confusion or altered mental state premonitory symptoms such as tingling, agitation

Haematological system:
- *Coagulopathy: in > 70% cases (CMACE, 2011)
- *Maternal haemorrhage

Fetus:
- Abnormalities of the fetal heart rate trace resulting in a pathological cardiotocograph and/or fetal bradycardia (occurrence in just under one-third AFE prior to onset of maternal symptoms)

Diagnosis

UKOSS have defined the diagnosis of AFE in terms of either a clinical diagnosis or by findings at autopsy

Clinically

- The occurrence of acute hypotension or cardiorespiratory arrest, acute hypoxia or DIC in the absence of other obstetric explanations such as eclampsia, septic or anaphylactic shock or pulmonary embolism
- There are certain diagnostic pointers such as fetal squames found in maternal sputum and also in blood aspirated from the right atrium, right ventricular strain on electrocardiograph (ECG) and also perihilar infiltrates on chest X-ray
- Coagulation failure occurs rapidly but the complete pulmonary shut down is the first sign. This results from amniotic fluid plugging the pulmonary vessels and the subsequent release of vasoactive substances leading to pulmonary vascular constriction. The coagulation abnormality is attributed to the thromboplastic activity of amniotic fluid.
- In DIC the normal regulatory mechanism of thrombin production is disturbed leading to uncontrolled production of thrombin which in turn leads to excessive intravascular fibrin deposition. This in turn may lead to end organ failure.

Pathologically at autopsy

- Identified by the presence of fetal squames or hair in the maternal lungs at autopsy. At autopsy the disorder can be confirmed using immunochemistry or in clinically classical cases where no squames can be found mucins should be searched for (CMACE, 2011).
- In the last maternal mortality report pathological conformation was confirmed in 11 cases and suspected in the remaining 2 women. Hence, it is of high importance that a maternal autopsy should occur as soon as possible after maternal death including immunochemistry or histochemistry to confirm whether fetal squames are present.

Management

As the clinical presentation of AFE may be similar to other obstetric emergencies (e.g. eclampsia). Resuscitation and the initial management is similar to other obstetric emergencies. The initial management is critical; the confidential enquiry into maternal deaths identified substandard care in 62% cases of AFE.

Management of AFE requires resuscitation and supportive care with immediate institution of cardiopulmonary resuscitation and Advanced Life Support (ALS) if necessary. The maintenance of a clear airway with intubation with immediate cricoid pressure to prevent regurgitation of stomach contents should be considered.

Immediate management

- Airway, breathing, circulation and obtain intravenous access
- Oxygenation and ventilation: 100% O_2 should be given to maintain normal saturation with intubation if necessary
- If the patient has a cardiac arrest, cardiac compressions should be commenced with the patient tilted to the maternal left (if antenatal). Cardiac output should be maintained with ongoing cardiac compressions until maternal cardiac output is restored or resuscitation is abandoned
- If patient does not respond to advanced life support timely perimortem caesarean section (CS) should be performed. CMACE 2011 identified perimortem CS within 5 minutes of witnessed cardiorespiratory arrest as an essential part of any resuscitation procedure in any pregnant woman of more than 20 weeks' gestation.
- Treat hypotension aggressively with intravenous fluid
- DIC: blood products such as fresh frozen plasma, cryoprecipitate and platelets as required. Massive transfusion is often required to address haemorrhage. Plasma exchange may be considered
- Activated recombinant factor VIIa has been described as treatment for heavy bleeding. Hysterectomy may also be required for haemostasis

Summary

AFE must be suspected in all cases of sudden maternal collapse. Death usually occurs as a result of cardiorespiratory collapse or disseminated intravascular coagulation. Improvements in maternal and perinatal mortality from AFE are achievable if the care is provided in a well-equipped environment with high-quality supportive care and improved approaches to resuscitation (CMACE, 2011). Clinicians should also evaluate the necessity for induction of labour (IOL) and CS as reductions in these two factors may lead to a decrease in incidence of AFE.

Further reading

Cantwell R, et al. Saving Mothers' Lives: Reviewing maternal deaths to make motherhood safer: 2006-2008. The Eighth Report of the Confidential Enquiries into Maternal Deaths in the United Kingdom. BJOG 2011; 118(1):1–203.

Knight M, et al. Incidence and risk factors for amniotic fluid embolism. Obstet Gynecol 2010; 115(5):910–917.

Gilbert WM, Danielsen B. Amniotic fluid embolism: decreased mortality in a population-based study. Obstet Gynecol 1999; 93(6):973–977.

Letsky EL. Coagulation defects in pregnancy. In: Turnbull Sir AC, Chamberlain GC (Eds). Obstetrics 1989; 568–569.

Related topics of interest

• Postpartum haemorrhage (p. 287)

• Pre-eclampsia and eclampsia (p. 290)

Anaemia in pregnancy

Around 30–50% of pregnant women develop anaemia and in 90% of cases the cause is iron deficiency. Other causes, including folate/vitamin B_{12} deficiency, haemoglobinopathy and surgical causes, should be excluded. The 2011 UK guidelines for the management of iron deficiency in pregnancy defined anaemia as:

- < 110 g/L in the first trimester
- < 105 g/L in the second and third trimesters
- < 100 g/L postpartum

Physiological changes during pregnancy

Pregnancy is associated with the following physiological changes which predispose women to anaemia:

- Plasma volume expands more than the red cell mass, resulting in a dilutional effect which is maximal at 32–34 weeks. This results in a fall in haemoglobin concentration, haematocrit and red cell count
- Iron requirements increase up to 3-fold and folate 10–20 times, because of increased synthesis of red blood cells and the fetal demands. In response, iron absorption increases
- Increased red cell synthesis leads to a stable or slightly increased mean cell volume (MCV). There is no change in mean cell haemoglobin concentration (MCHC)
- Serum iron and ferritin levels fall because of increased use and haemodilution

Iron-deficiency anaemia

All women should be screened for iron-deficiency anaemia at booking and at 28 weeks. Iron-deficiency anaemia is associated with unpleasant symptoms and poorer maternal and fetal outcomes; therefore it should be actively diagnosed and treated:

- A full blood count (FBC) will show a low haemoglobin, and low MCV, mean cell haemoglobin (MCH) and MCHC, although in milder cases the MCV may be normal. A normocytic or microcytic anaemia should be assumed to be due to iron deficiency
- Serum ferritin is the best test of iron stores in pregnancy in the absence of inflammation. A level of < 15 μg/L at any stage in pregnancy is diagnostic. Current guidelines suggest that levels < 30 μg/L should be treated as this indicates early iron depletion that will worsen during pregnancy
- As haemoglobinopathies can cause a similar FBC result, ferritin levels must be used to guide iron supplementation in these women
- In women with normocytic or microcytic anaemia oral iron treatment should be commenced as this is both therapeutic and diagnostic. Haemoglobin levels will rise within 2 weeks and this confirms diagnosis. In women who have not been screened for haemoglobinpathy, a sickle/thalassaemia screen should be conducted in line with the current guidelines. However, this should not delay treatment
- Treatment should initially be 100–200 mg of oral elemental iron per day (see **Table 28**). Higher doses should not be used as absorption is saturated at this dose and this increases side effects
- Absorption will be maximised if taken on an empty stomach with a vitamin C containing drink
- Side effects, in particular gastrointestinal irritation, occur in up to a third of patients. This can be managed by reducing the dose of elemental iron or using an alternative preparation
- Response should be checked in 2 weeks. A rise of haemoglobin of 20 g/L over 3–4 weeks should be expected

Parenteral iron supplementation

Intravenous iron supplementation can be considered in women who are intolerant or non-compliant of oral iron or in women with reduced absorption, such as inflammatory bowel disease.

Table 28 Content of commonly used iron and folic acid preparations				
Preparation name	Type	Iron salt dose per tablet	Elemental iron dose per tablet	Folic acid dose per tablet
Ferrous sulphate (dried)	Iron supplement	200 mg	65 mg	0
Ferrous fumarate	Iron supplement	200 mg	65 mg	0
Ferrous gluconate	Iron supplement	300 mg	35 mg	0
Ferrous Feredetate (Sytron)	Liquid iron supplement	190 mg/5 mL	27.5 mg/5 mL	0
Pregaday	Combined iron (fumerate) and folic acid	305 mg	100 mg	350 µg
Fefol	Combined iron (sulphate) and folic acid	325 mg	47 mg	500 µg
Glafer FA	Combined iron (fumerate) and folic acid	305 mg	100 mg	350 µg

- Ferritin level should be used to confirm the diagnosis of iron-deficiency anaemia
- Contraindications include the first trimester of pregnancy, previous anaphylaxis to parenteral iron, infection and chronic liver disease
- There may be a faster increase in haemoglobin and better replenishment of iron stores, although this may reflect compliance
- Adverse effects occur in 1–3% and administration must occur in a facility able to deal with anaphylaxis, which is the most serious side effect

Blood transfusion

This should be a treatment of last resort for iron-deficiency anaemia as although it results in a rapid increase in haemoglobin it has minimal impact on iron stores and is associated with risks.

Megaloblastic anaemia

Megaloblastic anaemia (raised MCV) is usually because of folate deficiency as vitamin B12 stores are usually adequate. Serum and red cell folate can be measured to confirm the diagnosis. A normal diet is associated with folate deficiency in up to 25% of pregnant women, socioeconomically deprived women at highest risk.

- All women should take 400 µg of folic acid daily preconceptually and in the first trimester to prevent neural tube defects

(NTD). High risk women (diabetics, previous NTD, on anticonvulsants) should take 5 mg/day
- Women previously taking B_{12} injections should continue these during pregnancy

Haemoglobinopathies

Haemoglobinopathies are inherited anaemias because of either abnormal synthesis of haemoglobin (thalassaemia) or structure (sickle cell disease).

Sickle cell disease

This is caused by a single amino acid substitution in the β-globin chain, resulting in the abnormally structured haemoglobin S. This is insoluble when deoxygenated causing the erythrocyte to form a sickle shape. These erythrocytes occlude vessels and cause haemolysis leading to sickle cell crises. Crises can be precipitated by hypoxia, infection, dehydration and acidosis.

- Sickle cell disease is autosomal recessive, so two carrier parents may opt for antenatal invasive testing
- Women with homozygous SS disease have marked chronic anaemia. Women with heterozygous SC disease have a milder anaemia but have the same risk of sickling. Heterozygous women with sickle cell trait are not at increased risk, but rarely exhibit sickling in extreme hypoxia
- Sickle in pregnancy causes an increased risk of pre-eclampsia, thrombosis, sickling

and crisis, infection and increased maternal mortality
- Fetal risks include an increased risk of miscarriage, stillbirth, growth restriction and prematurity
- Women with sickle cell disease should be managed in a specialist joint clinic
- They should be offered penicillin prophylaxis, 5 mg folic acid, vitamin D supplementation and 75 mg of aspirin antenatally

Thalassaemia

Thalassaemia is either α-thalassaemia, in which 1–4 genes of the α-globin gene are deleted or β-thalassaemia, in which 1 or 2 of the β-genes are deleted:
- α-thalassaemia trait: these women are usually asymptomatic as they have two or three normal α-globin genes but are at risk of anaemia during pregnancy.
- Haemoglobin H disease: these women have three faulty α-globin genes and have chronic haemolytic anaemia. Iron supplementation is not needed but folic acid is given

- Haemoglobin Barts (α-thalassaemia major): this is caused by four faulty α-globin genes and is incompatible with survival. A fetus with haemoglobin Barts will be hydropic and this may be associated with maternal severe early onset pre-eclampsia
- β-thalassaemia trait: these women have a single faulty β-globin gene and are usually asymptomatic but are at risk of anaemia in pregnancy
- β-thalassaemia major: these women have two faulty β-globin genes and are transfusion dependent. They usually therefore suffer from iron overload and pregnancy is rare. It is now treatable with a bone marrow transplant
- α- or β-thalassaemia trait causes a low MCV, low MCH and a normal MCHC. Often the haemoglobin will be normal or near-normal. Women should receive iron and folate supplements but not parenteral iron
- Prenatal diagnosis is available to couples at risk

Further reading

RCOG Green-top Guideline No. 61. Management of sickle cell disease in pregnancy. London: RCOG, 2011.
British Committee for Standards in Haematology. UK guidelines on the management of iron deficiency in pregnancy. London: BSCH, July 2011.

Leung TY, Lao TT. Thalassemia in pregnancy. Best Practice and Research in Clinical Obstetrics and Gynaecology 2012; 26:37–51.

Related topics of interest

- Blood transfusion (p. 192)
- Invasive fetal testing (p. 250)
- Changes to maternal physiology in pregnancy (p. 210)

Analgesia and anaesthesia in labour

Analgesia and anaesthesia are used in normal labour and for obstetric interventions; one-third of women had an epidural, spinal or general anaesthetic for labour or birth in 2002–2003. The different forms of analgesia and anaesthesia used in maternity care include:

- Non-pharmacological methods of pain relief
- Inhalational analgesics
- Narcotic analgesics [including patient-controlled analgesia(PCA)]
- Regional analgesia and anaesthesia (including epidural and spinal techniques)
- General anaesthesia

Women should be given information regarding methods of pain relief for use during labour, which discuss risks and benefits of individual strategies and should be encouraged to make an educated decision regarding the method(s) of pain relief they would like to use; women should be encouraged to ask for analgesia at any point during labour.

Non-pharmacological

A friendly atmosphere, patient education and one-to-one midwifery care all decrease the need for analgesia in labour. One advantage of using non-pharmacological measures is that they need limited professional oversight.

- Women should be encouraged to labour in water for pain relief
- Women who choose to use hypnosis, acupuncture, aromatherapy, relaxation and breathing methods should be supported to do so. These should not be provided by the maternity unit as there is no robust evidence that they provide analgesic effect
- A popular method of non-pharmacological analgesia is transcutaneous electrical nerve stimulation (TENS). In this technique electrodes are placed over the posterior primary rami of T10-L1 and S2-4

and a current passed between them. The level of current can be increased during a contraction. A systematic review found that there was no significant reduction in pain control using TENS in active labour. There have been no studies of TENS in latent labour

Inhalational analgesia

Nitrous oxide is the most widely used inhalational analgesic in the UK, and is recommended to be available in all birth settings as a 50:50 mixture of N_2O and O_2. Other volatile agents such as isoflurane and sevoflurane have all been investigated but show little advantage over nitrous oxide. However, nitrous oxide has limited analgesic qualities and can make women light-headed and nauseated.

Narcotic analgesics

Pethidine and diamorphine may be given by midwives for pain relief in labour. Both agents show a reduction in pain score, although diamorphine has greater analgesic properties than pethidine. Partial opioid agonists such as pentazocine, meptazinol and nalbuphine have all been used, but have not shown any greater analgesia effect or better side effect profile than pethidine or diamorphine.

Both pethidine and diamorphine can cause drowsiness, nausea and vomiting in the mother and respiratory depression and drowsiness in the neonate.

Because of these side effects, opiate analgesia should be combined with an antiemetic, e.g. prochlorperazine 12.5 mg. Women should be advised that they cannot use the birthing pool for two hours after administration of opioid analgesia.

PCA using a variety of therapeutic agents given intravenously including diamorphine and remifentanil has been used. Initial data found that diamorphine administered by PCA was less effective than intermittent administration. More recently, remifentanil – a short-acting synthetic opioid has been used for PCA in labour. Remifentanil is broken down by plasma esterases, so has a very short half-life (~4 min). Remifentanil PCA has been reported as superior to other forms opioid analgesia in labour. Trials have been proposed comparing remifentanil PCA and epidural analgesia.

Epidural analgesia

Epidural analgesia describes the technique of delivering a substance, usually a mixture of local anaesthetic and opiate analgesia into the epidural space (between the ligamentum flavum and the dura mater), using a catheter. In the UK, epidural analgesia is administered by anaesthetists and is only available in obstetric units. Epidural analgesia requires continuous electronic fetal heart rate monitoring and intravenous access. Epidural analgesia can be given by patient controlled epidural analgesia (PCEA) or intermittent boluses, which can be given by midwives.

Epidural analgesia provides more effective pain relief than opiates in labour, with significantly less respiratory depression in the neonate. The hypotensive effect of epidural analgesia can be beneficial in women with severe pre-eclampsia or maternal cardiac disease where swings of blood pressure would be undesirable.

Epidural analgesia increases the length of the second stage of labour with a commensurate increase in instrumental vaginal delivery. There is an increased need for augmentation of labour with oxytocin and an increased risk of caesarean section for fetal distress. Commonly experienced side effects include hypotension, lower limb muscular weakness for a period of time after the birth, fluid retention and fever. There are no data to support increased risk of backache for women who use epidural analgesia.

Epidural analgesia cannot be used if there is coagulopathy, sepsis, thrombocytopenia (platelets < 80), or within 24 hours of administration of therapeutic low-molecular heparin or 12 hours of prophylactic low-molecular weight heparin. Other contraindications are relative and include history of spinal injury/surgery and hypovolaemia.

Common complications include ineffective analgesia, accidental dural puncture leading to postdural puncture headache (1 in 200). Rare but serious complications include high-block/total spinal, neurological injury (temporary 1 in 1000, permanent 1 in 13,000), epidural abscess (1 in 50,000) and paraplegia (1 in 250,000).

The difference between analgesia and anaesthesia is the density of the neurological block. An epidural used for normal labour is analgesia; a 'topped-up' epidural for caesarean section is anaesthesia.

In anticipation of a complex caesarean section or a maternal condition, where a low-dose spinal is appropriate, epidural and spinal anaesthesia can be combined to give a rapid onset that can be augmented; this is known as combined spinal-epidural (CSE).

Spinal anaesthesia

Spinal anaesthesia describes regional anaesthesia where local anaesthetic or a mixture of local anaesthetic and opioid are injected into the subarachnoid space; this must be below L2 to avoid damaging the spinal cord. Spinal anaesthesia has a much faster onset than epidural anaesthesia. As with epidural anaesthesia, intravenous access and fetal monitoring should be in place.

Spinal anaesthesia is often used for operative procedures in obstetrics as the outcomes for the neonate are better than with general anaesthetic after caesarean section. Aorta-caval compression during anaesthesia is minimised by the use of left lateral tilt of the patient.

Contraindications are similar to epidural analgesia, although the risk of sepsis is decreased as there is no indwelling component.

Side effects include hypotension which may be treated with phenylephrine or a similar vasopressor (1 in 5), postdural puncture headache (1 in 500), nerve damage (1 in 13,000) and meningitis (1 in 100,000).

General anaesthesia

General anaesthesia may be used for operative procedures where regional techniques are contraindicated, there is insufficient time for their onset (Grade 1 emergency caesarean section) or regional analgesia/anaesthesia has failed to work effectively.

General anaesthesia carries increased risks for mother and infant, which remains a significant cause of maternal morbidity and mortality (although the risk of death is 1:100,000). This appears to be associated with inexperienced anaesthetists with a poor standard of help available.

To prevent aspiration of gastric contents oral ranitidine and sodium citrate are given preoperatively and cricoid pressure is applied at induction of anaesthesia. Aorta-caval compression during anaesthesia is minimised by the use of left lateral tilt of the patient.

Adverse effects of general anaesthesia include: lower respiratory tract infection (1 in 5), nausea (1 in 10), airway problems leading to hypoxia (1 in 300) and aspiration of gastric contents (1 in 300).

Failed endotracheal intubation may also occur and obstetric units should have an emergency protocol if this occurs, as the patient will not be able to breathe on their own after administration of a neuromuscular blocker (e.g. suxamethonium). This will usually involve bag and mask ventilation until an airway can be established.

Further reading

NICE. Clinical Guideline No. 55. Intrapartum Care. London: NICE, 2007.

Schnabel A, Hahn N, Broscheit J, et al. Remifentanil for labour analgesia: a meta-analysis of randomised controlled trials. Eur J Anaesthesiol 2012; 29(4):177–185.

Obstetric Anaesthetists' Association. Pain relief in labour. London: Obstetric Anaesthetists' Association, 2012.

Jenkins JG. Some immediate serious complications of obstetric epidural analgesia and anaesthesia: a prospective study of 145,550 epidurals. International Journal of Obstetric Anesthesia 2005; 14:37–42.

Jenkins JG, Khan MM. Anaesthesia for caesarean section: a survey in a UK region from 1992 to 2002. Anaesthesia 2003; 58:1114–1118.

Related topics of interest

Antenatal care

Overview

Antenatal care (care before birth) aims to improve maternal and fetal outcomes of pregnancy. It is a package of education, counselling, screening and monitoring, with the ethos being 'woman-centred care and informed decision making'. Women with risk factors for pregnancy complications should be identified early to enable appropriate management. Risk profiles may change during pregnancy and a key part is now thromboembolic risk assessment. For low risk women, antenatal care with a restricted number of visits provided in the community is as cost and clinically effective as more intensive packages.

Preconception counselling

Preconception counselling aims to address health issues prior to pregnancy, particularly in women with pre-existing medical disorders. There are no UK guidelines for general preconception counselling but optimisation of chronic disease prior to pregnancy is paramount. As around 25% of pregnancies in the UK are unplanned, many opportunities are currently missed. Women with complex conditions require the input of specialist hospital clinics. Issues to address in preconception counselling include:

General

- Folic acid supplementation should be taken for at least 3 months preconception and for the first 12 weeks of pregnancy to reduce the risk of neural tube defects by 50–70%. All women should take 400 µg folic acid daily and high risk women (enzyme-inducing drugs, diabetes) 5 mg daily
- Dietary deficiencies, such as iron deficiency and vitamin D deficiency should be treated
- Immunity to infections known to cause fetal abnormality should be confirmed. In particular, women without immunity to rubella should receive the measles, mumps and rubella (MMR) vaccination

- Advice relating to alcohol consumption, cigarette smoking and drug misuse should be given
- Overweight or obese women should be advised to lose weight as this reduces the risks of pregnancy complications

Women with chronic diseases

- Disease control should be optimised prior to conception as this improves outcome
- A medication review generally aims for disease control on the minimum number of drugs. For some disorders changing teratogenic medication preconception is optimal, whereas for some drugs changing as soon as a pregnancy is confirmed is preferable
- Women should be reassured regarding medication and advised not to suddenly stop medication if they find out that they are pregnant
- The impact of the disease on the pregnancy should be considered with consideration of outcomes so that women can make an informed choice about whether to attempt pregnancy
- The impact of the pregnancy on the disease should be assessed. Some women may wish to avoid pregnancy if long term prognosis may worsen
- Some chronic diseases impact on mode of delivery and anaesthesia, and this should also be addressed

Maternal screening

All pregnant women are offered screening for pre-existing disorders, and also for disorders that may develop during pregnancy.
- Screening offered at booking (usually first trimester) includes:
  - Anaemia (also at 28 weeks)
  - Red cell grouping and red cell alloantibodies (also at 28 weeks for Rhesus negative women)
  - Haemoglobinopathies
  - Asymptomatic bacteruria
  - Infections – hepatitis B and C, HIV, rubella, syphilis, women under 25 years

should be advised of the chlamydia screening programme

- – Risks of venous thromboembolism
- Screening offered on a ongoing basis includes:
  - – Screening for hypertension and proteinuria. More frequent blood pressure checks should be considered in women with specific risk factors for pre-eclampsia, including age ≥ 40 years, nulliparity, pregnancy interval > 10 years, family or personal history of pre-eclampsia, body mass index (BMI) ≥ 30 kg/m², pre-existing vascular or renal disease, or multiple pregnancy
  - – Screening for gestational diabetes using a urine dipstick. Women at high risk are offered a glucose tolerance test (GTT) at 24–28 weeks' gestation. High risk women are those with a BMI ≥ 30 kg/m², previous baby ≥ 4.5 kg, previous gestational diabetes (require blood glucose monitoring or a GTT at 16–18 weeks), first-degree relative with diabetes, or women of South Asian, black Caribbean or Middle Eastern origin

Screening for fetal abnormality

All pregnant women are offered screening for chromosomal abnormalities and ultrasound to detect structural defects. In the third trimester, the fetus is screened for fetal growth restriction using symphysis-fundal height measurements.

Screening for chromosomal abnormality

All women in the UK are offered screening for trisomy 21. Women are currently offered combined screening or serum screening.

- Combined screening is offered at 10^{+0} to 13^{+6} weeks (usually 11+ weeks) and includes an ultrasound scan (USS) for nuchal translucency (NT) measurement and serum beta-human chorionic gonadotrophin (β-HCG), and pregnancy-associated plasma protein A. The aim is a detection rate of over 90%
- Serum screening is offered to women who attend too late in pregnancy (from 14^{+2} to 20^{+0} weeks) for combined testing,

or in whom NT measurement was not possible. This measures serum β-HCG, α-fetoprotein, unconjugated oestriol (triple test) and inhibin A (Quad test). The aim is a detection rate of over 75%

- Since 2011, women with a risk greater than 1:150 are offered invasive testing. It is personal choice after counselling whether to undergo testing
- Technology now exists to test fetal DNA in maternal plasma and is likely to replace current screening strategies in the future

Detection of structural defects

All women are offered an USS at the end of the first trimester, and again at 18^{+0}–20^{+6} weeks of gestation (anomaly scan). The first trimester scan aims to confirm a viable intrauterine pregnancy, number of fetuses and gestation (as ultrasound dating should be used rather than menstrual dates). Some serious structural defects are also detectable, e.g. anencephaly. The anomaly scan is a systematic fetal survey that aims to detect serious abnormality, which would cause significant disability or be life-threatening, or which would require additional intervention with monitoring or delivery in a specialist centre. It is important that women are advised of the purposes of the scan, and that consent is documented. Not all abnormalities are

Table 29 Detection rates by ultrasound at 18–20 + 6 weeks of the common structural abnormalities	
Abnormality	Detection rate (%)
Anencephaly	98
Open spina bifida	90
Cleft lip	75
Diaphragmatic hernia	60
Gastroschisis	98
Exomphalos	80
Serious cardiac abnormality	50
Bilateral renal agenesis	84
Lethal skeletal dysplasia	60
Trisomy 18 (Edwards syndrome)	95
Trisomy 21 (Patau syndrome)	95

detectable on ultrasound, and detection rates are between 50% and 98% (**Table 29**).

Management of low risk pregnancy

As per National Institute for Health and Clinical Excellence (NICE) guidelines primiparous women should be offered 11 antenatal appointments (including USS), largely in the community, at 10, 16, 20, 25, 28, 31, 34, 36, 38, 40 and 41 weeks' gestation. Multiparous women are offered eight visits at 10, 16, 20, 28, 34, 36, 38 and 41 weeks. The need for iron, vitamin D and aspirin should be assessed:

- All women should be advised about the importance of vitamin D in the diet and $10\,\mu g$/day vitamin D should be offered, especially to those:
  - Of South Asian, African, Caribbean or middle Eastern origin
  - With limited exposure to sunlight or whose diet is low in vitamin D (e.g. no eggs, meat, oily fish or fortified cereal/ margarine)
  - With a BMI $> 30\,kg/m^2$
- Indications for aspirin 75 mg:
  - Those with at least two of:
    - First pregnancy
    - Age 40 years or older
    - Pregnancy interval > 10 years
    - BMI $> 35\,kg/m^2$
    - Family history of pre-eclampsia
    - Multiple pregnancy
  - Those with one of:
    - Hypertension in a previous pregnancy
    - Chronic kidney disease
    - Systemic lupus erythematosus or antiphospholipid syndrome
    - Type 1 or type 2 diabetes
    - Chronic hypertension

Management of high risk pregnancy

High risk women should be identified early and referred for an early consultant opinion. An individualised plan of care should be formulated and clearly documented.

Planning for delivery

For all women, this will involve planning place of delivery, pain relief options, management of the third stage and postnatal plans for the baby, including benefits of breastfeeding and use of vitamin K. For high risk women, this may include a review by an obstetric anaesthetist, formulation of a specific delivery plan and plans for the postnatal period. This should be in place by 36 weeks.

Further reading

National Institute for Health and Clinical Excellence. NICE Clinical Guideline 62. Antenatal Care. London: NICE, 2010.

NHS Fetal Anomaly Screening Programme (FASP). The 18+0-20+6 Fetal Anomaly Scan. Exeter: NHS FASP, 2010.

Nicolaides KH, Syngelaki A, Ashoor G, et al. Noninvasive prenatal testing for fetal trisomies in a routinely screened first-trimester population. American Journal of Obstetrics and Gynecology 2012; 207:374e1–374e6.

Related topics of interest

Antepartum haemorrhage

Overview

Antepartum haemorrhage (APH) is defined as bleeding from the genital tract after 24 weeks' gestation and prior to the delivery of the baby. It is the leading cause of perinatal and maternal mortality worldwide. 3–5% of pregnancies are affected by APH. A suggested algorithm for the management of a major APH is shown in **Figure 19**. The management is dependent on the precise cause of the bleeding. Although placenta praevia and placental abruption are not the most common cause they are the most important, as they are associated with maternal and perinatal morbidity and mortality.

Placenta praevia

Placenta praevia occurs (covered in more depth in Topic 91) when the placenta is partly or wholly inserted in the lower uterine segment. Traditionally placenta praevia was divided into four grades by the Dewhurst classification:
- Grade I: placenta just encroaches into lower segment
- Grade II: placenta reaches the margin of the cervical os

- Grade III: placenta covers the os but not at full dilatation
- Grade IV: placenta covers the cervical os completely (centric)

More recently, however, it has been classified by ultrasound imaging. A major placenta praevia is one that lies over the internal cervical os and a minor or partial placenta praevia is one where the leading edge of the placenta is located in the lower uterine segment.

Despite not being evidence-based, the majority of UK hospitals document placental site at the 20 weeks anomaly ultrasound scan (USS). This is supported by the Royal College of Obstetricians and Gynaecologists (RCOG). Following the USS 5–28% of women will have low implantation of the placenta, reducing to 3% at term as the lower uterine segment forms. Only 0.4–0.8% will be symptomatic.

Risk factors include multiple pregnancy, age (> 40 years), multiparity, cigarette smoking, uterine surgery, e.g. dilatation and curettage, and previous caesarean section. The latter is also associated with increased incidence of placenta accreta. Placenta accreta, increta and percreta describe a morbidly adherent placenta that penetrates

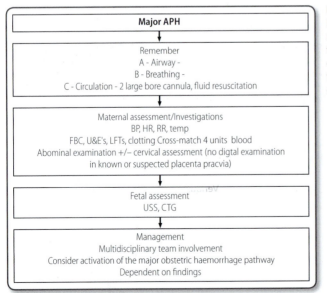

Figure 19 Major APH algorithm. BP, blood pressure; HR, heart rate; RR, respiratory rate; FBC, full blood count; U&E, urea and electrolytes; LFT, liver function tests; USS, ultrasound scan; CTG, cardiotocography.

through the deciduas into the myometrium. If a placenta praevia or anterior placenta is diagnosed in a woman with a previous caesarean section, there should be a high index of suspicion of placenta accreta. Magnetic resonance imaging (MRI) can be used in such cases to aid diagnosis.

Signs and symptoms

Placenta praevia may be asymptomatic or present with painless bleeding per vagina (PV) of varying amounts. Bleeding may recur throughout pregnancy. The fetus is usually unaffected. Clinically the mother may be well or if the bleeding is heavy she may be haemodynamically compromised. On examination the uterus is usually non-tender and soft, with a high presenting part or malpresentation. The diagnosis can be confirmed by ultrasound or MRI. Digital vaginal examination is contraindicated as this may disrupt the placenta precipitating further bleeding.

Management

Antenatal care

Following diagnosis at 20 weeks, women with asymptomatic minor placenta praevia should be offered a repeat USS at 36 weeks' gestation. An USS at 32 weeks should be offered to those with asymptomatic placenta praevia major. Transvaginal scanning (TVS) in cases of suspected placenta praevia is safe and may aid diagnosis. If the placental edge is < 2 cm from the internal os, a woman is likely to require caesarean section. TVS is useful in these scenarios.

Women should be advised to avoid penetrative sexual intercourse.

The asymptomatic patient does not require total inpatient care; however, women should be aware of the risk associated with placenta praevia and to seek immediate medical advice with any abdominal pain, bleeding PV or contractions. Expectant management should be followed postponing delivery until at least 38 weeks unless earlier intervention is indicated for fetal or maternal reasons.

Symptomatic women should be managed according to their clinical condition. Intramuscular corticosteroids should

be administered if preterm delivery is considered likely.

Delivery

Delivery is usually by caesarean section after 38 weeks' gestation and in cases of suspected placenta accreta after 36–37 weeks' gestation. Women should be counselled and consented regarding the potential complications of massive haemorrhage, the interventions that may be required (including cell salvage and interventional radiology where available) and the possibility of requiring a hysterectomy. A consultant obstetrician should be present at the caesarean section. A consultant anaesthetist should be present and the decision regarding anaesthetic technique used is made by the anaesthetist involved on an individual basis. There is no evidence to support the use of one type of anaesthetic over another. Cross-matched blood should be readily available along with the use of a cell saver.

Placental abruption

Placental abruption is defined as premature separation of the placenta from the uterine wall. It occurs in 0.49–1.8% of pregnancies and has a recurrence rate of about 6%. Risk factors include a raised alpha-fetoprotein on first or second-trimester serum screening, maternal thrombophilia, abdominal trauma, pre-eclampsia, cigarette smoking, cocaine and amphetamine use and sudden uterine decompression after membrane rupture in women with polyhydramnios. Bleeding starts in the decidua basalis and causes separation of the placenta from the uterine wall. It may be small and self-limiting or major with signs of maternal shock and fetal demise.

Signs and symptoms

Placental abruption classically presents as bleeding and severe abdominal or back pain, with or without uterine contractions. The (revealed) vaginal bleeding may be minimal in comparison to the abruption. Examination findings include uterine tenderness, vaginal bleeding, maternal shock, fetal compromise or fetal death. In severe abruption a coagulopathy can occur. Diagnosis is usually clinical.

Management

Management depends on the severity and presence or absence of complications.

If minor abruption is confirmed clinically before 37 weeks with no maternal or fetal compromise then expectant management should be followed, with close monitoring of fetal growth. Corticosteroids should be administered to aid fetal lung maturity in preterm infants.

If there is maternal or fetal compromise delivery should be immediate.

Vaginal birth in the absence of maternal compromise is the recommended delivery mode for fetal death in utero.

A multidisciplinary team approach is essential with involvement of anaesthetists and haematologists.

Massive abruption is associated with ischaemia of the overlying myometrium – the so-called couvelaire uterus.

Other sites/causes of APH
- Unclassified (47%)
- Lower genital tract, e.g. cervical polyps, trauma
- Coagulation defects, e.g. von-Willebrand's disease
- Vasa-praevia occurs where a placental blood vessel lies in front of the presenting part of the fetus – usually because of a velamentous insertion of the cord into the placenta. Bleeding from this causes vaginal bleeding but also exsanguination of the fetus
- Rarely, carcinoma of the cervix

Further reading

RCOG Green-top Guideline No. 63. Antepartum haemorrhage. London: RCOG Press, 2011.

RCOG Green-top Guideline No. 27. Placenta Praevia, Placenta Praevia Accreta and Vasa Praevia: Diagnosis and Management. London: RCOG Press, 2011.

James DK, Steer, PJ, Weiner CP, et al. High Risk Pregnancy, Management Options. Philadelphia: Elsevier, 2006.

Related topics of interest

Asthma in pregnancy

Overview

Pregnancy is associated with significant changes to respiratory physiology (discussed in Topic 66 – Changes to Maternal Physiology in Pregnancy).

During pregnancy there is equilibrium between bronchodilator ($\uparrow$progesterone, cortisol and PGE_2) and bronchoconstrictor ($\uparrow PGF_2$ and $\downarrow$lung volume ($\downarrow$residual volume and PaO_2) influences, such that there is no overall change in airway resistance.

Asthma is one of the most common chronic medical disorders encountered in pregnancy, affecting at least 5% of women of reproductive age.

However, the effect of pregnancy on maternal asthma is difficult to predict, and may be influenced by exposure to allergens, season, infection, emotional state and, probably most important, drug compliance.

Clinical features

Maternal asthma is frequently missed and the condition is undertreated; typical presentations include: dyspnoea, cough, chest pain and/or wheeze. Symptoms are typically worse at night and/or early morning – early morning dip.

The severity of asthma before pregnancy alters the risk that symptoms will worsen during pregnancy. Approximately, 25–33% of women with asthma will notice deterioration in their symptoms; deterioration is more frequent in women with severe asthma.

Triggers include pollen, animal hair and upper respiratory tract infection. Pregnancy itself is not a trigger but may worsen the condition because of reduced drug compliance. Symptoms are typically worse in the third trimester or postnatally. Drug maintenance throughout pregnancy is vital and should be encouraged.

At booking, a history of asthma should be taken including: previous attacks, admissions to hospital or critical care, current treatment and exacerbating factors. A peak expiratory flow rate (PEFR) should be measured.

Chronic and/or intermittent hypoxaemia, associated with severe and/or uncontrolled asthma may have adverse effects on the fetus.

Data, albeit from retrospective, uncontrolled and/or small studies, have reported an association between asthma and preterm labour/birth, intrauterine growth restriction and pre-eclampsia/pregnancy induced hypertension. Similarly potential neonatal risks have been highlighted – to include transient tachypnoea of the newborn (TTN), hypoglycaemia, seizures and/or admission to Neonatal Intensive Care Unit (NICU).

The feeling of breathlessness is very common, particularly between 28 and 31 weeks gestation. In the absence of other symptoms of cardiorespiratory disease and normal examination, chest X-ray and oxygen saturations of $\geq 95\%$, no further investigation is required. However, bronchospasm is a feature of pulmonary embolism and should be excluded in women who present with their first attack of apparent severe asthma in pregnancy.

Diagnosis

Diagnosis is suggested by symptoms of cough, wheeze and dyspnoea which may be precipitated by acknowledged triggers.

Airway bronchoconstriction is measured by either a PEFR and/or a forced expiratory volume in one second (FEV1). Variable and reversible airway obstruction, as indicated by a $\geq 15\%$ improvement in these parameters following a β-sympathomimetic bronchodilator, is diagnostic.

Management

Prevention is the key focus of management of asthma in pregnancy and most women with asthma should be prescribed and maintained on regular inhaled anti-inflammatories.

Pregnancy is an opportunity for inhaler technique to be checked and to eradicate symptoms.

In women with severe and/or poorly controlled disease preconceptual joint counselling (between the respiratory physician and obstetrician) would provide an opportunity to optimise therapy before pregnancy is considered. Use of daily home PEFR monitoring should be encouraged as a means of optimising therapy.

Self-management plans, to include information regarding when to increase the dose and/or frequency of inhaled steroids, in addition when to commence oral steroids and seek medical advice should be agreed.

Women should be advised that labour is unlikely to precipitate a severe exacerbation.

Breastfeeding is safe and may reduce the risk of asthma and other atopic manifestations by 20% in offspring. Drugs required to control asthma should be continued.

Drug therapy

Treatment is the same as that outside pregnancy. No drug is contraindicated.

Corticosteroids

Inhaled as first line prevention. Inhaled steroids are minimally absorbed, and are safe in pregnancy. Oral steroids are used to treat acute exacerbation. These are metabolised by the placenta such that < 10% active drug reaches the fetus. There do not appear to be any teratogenic effects, but steroids increase the risk of fetal growth restriction. While the potential for adrenal suppression in the neonate has been postulated this has not been confirmed. Maternal use can be associated with gestational diabetes and blood sugar monitoring should be introduced until oral steroid discontinued. Insulin may be required.

Beta-agonists

Minimal amounts of inhaled drug reach the fetus. No adverse fetal/neonatal side effects with short (salbutamol, terbutaline) or long-acting (salmeterol) drugs. Use should therefore continue in pregnancy.

Methylxanthines

For example theophylline, aminophylline. These are no longer recommended as fist line therapy. For women stable on these drugs, the dose may need increasing in pregnancy. Both drugs freely cross the placenta and are therefore potential teratogens if used in the first-trimester. Animal data suggests theophylline is cardiotoxic, an association that has not been shown in humans.

Other agents

Inhaled anticholinergic drugs (ipratropium), nedocromil, leukotriene receptor antagonists (montelukast, zafirlukast) and disodium cromoglycate are all safe for use in pregnancy.

Acute severe asthma

Women presenting with acute exacerbation of asthma or symptoms suggestive of asthma should have a history and clinical examination including: respiratory rate, pulse rate, PEFR, oxygen saturations. Where symptoms are severe an arterial blood gas should be performed. For diagnosis of severe and life-threatening asthma (see **Table 30**). Differential diagnoses include: lower respiratory tract infection (bacterial or viral), pulmonary embolism or pneumothorax.

Table 30 Factors present to define severe acute and life-threatening asthma	
Criteria for diagnosis of severe acute asthma	Criteria for diagnosis of life-threatening asthma
PEFR 33–50% best or predicted Respiratory rate ≥ 25/min Heart rate ≥ 110/min Inability to complete sentences in one breath	PEFR < 33% best or predicted SpO_2 < 92% PaO_2 < 8 kPa Normal $PaCO_2$ (4.6–6.0 kPa) Silent chest Cyanosis Poor respiratory effort Arrhythmia Exhaustion, altered conscious level

Treatment of severe asthma is the same as in the non-pregnant population – and includes high flow oxygen (to maintain PO_2 94–98%), nebulised β-agonists (e.g. salbutamol 5 mg) and oral steroids (usually 40–50 mg daily for approximately 5 days). Intravenous therapy is reserved for those failing to respond to first line therapy. IV magnesium sulphate is now the recommended second line therapy, given at a dose of 1.2–2 g over 20 minutes. The routine prescription of antibiotics is not required. A chest X-ray is not routinely recommended, but should be considered in specific circumstances (see **Table 31**).

Table 31 Indication for chest X-ray in severe acute asthma
Indications for chest X-ray
Suspected pneumomediastinum or pneumothorax
Suspected consolidation
Life-threatening asthma
Failure to respond to treatment satisfactorily
Requirement for ventilation

Continuous electronic fetal monitoring is recommended for women with severe acute asthma. Early referral to and liaison with the critical care team is important.

Further reading

The British Thoracic Society. Scottish Intercollegiate Guidelines Network British Guideline on the Management of Asthma. London: BTS, 2011.

M de Swiet. Respiratory disease. Chapter 1. In: De Swiet M (Ed). Medical Disorders in Obstetric Practice, 4th edn. Oxford: Blackwell Scientific Publications, 2002:513–531.

Related topics of interest

Blood transfusion

Overview

Complications in pregnancy, from miscarriage and ruptured ectopic pregnancy in the first trimester, to antepartum haemorrhage, placenta praevia and postpartum haemorrhage, can lead to the requirement of emergency blood transfusion.

In the last Triennial report (Centre for Maternal and Child Enquiries, CMACE, 2011), there were nine maternal deaths from haemorrhage in the UK between 2006 and 2008. The mortality rate was 0.39 per 100,000 maternities. Five deaths were from postpartum haemorrhage, two deaths from placenta praevia and two deaths from placental abruption. One woman refused blood products. There were six deaths from ectopic pregnancy, giving a death rate of 16.9 per 100,000 estimated ectopic pregnancies. The majority of these women collapsed at home, and four of the six presented with gastrointestinal symptoms, leading to delay in diagnosis and resuscitation.

Blood transfusion is associated with risks including: transfusion reactions, infection, red cell alloimmunisation, and incorrect sampling or labelling of cross-matched blood leading to incorrect blood components being administered.

To reduce the risk of transfusion, anaemia should be treated with oral ferrous sulphate tablets, if the haemoglobin (Hb) level is less than 105 g/L. Parenteral iron is the second line treatment and should be used if there is a lack of compliance or inability to tolerate oral medication. Iron sucrose is administered in multiple doses, whereas iron dextran is a single dose. Recombinant human erythropoietin should not be used routinely. Management should aim to minimise blood loss at delivery, by adopting an active management of the third stage of labour, encourage women at increased risk of haemorrhage to have a hospital delivery and to ensure women on anticoagulation therapy have an appropriate management plan for delivery in their notes.

A full blood count (FBC) and blood group and antibody screen should be performed on all pregnant women both at the booking visit and at 28 weeks. If there is an increased risk of haemorrhage anticipated, FBC and group and save blood samples should be sent to the laboratory on admission to the maternity unit.

Indications for transfusion

- The indication for blood transfusion should be made on both a clinical basis in conjunction with the blood results
- This is generally required with a Hb level of < 60 g/L, or in the presence of a massive or ongoing haemorrhage
- Massive blood loss has multiple definitions; some examples include a rate of blood loss of 150 mL/min, or loss of 50% of total blood volume within 3 hours
- When requesting red cells to be cross matched, blood samples from the patient should be fresh, but certainly no older than 3 days. Only cytomegalovirus (CMV) seronegative and Kell negative red cells should be used for transfusion in women of childbearing age to prevent CMV infection or alloimmunisation
- It is very important that FBC and coagulation screens are taken regularly during the acute emergency

Cross-matched versus group specific transfusion

- In an emergency situation where speed is essential and immediate transfusion is required, O Rhesus D negative red cells should be administered. However, it is important to be aware that if the patient has irregular antibodies these red cells may be incompatible
- If no irregular antibodies are present, determined both from the history and screening results, then group specific red cells can be available within 10 minutes of a sample received in the laboratory, or up to 30 minutes including transport time
- If irregular antibodies are present, then cross-matched blood must be administered. This can take up to 1 hour for availability

- Thus, the seriousness of the medical emergency and the speed of blood requirement will determine which type of red cells is required

Other blood products

In the presence of massive haemorrhage, when disseminated intravascular coagulation (DIC) is present or suspected, then fresh frozen plasma (FFP), platelets and cryoprecipitate should also be administered. DIC is suspected if there is oozing from multiple areas including: intravenous access lines, previous venepuncture and surgical/ trauma sites.

Many hospitals have a major haemorrhage protocol to ensure sufficient red cells, platelets and blood products are available in a timely manner.

FFP takes 30 minutes to thaw and be available after being requested. The cryoprecipitate and FFP administered should be of the same blood group as the patient; however, a different blood group can be administered if a high titre anti-A or anti-B is not present. If a Rhesus D negative woman has Rhesus D positive FFP or cryoprecipitate administered, anti-D prophylaxis is not required.

FFP is administered at 12–15 mL/kg to maintain the activated partial thromboplastin time (aPTT) and prothrombin time ratios less than 1.5. FFP and cryoprecipitate should maintain Fibrinogen levels above 1.0 g/L.

Platelet count should be maintained above 50×10^9/L in a patient with massive haemorrhage. Platelet transfusion should be requested when levels fall to 75×10^9/L and the transfusion laboratory should be warned in advance as some hospitals do not have available units on site. Platelets administered should be group compatible and Rhesus D negative for Rhesus D negative women. Anti-D immunoglobulin (250 IU) is required if Rhesus D positive platelets are administered to a Rhesus D negative woman.

Transfusion reactions

Early transfusion complications are rare, occurring in less than 1 in 1000 transfusions. UK data from the Serious Hazards of Transfusion (SHOT) give an incidence of error of 11.4 per 100,000 components transfused. The SHOT report in 2009 reported 13 deaths related to transfusion.

Patient observations of temperature, pulse, respiration and blood pressure must be documented before the transfusion commences, and at 15 and 29 minutes after commencement.

Symptoms and signs of a transfusion reaction include:
- Flushing
- Shivering
- Rashes
- Shortness of breath
- Loin pain

If this occurs the transfusion must be stopped immediately, the details checked, the blood removed and sent back to the laboratory, with notification of the incident.

Early complications include:
- Acute haemolytic transfusion reaction
- Infective shock from bacterial contamination
- Transfusion related acute lung injury (TRALI)
- Fluid overload

Febrile reactions occur in 1–2% of patients, and are more common in multiparous women and those with multiple previous transfusions. This normally develops at the end of the transfusion or 2 hours later; most treatment is by stopping the transfusion and paracetamol.

Anaphylaxis can be treated by slowing down the transfusion and administering antihistamines.

Delayed reactions include:
- Delayed red cell haemolysis
- Alloimmunisation
- Post-transfusion purpura
- Graft versus host disease
- Iron overload
- Infection

The risk of HIV, hepatitis C and hepatitis B transmission is 1 in 4 million, 1 in 400,000 and 1 in 100,000 respectively.

Jehovah's Witnesses

Individuals have a right to decline transfusion of blood and its components, and this must be respected. These patients must take full legal responsibility for their actions. They must provide an 'advance decision' document (Advance Directive), which must be witnessed, signed and kept in their handheld notes. This must be discussed at each attendance. This is legally binding, unless the patient changes their mind or is under undue influence; clear documentation is vital.

Usually, transfusion of red cells, white cell, platelets and FFP are unacceptable. However, autologous transfusion, albumin, cryoprecipitate and coagulation factors may be acceptable. Antenatally, haemoglobin should be checked and treated if < 105 g/L.

Cell salvage

Intraoperative cell salvage (IOCS) is the transfusion of salvaged blood during surgery. The machine retrieves, washes, centrifuges and resuspends the red cells to transfuse back to the patient in theatre. Its use is recommended in women predicted to lose more than 1500 mL of blood (e.g. planned caesarean section for placenta praevia). Only health care teams, with appropriate expertise, and regular use, should operate it. National Institute for Health and Clinical Excellence (NICE) guidance on IOCS in obstetrics suggests using two suctions, one for liquor and one for blood, and a leucodepletion filter to reduce the risk of amniotic fluid embolism.

Further reading

Cantwell R, et al. Saving Mothers' Lives: Reviewing maternal deaths to make motherhood safer: 2006 -2008. The Eighth Report of the Confidential Enquiries into Maternal Deaths in the United Kingdom. BJOG 2011; 118(1):1–203.

RCOG Green-top Guideline No. 47. Blood transfusion in obstetrics. London: RCOG, 2008.
Taylor C, et al, on behalf of the Serious Hazards of Transfusion (SHOT) Steering Group. The 2009 Annual SHOT Report, 2010.

Related topics of interest

Breech presentation

Overview

The incidence of breech presentation reduces with gestation from 20% at 28 weeks, 16% at 32 weeks to 3–4% by term. Irrespective of mode of delivery, breech babies experience a higher rate of developmental delay, suggesting that failure to spontaneously adopt the cephalic presentation at term may reflect underlying fetal abnormality. There are three types of breech presentation:
- Extended (or frank) breech (65%) with flexed hips, knees extended
- Flexed breech (25%) with flexed hips and flexed knees, but with buttocks below the feet
- Footling breech (10%) with feet presenting

Aetiology

In many cases, the cause of breech presentation is unknown, but it is associated with the following factors:
- Fetal factors: extended legs preventing spontaneous version, fetal anomaly (e.g. hydrocephalus, anencephaly and cystic hygroma), prematurity and twins.
- Maternal factors: uterine anomaly, e.g. bicornuate uterus, placenta praevia, pelvic tumours, e.g. ovarian cyst, cervical fibroid, polyhydramnios, previous breech presentation

Clinical features and diagnosis

Breech presentation may initially be indicated on abdominal palpation after 36 weeks' gestation, when the head may be palpable in the upper part of the uterus. Auscultation of the fetal heart above the umbilicus in late pregnancy may also be indicative. Earlier assessment of presentation is inaccurate and does not alter management, so it is not recommended in the setting of routine antenatal care. During labour, a breech presentation is usually obvious after the membranes have ruptured and is commonly associated with the passage of frank meconium.

In the antenatal setting, breech presentation should always be confirmed with an ultrasound scan. This should also assess placental site, fetal growth, liquor volume and Doppler, presence of fetal abnormality (inaccurate in late gestation), presence of a nuchal cord or an extended head. The type of breech (extended, flexed or footling) should also be described.

Management

External cephalic version (ECV)

- Women with a breech presentation after 36 weeks of gestation should be offered an ECV as this almost halves the risk of caesarean section. ECV should be offered at 36 weeks in primiparous women and at 37 weeks in multiparous women, but there is no upper limit of gestation at which ECV can be offered. It can be performed in early labour with intact membranes
- ECV is a safe procedure rarely associated with complications, but should be performed after informed consent and ultrasound assessment as above. Guidelines suggest that cardiotocograph (CTG) should also be performed before the procedure
- Reported complications include maternal discomfort, transient CTG abnormalities, uterine rupture, fetomaternal haemorrhage and placental abruption. There is a 1:200 chance of an emergency caesarean section after EVC; therefore it should only be offered in a unit where immediate delivery is possible
- Absolute contraindications are:
  - Where caesarean delivery is required for another reason
  - Antepartum haemorrhage within the last 7 days
  - Abnormal CTG
  - Major uterine anomaly
  - Ruptured membranes
  - Multiple pregnancies, except delivery of second twin
- Relative contraindications are:
  - Small-for-gestational-age fetus with abnormal umbilical artery Doppler parameters

- Pre-eclampsia
- Oligohydramnios
- Major fetal anomalies
- Scarred uterus
- Unstable lie

- Success rates with a trained operator are around 50%, with rates being higher in multiparous women (60%) compared with primiparous women (40%). Success rates are higher if the patient is slim, the fetal head easily palpable and the breech is not engaged, the fetal back lateral and in non-white women. Use of tocolysis, usually with terbutaline (250 μg subcutaneously), results in an increased success rate
- After ECV, spontaneous reversion to breech occurs in < 5%. After an unsuccessful ECV, spontaneous version in primps occurs in < 5%. A further attempt can be offered
- After an ECV attempt, a CTG should be conducted, and Rhesus negative women should be given anti-D
- Labour after a successful ECV is associated with a 2-fold increase in intrapartum caesarean section rate and small increase in instrumental deliveries

Mode of delivery

The risks and benefits of the options of a planned vaginal breech delivery compared with an elective caesarean section should be discussed with the parents.

An elective caesarean section is associated with reduced perinatal/neonatal morbidity and mortality compared to a planned vaginal breech birth.

- A systematic review of trials comparing planned modes of delivery (most data was from the Term Breech Trial), showed the relative risk of perinatal/neonatal mortality and morbidity was 0.33 (95% confidence interval 0.19–0.56) with caesarean section
- After exclusion of cases in which risk factors for labour were identified (e.g. augmentation with oxytocin), the risk of the combined outcomes of perinatal/neonatal mortality and early neonatal morbidity was 3.3% for planned vaginal birth, compared with 1.6% for planned

caesarean section (p = 0.02). In contrast, a more recent observational study reported no difference in these outcomes between planned modes of delivery in units where a strict selection procedure is followed and vaginal breech birth is common practice
- There is no evidence of long term benefit to the infant from caesarean section as the 2 years follow up study for the term breech trial showed no difference in neonatal outcomes. The reduction in deaths in the caesarean section group was balanced by an increase in neurodevelopmental delay

A planned caesarean section is associated with a small increase in maternal complications compared with vaginal birth.

- The risks of a scarred uterus in subsequent pregnancy should be considered
- Although there are no good trials assessing the magnitude of these risks, authors have estimated that for every infant death avoided from planned caesarean section, one woman will suffer a ruptured uterus in a subsequent pregnancy

The Term Breech Trial focussed on planned vaginal delivery so should not be used to inform decision making in women in whom a breech presentation is diagnosed for the first time during labour. Diagnosis during labour is not a contraindication to a vaginal birth. Factors considered relative contraindications to a vaginal breech birth include:

- A footling or kneeling presentation (feet below the buttocks)
- Large baby > 3.8 kg
- Inadequate pelvis
- Growth restricted baby < 2 kg
- Hyperextended fetal neck
- Lack of a clinician trained to conduct vaginal breech births
- Previous caesarean section
- Augmentation of vaginal breech labour should not be used, as failure to progress in labour may suggest pelvic disproportion
- Options for labour analgesia in a vaginal breech birth should be the same as for labours with a cephalic presentation, as there is no specific evidence of benefit from an epidural
- The fetus should have continuous electronic fetal monitoring during a

planned vaginal breech birth. Although fetal blood sampling is possible it is not recommended practice
- There is currently no good evidence regarding the delivery of a preterm uncomplicated labour with a breech presentation, therefore decisions should be made on an individual basis. There is a particular risk of head entrapment caused by descent of the body through an incompletely dilated cervix. This should be managed using cervical incisions (at 10 and 2 o'clock)

Further reading

RCOG Green-top guideline No. 20a. External cephalic version and reducing the incidence of breech presentation. London: RCOG, 2006.

RCOG Green-top guideline No. 20b. Management of breech presentation. London: RCOG, 2006.

Hannah ME, Hannah WJ, Hewson SA, et al. Planned caesarean section versus planned vaginal birth for breech presentation at term: a randomised multicentre trial. Lancet 2000; 356:1375–1383.

Related topics of interest

- Multiple pregnancy (p. 265)
- Monitoring in labour (p. 262)
- Normal labour (p. 271)

Caesarean section

Overview

The caesarean section rate in England in 2010–2011 was 24.8% which has remained stable over the past few years. However, rates above 13–15% have not been shown to improve perinatal mortality. There can be associated maternal morbidity with such a delivery with impact for future deliveries. With an increasing number of repeat caesarean sections there is a significant increase in need for blood transfusion and risks of placenta accreta, injury to bladder, bowel or ureters, admission to the intensive care unit (ICU) and hysterectomy. The case fatality rate for all caesarean sections is at least 5 times that of a normal vaginal delivery and for emergency caesarean section it may be 12 times greater.

Delivery by elective caesarean section can confer some benefits – safer delivery for some babies, reduced incidence of pelvic floor trauma, avoidance of labour pain and convenience with the ability to plan the delivery date in advance.

Most caesarean sections are now performed under regional anaesthesia with administration of H_2-antagonists (ranitidine) and anti-emetic/gastric emptying (metoclopramide) medication prior to the operation.

Lower segment caesarean section

The majority of caesarean deliveries are performed via a transverse lower segment uterine incision. The skin incision is usually a transverse abdominal incision as this is associated with less postoperative pain and achieves better cosmetic results than a midline incision. A Joel-Cohen transverse skin insicion is now favoured over a pfannenstial incision as this appears to have less blood loss, a shorter operating time, a shorter duration of postoperative pain and a shorter time from skin incision to delivery. Delivery of the baby and placenta is followed by closure of the uterus in two layers with a continuous absorbable suture, the first layer commonly being locked. There is evidence for improved short term postoperative outcome if the peritoneum is not closed. Oxytocin 5 IU intravenous should be administered to encourage contraction of the uterus and minimise blood loss. The placenta should be delivered where possible with cord traction rather than manual removal. This reduces the incidence of blood loss and endometritis. The subcutaneous layer should be sutured if there is > 2 cm of fat. It is acceptable to use both absorbable and non-absorbable methods for skin closure.

Antibiotics should be administered prior to the skin incision to reduce the incidence of postoperative infection – broad spectrum cover is recommended for both aerobic and anaerobic microbes. Women having a caesarean section should be offered thromboprophylaxis because of the increased risk of venous thromboembolism. The method of choice, e.g. graduated stockings, low molecular weight heparin, should take into account risk factors and guidelines.

Indications

Scheduled/elective (grade 3 or 4)

- Maternal
  - Low lying placenta, obstruction in the lower uterus, e.g. fibroids, prior caesarean section delivery (with up to two prior caesarean sections vaginal delivery can be considered), prior classical caesarean delivery or uterine surgery entering the uterine cavity (e.g. open myomectomy), carcinoma of the cervix, maternal request secondary to tocophobia – an intense fear of childbirth, true cephalopelvic disproportion, prior pelvic floor repair
- Fetal
  - Transverse lie, breech presentation (if the mother wishes to avoid a vaginal delivery), high maternal HIV viral load, maternal coinfection with HIV and hepatitis C, multiple pregnancy (triplets of higher order or twins if the presenting twin is not cephalic),

if iatrogenic delivery is required at premature gestation or with severe intrauterine growth restriction, previous severe shoulder dystocia, monoamniotic twins

Emergency/urgent (grade 1 or 2)

- Maternal
  - Maternal illness requiring expedition of delivery – severe sepsis, fulminating pre-eclampsia
  - Failure to progress in labour
  - Failed induction of labour
  - Absolute cephalopelvic disproportion, e.g. a brow presentation
- Fetal
  - Possible fetal compromise – pathological cardiotocograph tracing (CTG) where a fetal blood sample (FBS) cannot be obtained, abnormal fetal pH result on FBS, prolonged fetal bradycardia
  - Cord prolapse
  - Uterine rupture
  - Placental abruption
  - Failed instrumental delivery

With some indications the need for caesarean delivery may influenced by the parity, gestation, presence of other risk factors, e.g. meconium, progress in labour and dilatation of the cervix. It is recommended that consultant obstetricians are involved in the decision making for non-elective caesarean sections as it can reduce the incidence of caesarean delivery.

Classical caesarean section

This procedure, where a midline longitudinal incision involving the upper segment of the uterus is now rarely performed. Compared to the lower segment technique there is a higher rate of maternal morbidity (infection, need for transfusion, hysterectomy, ICU admission). Subsequent delivery should always be by elective caesarean section as there is a significantly increased risk of uterine rupture during labour – up to 9%.

The abdomen is entered via a lower midline or transverse incision. The uterus is incised vertically and is normally repaired in three layers, particularly at the fundus, where the myometrium is thickest.

Indications

There are few indications for a classical incision, e.g. extreme prematurity, lower segment obliterated by fibroids or scar tissue, consideration if there is a transverse lie with ruptured membranes.

Rarely the lower segment incision needs to be converted to a 'J' or a 'T'-shaped incision to facilitate a difficult delivery (approximately a 2% risk of uterine rupture in a future labour).

Complications of a caesarean section

Maternal   The frequent risks are bleeding, infection and need for readmission to hospital. The rarer risks include thromboembolic disease, organ damage, hysterectomy, ICU admission, need for further surgery and maternal death. Certain factors can increase such risks, e.g. delivery at full dilatation, placenta praevia/accreta, increased maternal body mass index, multiple repeat prior surgeries.

Fetal   Fetal laceration can occur in 1–2% of caesarean deliveries. With elective caesarean section there is an increased risk of respiratory distress syndrome. This decreases with increasing gestational age – 37 weeks $\approx$ 8%, 38 weeks $\approx$ 5%, 39 weeks $\approx$ 1–2%. Thus, planned caesarean section should not be carried out before 39 weeks' gestation unless there are specific clinical indications. The Royal College of Obstetricians and Gynaecologists recommend the administration of corticosteroids to reduce respiratory morbidity if an elective caesarean is to be performed at $< 38^{+6}$ weeks' gestation.

Procedural aspects of a caesarean section

Caesarean sections should be graded/categorised as to the degree of urgency.
1. Immediate threat to the life of the woman or fetus

2. Maternal or fetal compromise which was not immediately life-threatening
3. No maternal or fetal compromise but needs early delivery
4. Delivery timed to suit woman or staff

Grade 1 and 2 caesarean sections should be performed as quickly as possible after the decision has been made – particularly for grade 1. A decision to delivery time of 30 minutes is often used as an audit standard. Grade 2 should be performed in most situations within 75 minutes of making the decision.

Full consent should be obtained prior to surgery where at all possible, although in some emergency obstetric situations this can be difficult to achieve. Resistance to a recommended caesarean section is rare; however, if refusal occurs then no health care provider can force a competent adult to undergo surgery against her will. If time allows then a psychiatric opinion would be mandatory. In the UK, the fetus has no legal rights.

Further reading

National Institute for Health and Clinical Excellence. Clinical Guideline 132 – Caesarean Section. London: NICE, 2011.

Royal College of Obstetricians and Gynaecologists. RCOG consent advice no 7: Caesarean section. London: RCOG, 2009.

Walsh CA. Evidence-based cesarean technique. Curr Opin Obstet Gynecol 2010; 22(2):110–115.

RCOG Green-top Guideline No. 45. Birth after previous caesarean birth, London: RCOG, 2007.

RCOG Green-top Guideline No. 27. Placenta praevia, placenta praevia accreta and vasa praevia: diagnosis and management. London: RCOG, 2011.

Nama V, Wilcock F. Caesarean section on maternal request: is justification necessary? The Obstetrician & Gynaecologist 2011; 13(4):263–269.

Related topics of interest

Cancer and pregnancy

Overview

A new diagnosis of cancer occurs in approximately 1 in 1000 pregnancies. Diagnosis and management should be individualised, taking into account the site and stage of the disease, gestation and the health of both mother and fetus. Investigation and treatment may affect the fetus, leading to conflict between the need to treat the mother and potential fetal harm.

Clinical features

The clinical features of cancer match those outside pregnancy, although symptoms of pregnancy may delay diagnosis.

Aetiology

Aetiology of individual cancers is as outside pregnancy, and the distribution of the disease maps that seen in women of reproductive age. Cervical screening has reduced the risk of cervical cancer such that it is no longer the commonest cancer in pregnancy (0.3/1000). Malignant melanoma may now be the commonest cancer diagnosis (between 0.2 and 2.6/1000). As the average age of childbearing increases, the incidence and pattern of cancer in pregnancy will change to reflect this.

Diagnosis

Cervical cancer in pregnancy

- False positive smears are more likely, so are usually delayed until postpartum
- Abnormal smears in pregnancy should be referred for colposcopy as usual. Treatment is usually deferred until postpartum as some lesions may regress and pregnancy does not alter progression. Assessment should be individualised but may consist of colposcopic surveillance in each trimester
- Cervical cancer presenting in pregnancy should be staged in the usual way, with magnetic resonance imaging (MRI) preferable to computed tomography (CT) scanning

- Traditionally, a diagnosis before 20 weeks is treated immediately by termination (which may be by hysterectomy), surgery and chemotherapy/radiotherapy as appropriate
- After 20 weeks, delaying treatment until fetal viability is possible. Delivery by caesarean section is usually recommended as vaginal delivery may risk bleeding from the lesion and increase the risk of metastasis. Radical hysterectomy may be conducted at the same time as a caesarean section
- Neoadjuvant chemotherapy may be used in the second and third trimesters to limit disease until whilst waiting for fetal maturity

Ovarian cancer in pregnancy

- Adnexal masses identified in pregnancy on ultrasound are relatively common (1 in 100), but carcinoma of the ovary is rare (1 in 5000–18,000).
- Management of adnexal masses is as outside of pregnancy. Simple cysts < 6 cm usually resolve but larger or more complex masses should be discussed with a gynaecological oncologist who may suggest additional imaging/monitoring and the use of tumour markers such as Ca-125
- If possible, any necessary surgery is best performed in the second trimester of pregnancy

Breast cancer and pregnancy

- The incidence of breast cancer in pregnant women is 1.3–2.4/10,000 live births
- Pregnancy itself does not alter the prognosis, but may delay diagnosis
- Women with breast lumps during pregnancy should be referred to the specialist breast team. First line investigation is ultrasound followed by mammography with fetal shielding. Tissue diagnosis is by ultrasound guided biopsy for histology as cytology is difficult to interpret due to proliferation
- Pelvic CT scanning and isotope bone scanning are usually used to identify

metastases outside pregnancy but these should be delayed until postpartum Concern about bone involvement should be investigated with plain X-ray or MRI. Disease is staged using chest X-ray and liver ultrasound

- Surgical treatment can be used in all trimesters of pregnancy, with reconstruction delayed until postpartum
- Radiotherapy is usually delayed until after delivery unless it is life-threatening
- Chemotherapy can be used from the second trimester onwards
- Tamoxifen and trastuzumab (HER2 receptor antibody/herceptin) should not be used in pregnancy or lactation due to concerns about fetal effects
- Most women with breast cancer can progress almost to term and have a normal delivery

Pregnancy after breast cancer

- Pregnancy should be delayed until at least 2 years after completing treatment. This may necessitate a discussion of risks and benefits in older women
- There is no evidence of an increased risk of malformation or miscarriage and most pregnancies progress to a live birth
- Women with oestrogen receptor positive disease taking tamoxifen usually need to take this treatment for 5 years and this medication is contraindicated during pregnancy
- There is no affect on long term prognosis
- Pregnancy should be managed by a multidisciplinary team including the breast team
- Women who received anthracycline chemotherapy require echocardiography as these drugs can rarely cause cardiomyopathy
- Women can breastfeed from the unaffected breast
- Adjuvant chemotherapy may adversely affect fertility, with 20–70% of premenopausal women being amenorrhoeic post-therapy. These rates are lower in younger women, with only 5% of women under 30 being amenorrhoeic

Other cancers

- Leukaemias and lymphomas (especially Hodgkin's disease) are relatively common in women of childbearing years. This is treated with chemotherapy which can be used from the second trimester with careful selection. Fertility is often preserved and subsequent pregnancy is safe after a reasonable interval of about 2 years
- Older data suggested that a diagnosis of melanoma in pregnancy was associated with a poor prognosis but recent series suggest there is no difference in survival rates. Melanoma is the cancer most likely to metastasise to the fetus but this is rare. If metastases are found in the placenta 30% of fetuses will be affected
- Hormone-dependent thyroid cancers are stimulated by the thyroid-stimulating hormone (TSH) effect of the gonadotrophins and prompt termination should be recommended

Management

- Management should be individually tailored involving a multidisciplinary team (often in specialist centres), including obstetric, neonatal, oncology and surgical teams, with parents involved in decisions
- In general (dependent on disease), it may be necessary to terminate early pregnancies to optimise outcomes for the mother. A diagnosis in later pregnancy may permit delay of treatment until fetal maturity
- Surgery is possible at any gestation, with pregnancy increasing risks for general anaesthesia. General anaesthesia is associated with a small risk of miscarriage or preterm labour
- Chemotherapy can be used during pregnancy:
  - During the first trimester of pregnancy (especially between 5 and 10 weeks) there is a 10–20% risk of fetal malformations
  - In the second and third trimesters there is no increased risk of malformations

although there is an up to 40% risk of fetal growth restriction and an increased risk of stillbirth and preterm labour
- There is a risk of fetal myelosuppression; therefore delivery should be planned 2–3 weeks after the last chemotherapy. This also reduces maternal complications at delivery associated with neutropenia from myelosuppression
- Breastfeeding should be avoided during chemotherapy, but may be possible for a brief period in between regimes, if

delivery is timed 3 weeks after a dose
- Data suggests there are no long term complications to the infant from in utero exposure to chemotherapy
- Radiotherapy can be used after the first trimester of pregnancy with fetal shielding. Therefore, pelvic radiotherapy is not possible as the fetus cannot be protected
  - Effects on the fetus from exposure to radiotherapy are miscarriage (especially in the first trimester), stillbirth, congenital malformations, growth restriction and childhood malignancy

Further reading

RCOG Green-top Guideline no 12. Pregnancy and breast cancer. London: RCOG, 2011.

Selig BP, Furr JR, Huey RW, et al. Chemotherapeutic agents as human teratogens. Birth Defects Res A Clin Mol Teratol 2012; 94(8):626–650.

Goncalves CV, Duarte G, Costa JS, et al. Diagnosis and treatment of cervical cancer during pregnancy. Sao Paulo Med J 2009; 127(6):359–365.

Related topics of interest

- Cervical cancer (p. 12)
- Ovarian cancer (p. 97)
- Cervical screening (p. 16)

Cardiac disease

Overview

The impact of cardiac disease in pregnancy is significant; it is the leading cause of death in pregnancy in the UK with 2.31 deaths per 100,000 maternities. There were 53 deaths in 2006–2008 due to cardiac disease in pregnancy. The vast majority of the deaths were due to acquired cardiac disease with sudden adult death syndrome, aortic dissection, myocardial infarction and ischaemic heart disease and cardiomyopathy being the most common causes. Congenital heart disease accounted for 5.7% of the deaths. Substandard care was present in 51% of these deaths. By way of comparison the prevalence of cardiac disease in high income countries is of the order of 1%.

Clinical features

Shortness of breath initially with exertion worsening with pregnancy, orthopnoea, paroxysmal nocturnal dyspnoea, cough and pedal oedema are symptoms of cardiac failure; symptoms will be specific to the particular heart disease. Cyanosis can be due to pulmonary atresia, tetralogy of Fallot or Eisenmenger's syndrome. Palpitations, angina, dizziness and syncope can result from arrhythmias, acute coronary syndromes and aortic dissection.

Clinical signs include heart murmur (although many pregnant women have a systolic flow murmur due to hyperdynamic circulation), tachycardia, wheeze, raised jugular venous pressure and worsening pedal oedema.

Aetiology

- Myocardial infarction: rare (frequency 1:10,000 pregnancies), with a 40% mortality. Associated with pre-eclampsia
- Cardiomyopathy: may be pregnancy specific (e.g. peripartum cardiomyopathy)
- Coarctation of the aorta and Marfan's disease: risk of aortic dissection. Delivery

by caesarean section is probably best if there significant aortic disease
- Aortic and mitral stenosis with risk of restenosis and dissection after repair in the former and left heart failure in the latter
- Regurgitant valve diseases: are well tolerated if there is no significant left ventricular dysfunction
- Heart block: this is generally not a problem, but pacing may be necessary
- Arrhythmia: supraventricular tachycardia being most common. This usually predates the pregnancy but may become more frequent and symptomatic in pregnancy
- Patent ductus arteriosus (most would have undergone correction in childhood); atrial septal and ventricular septal defects are usually well tolerated in pregnancy unless Eisenmenger's syndrome has developed

Diagnosis

- Electrocardiograph, 24-hour electrocardiograph and/or cardiomemo to assess for arrhythmias. (NB: the heart is rotated in pregnancy, which needs to be accounted for when interpreting an ECG in pregnancy.)
- Echocardiogram to assess valvular size and function, ventricular morphology and function and the great vessels. Cardiac magnetic resonance imaging (MRI) is becoming increasingly useful for assessing the size of vessels
- Troponin I is not changed in normal pregnancy but is elevated in pre-eclampsia, atrial fibrillation, pulmonary embolism, myocarditis and myocardial infarction/acute coronary syndromes

Management

Management should be multidisciplinary involving a cardiologist with experience of looking after pregnant women, an obstetrician, an obstetric anaesthetist, a midwife (and a haematologist for those that are at significant risk of thrombosis or require therapeutic anticoagulation).

The identification, assessment with risk stratification, counselling and modification of treatment of women with cardiac disorders should ideally be made prepregnancy.

Patients can be assessed based on the presence of pulmonary hypertension and cyanosis, the haemodynamic significance of the particular lesion and the use of formal functional classification schemes such as the New York Heart Association (NYHA) and World Health Organization (WHO) classifications (**Tables 32** and **33**). Class I patients have no discernible increase in risk while class II has a small increase in mortality and a moderate increase in morbidity risk. Those with class III are at significantly increased mortality and severe morbidity risk and require expert counselling and intensive specialist monitoring. Class IV patients are at extremely high risk and pregnancy is contraindicated. The relationship between specific conditions to the WHO classifications of morbidity is shown in **Table 34**.

These known cardiac patients (and those newly diagnosed) are reassessed in the first trimester and a plan for follow-up in the pregnancy devised. The disease might worsen in the late second and third trimesters and decisions for the timing, mode and management of delivery made at this stage. The greatest risk is at delivery and the immediate postpartum period because of the significant changes in maternal haemodynamics. The aim is to minimise sudden changes in blood volume and cardiac output secondary to uterine contraction, vasodilatation and haemorrhage.

Table 32 New York Heart Association functional classification of heart disease	
Class I	No breathlessness/uncompromised
Class II	Breathlessness on severe exertion/slightly compromised
Class III	Breathlessness on mild exertion/moderately compromised
Class IV	Breathlessness at rest/severely compromised

Table 33 Modified WHO classification of maternal cardiovascular risk: principles	
Risk class	Risk of pregnancy by medical condition
Class I	No detectable increased risk of maternal mortality and no/mild increase in morbidity
Class II	Small increased risk of maternal mortality or moderate increase in morbidity
Class III	Significantly increased risk of maternal mortality or severe morbidity. Expert counselling required. If pregnancy is decided upon, intensive specialist cardiac and obstetric monitoring needed throughout pregnancy, childbirth and the puerperium
Class IV	Extremely high risk of maternal mortality or severe morbidity; pregnancy contraindicated. If pregnancy occurs termination should be discussed. If pregnancy continues, care as for class III

Table 34 Modified WHO classification of maternal cardiovascular risk: application	
Risk Class	Conditions
WHO Class I	Uncomplicated pulmonary stenosis, PDA, mitral valve prolapse, successfully repaired ASD, VSD, PDA, atrial or ventricular ectopic beats
WHO Class II	Unoperated, uncomplicated VSD, ASD; repaired tetralogy of Fallot; most arrhythmias
ASD, arterial septal defect; PDA, patent ductus arteriosus; VSD, ventral septal defect	
WHO Class II-III	Mild left-ventricular impairment, hypertrophic cardiomyopathy, tissue valve replacements, Marfan syndrome with no aortic dilatation
WHO Class III	Mechanical heart valves, systemic right heart, fontan circulation, cyanotic heart disease, Marfan syndrome with aortic diameter 40–45 mm
WHO Class IV	Pulmonary hypertension, severe left heart dysfunction, severe mitral stenosis, severe symptomatic aortic stenosis, Marfan syndrome with aortic diameter > 45 mm, previous peripartum cardiomyopathy with residual left heart impairment, severe aortic coarctation
ASD, arterial septal defect; PDA, patent ductus arteriosus; VSD, ventral septal defect	

Induction of labour should be evaluated on merit. Most cardiac patients in pregnancy will tolerate epidural analgesia. The second stage should not exceed the normal parameters, but elective forceps deliveries are not always necessary. Syntocinon is the drug of choice in the third stage (to avoid the 500 mL bolus of blood 'squeezed' into the maternal systemic circulation from the use of ergometrine), but in a postpartum haemorrhage use of ergometrine is essential. The addition of IV furosemide may counteract the tendency to pulmonary oedema in such cases. Endocarditis is a risk in some cases, and this has been specifically targeted by the Confidential Enquiries into Maternal Deaths. Ampicillin 500 mg intramuscular at 8-hourly intervals for three doses and gentamicin 80 mg IM at 8-hourly intervals for three doses (check renal function and monitor levels) are the drugs of choice, with vancomycin 500 mg intravascular in two doses at 12-hour intervals being reserved for the penicillin-sensitive patient.

Artificial heart valves

The pregnant patient with certain types of artificial heart valve deserves special mention, the main problem being one of anticoagulation. Fetal and maternal morbidity and mortality are significantly higher in this group of patients. There is the dilemma of high risk of thrombosis with low molecular weight heparin, low molecular weight heparin (LMWH) versus warfarin embryopathy. Despite the associated embryopathy (which is dose-dependent), warfarin is becoming the drug of choice in such patients because of the high risk of thrombosis with LMWH. Warfarin is converted to LMWH before 6 weeks, restarted after 12 weeks and then changed to LMWH at 36 weeks.

Further reading

The Task Force on the Management of Cardiovascular Diseases during Pregnancy of the European Society of Cardiology (ESC). ESC Guidelines on the management of cardiovascular diseases during pregnancy. Eur Heart J 2011; 32(24):3147–3197.

Nelson-Piercy C. Handbook of Obstetric Medicine, 4th edn. London: Informa Healthcare, 2010; 19–38.

Related topics of interest

Cervical incompetence and cervical suture

Overview

Preterm birth before 37 weeks of gestation accounted for 7.6% of all live births in England and Wales in 2005. Preterm birth is the single most important factor in neonatal mortality. Mortality increases from about 2% for infants born at 32 weeks of gestation to more than 90% for those born at 23 weeks of gestation.

In its simplest form cervical incompetence refers to a 'weakness' within the cervical canal resulting in painless cervical dilation and late second trimester/preterm fetal loss. However, cervical incompetence is an imprecise clinical diagnosis and recent evidence would suggest that far from being a two point variable (normal/abnormal), cervical 'competence' is likely to be a 'continuum' influenced by factors related not just to the inherent structure of the cervix but also to other processes causing premature effacement and dilatation which include inflammation, infection and/or uterine irritability (see topic 94 premature labour).

Clinical features

Typically presents with painless cervical dilatation and/or second trimester/preterm delivery. Signs include:
- Increased vaginal discharge
- Bleeding (spotting)
- Sensation of pressure in vagina or urge to push
- Preterm prelabour rupture of membranes

Aetiology

Possible risk factors for cervical weakness include:
- Previous late second trimester loss and/or preterm delivery (particularly < 32 weeks of gestation)
- Surgical termination of pregnancy and/or greater than one dilatation and curettage
- Cervical surgery - including cone biopsy and/or large loop excision of the transformation zone (LLETZ), trachelectomy
- Cervical shortening on transvaginal scan with a history of spontaneous preterm delivery or second trimester loss

Management

Routine surveillance of cervical length in low risk women is not recommended. Likewise, there is no evidence to support measurement of cervical length and/or history directed cervical cerclage in women with multiple pregnancies as there is no evidence of benefit and some evidence of harm.

A full history should be taken from all women at booking, although there is no evidence that clinical history is a good way of telling if there is cervical weakness. Women with a history of late second trimester and/or preterm delivery (≤ 32 weeks) should be offered review in a preterm labour clinic.

Women at risk may be offered cervical scan surveillance. In those that opt for surveillance this usually begins at 16 weeks of gestation, but may start as early as 14 weeks if history dictates, although the upper portion of the cervix is difficult to distinguish at gestations below 16 weeks of gestation (**Figure 20a**). Accurately measured ultrasound cervical length has an inverse relationship with the risk of preterm birth. In women at a high risk of cervical incompetence a cervical length of ≤ 2.5 cm (**Figure 20b**) would usually justify suture (**Figure 20c**). Funnelling without shortening is not significant.

Any signs of infection should be treated appropriately. Bacterial vaginosis requires therapy until 34 weeks' gestation (vaginal cream - 2% Clindamycin daily).

A transvaginal suture is usually inserted as a day case under regional (spinal) anaesthetic. Mersilene tape on a round bodied needle is frequently used, although the choice of suture type and material is surgeon dependant. A catheter (inserted because of the spinal) is removed after 6 hours, when the woman may be discharged. Bed rest may be offered for 24–48 hours dependant on suture type, cervical length/dilatation and previous history. Tocolysis (indomethacin 100 mg PR given 12 hourly for 48 hours) can be offered. Follow up scan surveillance to assess integrity of the suture may be undertaken 7–10 days following insertion (see **Figure 20d**).

Routine fibronectin is not recommended although a negative result can be very reassuring, a high false positive result is to be expected following suture insertion.

Prophylactic corticosteroids, to accelerate fetal lung maturation, may be considered – particularly for salvage sutures placed at the cusp of viability.

Risks (< 1%) associated with insertion include miscarriage, bleeding, spontaneous rupture of membranes, preterm delivery, maternal pyrexia and/or possible bladder injury (depending on suture type).

When referring to cervical sutures the following terms below are increasingly used in the scientific literature.

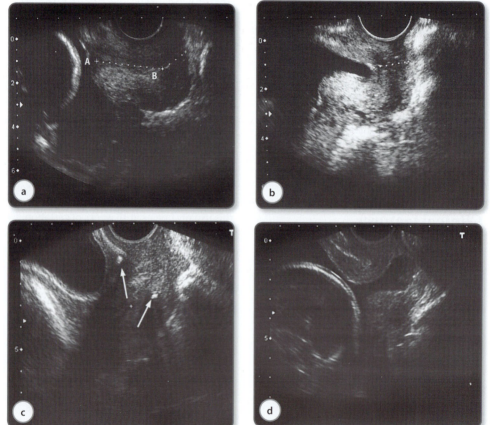

Figure 20 (a) Transvaginal scan of the cervix demonstrating a normal cervical length of 4.4 cm (43 mm). (b) Transvaginal scan of the cervix demonstrating a short cervix 1.4 cm (14 mm) with funnelling. (c) Transvaginal scan of the cervix postcervical cerclage (McDonald). The suture can be clearly seen (arrows) and the original funnelling (Figure b) has been corrected. (d) Transvaginal scan demonstrating extensive funnelling extending to the external os. On speculum the membranes were clearly visible and would require a rescue suture.

History-indicated cerclage   Insertion of a cervical suture based on risk factors identified in a woman's obstetric and/or gynaecological history. This prophylactic suture is usually inserted electively at 12–14 weeks of pregnancy, following nuchal translucency screening. Subgroup analysis of largest multicentred randomised controlled trial to date only indicated a benefit in those women with a history of three or more pregnancies ending before 37 weeks of pregnancy.

Ultrasound-indicated cerclage   Insertion of a cervical suture as a therapeutic measure after cervical length shortening (≤ 2.5 cm) has been identified on transvaginal ultrasound (usually undertaken between 16 and 23 weeks).

Rescue cerclage   Insertion of cervical suture as a salvage measure when premature cervical dilatation with exposed fetal membranes has been identified – either via vaginal/speculum examination or transvaginal scan (**Figure 65.1d**). Insertion may facilitate delay in delivery by 4–5 weeks. However, cervical dilatation of ≥ 4 cm and/or membranes beyond the level of the external os is associated with greater risk of suture failure. Data demonstrating improved neonatal morbidity/mortality is limited.

Transvaginal cerclage (McDonald)   A transvaginal purse-string suture placed tansvaginally at the cervicovaginal junction, without bladder mobilisation. This technique is most frequently adopted first line approach.

High transvaginal cerclage (Shirodkar)   A purse-string suture is inserted transvaginally after first mobilising the bladder, thereby permitting insertion above the level of the cardinal ligaments.

Transabdominal cerclage   A suture is inserted at the level of the cervicoisthmic junction, performed via a laparotomy or laparoscopy. This is usually inserted after a failed vaginal suture. There is, to date, no RCT comparing abdominal with transvaginal sutures. It may be inserted preconceptually, when access to the uterus is technically easier.

Successful sutures are usually removed at approximately 37 weeks of gestation. Preterm labour and/or SROM would be indications for immediate and delayed (48 hours latency in the absence of sepsis to facilitate steroids and/or in utero transfer) removal. In those with abdominal sutures delivery is by elective lower segment caesarean section, leaving the suture in place.

Further reading

RCOG Green-top Guideline No. 60. Cervical cerclage. RCOG: London, 2011.

Lim K, Butt K, Crane JM. Ultrasonographic cervical length assessment in predicting preterm birth in singleton pregnancies. J Obstet Gynaecol Can 2011; 33(5):486–499.

Iams JD, Goldenberg RL, Meis PJ, et al. The length of the cervix and the risk of spontaneous premature delivery. National Institute of Child Health and Human Development Maternal Fetal Medicine Unit Network. N Engl J Med 1996; 334:567–572.

Related topics of interest

Changes to maternal physiology in pregnancy

Overview

In a normal, singleton pregnancy the physiological changes of pregnancy are positive and adapt to meet fetal demands in a favourable way, are reversible and cause no permanent damage to the mother. However, physiology may turn into pathophysiology. The magnitude of adaptation is greatest in first pregnancies than subsequent ones. Physiological changes in pregnancy begin soon after conception.

General

Average weight gain in pregnancy is 12.5 kg, with most of the weight gain occurring and the rate of gain being fairly constant throughout the second and third trimesters. There is a positive correlation between maternal weight gain and birthweight. The main factor in weight gain is water (62%), fat (30%) and protein (8%). The fetal component (everything contained within the gravid uterus) at term is responsible for almost 5 kg (40%) of the weight gained.

Joint laxity and postural change, secondary to the alteration in the axis and position of the maternal centre of gravity, are very common, and lead to an altered gait at term and many of the aches and pains in pregnancy, including hip and back pain.

Oedema is ubiquitous and may lead to tracheal and intubation problems.

The exact calorific requirements of a pregnancy are in dispute, but are of the order of 100 kcal/day up to 10 weeks and 200–300 kcal/day thereafter.

There is an increased blood flow to the skin, sweat and sebaceous glands are more active and there may be increased body and facial hair. The subcutaneous tissue is thickened, leading to the coarsened facial features seen in many at term, and pigmentation of the face (chloasma or 'mask of pregnancy'), nipples, umbilicus, vulva and scars may increase. Striae gravidarum, especially of the abdominal wall, buttocks and thighs, occurs secondary to the rapid and excessive skin stretching in these areas. Breast development is accentuated after 8 weeks and is mainly the result of glandular hyperplasia and hypertrophy and fat deposition. Colostrum may be expressed from the second trimester.

Cardiovascular

Blood volume increases by 1250–1500 mL, reaching a zenith at 34–36 weeks. As more of this is due to an increase in plasma volume than by an expansion in red cell mass, physiological haemodilutional anaemia occurs; the haematocrit declines correspondingly. Mean cell volume (MCV) is steady or increases slightly with a normal range of 80–100 fl.

Stroke volume rises by 10% and pulse rate by 10–20 beats per minute. Cardiac output is increased by 1.5 L/min to 6.5–7.0 L/min at 20–28 weeks and remains at this level until term. Cardiac output increases by about 15% to 8 L/min in the first stage of labour and by 50% to 9 L/min in the second stage. There is a further increase of 60–80% immediately after delivery, returning to prelabour values within 1 hour. These increases are due to uterine autotransfusion with contraction and delivery, increased sympathetic tone from pain and anxiety, relieved uterine pressure on the inferior vena cava (IVC) and return of extravascular fluid to the intravascular compartment.

Arterial blood pressure does not rise in parallel with the increase in cardiac output, because of the drop in hormonally mediated peripheral vascular resistance and vessel dilatation and the development of a high capacitance, low pressure placental circulation. Blood pressure normally falls on average by 5 mmHg systolic and 15 mmHg diastolic prior to 20 weeks, rising to prepregnancy levels at term. The effect of the gravid uterus on the IVC may drastically alter maternal haemodynamics, e.g. supine hypotension and syncope, so it is important to measure blood pressure with a correctly sized cuff on a relaxed patient sitting or semirecumbent and tilted to the left. The fifth Korotkoff sound should be used. Venous blood pressure is only slightly raised in pregnancy in most parts of the body, but it is significantly raised in the dependent lower limbs.

As a consequence of the hyperdynamic circulation of pregnancy many women develop cardiac murmurs. In the absence of symptoms or signs of cardiac compromise they do not warrant investigation.

Respiratory

The thoracic cage is lifted up and the ribs flare, there is an increased anteroposterior diameter, an elevation and increased excursion of the diaphragm, except towards term where it reduces.

The respiratory rate does not generally increase, but the tidal volume increases by 200 mL and the vital capacity by 100–200 mL. This hyperventilation causes a mild alkalosis; arterial pH ≥ 7.44. These changes, plus the reduction of the maternal respiratory centre threshold to PCO_2 stimulus (probably due to progesterone) by a rise of 1 mmHg, increase the maternal minute volume to 6 L/min. It also facilitates gas exchange from the fetus to the mother and, in conjunction with increased maternal respiratory centre sensitivity caused by high levels of oestrogen, makes the mother prone to dyspnoea and dizziness. These physiological changes have a significant effect on anaesthesia during pregnancy.

Renal

The osmoregulatory system for diuresis and thirst is set 6–8 mosmol/kg lower than before pregnancy. Aldosterone is raised, being 8- to 10-fold greater at 36 weeks than in the non-pregnant state. The increase in progesterone and glomerular filtration rate (GFR) causes sodium loss and potassium retention, but the 2- to 3-fold increase in plasma renin substrate resulting from increased oestrogen and progesterone activates the renin-angiotensin-aldosterone cascade, thereby balancing the sodium loss and volume depletion effects of progesterone. It is this renal retention of sodium that causes the water retention noted above. Angiotensin is raised 2- to 4-fold, but its pressor effects are checked by increased synthesis of the vasodilator prostaglandins (PGE2) and prostacyclin (or PGI2).

In addition, please see renal disease in pregnancy (Topic 100).

Gastrointestinal

Appetite may change, nausea and vomiting is very common, along with cravings for unusual substances (pica). Salivary excretion is increased and gastric secretion and motility are decreased. Gut transit times are increased, and water retention (whether or not due to iron supplementation) promotes constipation in conjunction with the physical obstruction from the growing uterus and fetus. Gastro-oesophageal reflux is common owing to increased gastric pressure and loss of tone at the cardia c sphincter. Alkaline phosphatase rises, but it originates mostly from the placenta. The normal range for liver function tests vary with trimester of gestation and are less than non-pregnant levels. Although hepatic function is relatively unchanged, other changes (such as those seen in the kidneys) may significantly alter maternal drug metabolism. All lipids rise in pregnancy, predominantly cholesterol and triglycerides.

Endocrine

See Diabetes and Pregnancy (Topic 69) and Thyroid and Pregnancy (Topic 106).

Further reading

Nelson-Piercy C. Handbook of Obstetric Medicine, 4th edn. London: Informa Healthcare, 2010.

Davey DA. Normal pregnancy: physiology and antenatal care. In: Whitfield CR (Ed.). Dewhurst's Textbook of Obstetrics and Gynaecology for Postgraduates, 4th edn. Oxford: Blackwell Scientific Publications, 1988; 126–158.

Related topics of interest

- Anaemia in pregnancy (p. 177)
- Cardiac disease (p. 204)
- Renal disease in pregnancy (p. 311)

Coagulation and pregnancy

Overview

To prevent substantial blood loss during pregnancy, particularly at delivery, the coagulation system shifts to a procoagulant state. Hence, women with underlying coagulation disorders may be at risk of thrombosis, or bleeding dependent on the disorder.

Clinical features

Disorders have usually been diagnosed before pregnancy due to an unexpected thrombosis or bleeding, or similar event in a family member.

Aetiology

Blood clotting is determined by three factors (Virchow's triad): blood flow, blood vessel wall integrity and coaguability of the blood. Coaguability is dependent on platelets, the clotting cascade and the fibrinolytic pathway. The procoagulant state in pregnancy is due to:

- Increases in the clotting factors VII, VIII, X, XII, von Willebrand factor (vWF), and fibrinogen. Others remain constant
- Fibrinolytic activity falls, due to a reduction in the anticoagulant protein S and low activity of tissue plasminogen activator (tPA). Antithrombin III, which is required for the action of heparin, and protein C remain approximately the same
- Blood vessels are generally dilated and pressure from the gravid uterus causes stasis of venous blood in lower limbs. Vessel walls do not change
- Platelet counts may fall by up to 10% but this does not affect clot formation. D-dimers increase
- Prothrombin time, international normalised ratio and activated partial thromboplastin time may be shortened but remain within the normal range

Bleeding disorders during pregnancy

Platelet disorders

- Thrombocytopenia is common affecting 6–10%
- Underlying causes, such as systemic lupus erythematosus (SLE), antiphospholipid syndrome, HIV, von-Willebrand disease (vWD), bone marrow disease and pregnancy related causes such as haemolysis, elevated liver function and low platelets (HELLP) syndrome should be considered
- In most (around 80%) the reduction in platelets is gestational thrombocytopenia (GTP) and platelets remain above $90–100 \times 10^9/L$. This is a benign condition not associated with risks of bleeding. However, documentation of a return to a normal platelet count postnatally is required for confirmation. Therefore, many women may need to be managed as for immune thrombocytopenic purpura (ITP), as this can arise during pregnancy
- ITP occurs in 1–2/10,000 pregnancies and should be suspected with low platelets occurring before 20 weeks of pregnancy. It is associated with antiplatelet (IgG)
- Patients with ITP may present with bleeding or bruising. Spontaneous haemorrhage is unlikely with platelet counts above $20 \times 10^9/L$, and surgical bleeding is unlikely if the platelet count is greater than $50 \times 10^9/L$. Anaesthetists usually require a platelet count $>80 \times 10^9/L$ prior to administering regional analgesia
- Antiplatelet IgG can cross the placenta, resulting in fetal thrombocytopenia in 5–10% of cases. Therefore, caution should be employed during labour to avoid procedures which may increase the risk of neonatal bleeding, such as repeated fetal blood sampling, the use of fetal scalp electrodes, ventouse or rotational instrumental deliveries

- First line treatment for women with very low platelet counts in pregnancy is oral corticosteroid at high doses (usually 60–80 mg/day). Alternatives include intravenous immunoglobulin or azathioprine
- Platelet transfusions are reserved for emergency situations or to cover delivery in resistant cases, as they increase antibody titres and have a short half-life in the circulation

Clotting factor disorders

There are several genetic disorders causing deficiency of individual clotting factors, the commonest being vWD. Such women require joint management with the input of specialist haematologists.

- vWD occurs in around 1% and is autosomal dominant
- There are several types, with the commonest, type 1, being associated with a deficiency of vWF and is usually mild
- vWF is a large protein needed for the binding of platelets to endothelium and also protects factor VIII in the circulation from breakdown
- vWD is diagnosed by a prolonged activated partial thromboplastin time (APTT) and low levels of vWF and factor VIII. The ristocetin cofactor assay provides a functional assessment of vWF
- Pregnancy increases levels of factor VIII and vWF so women with mild–moderate type 1 disease usually normalise by the late second trimester, so are not at risk of bleeding. However, levels fall rapidly postpartum

- Women with more severe disease may need treatment with desmopressin (DDAVP) or factor replacement. Tranexamic acid may also reduce the risk of bleeding
- Haemophilia A (factor VIII deficiency) and haemophilia B (factor IX deficiency) are rare X linked recessive disorders. However, some carrier females have low levels so should be assessed as they may be at risk of bleeding if low levels do not correct
- The risk of inherited bleeding disorders in the fetus should be remembered and managed as for ITP above

Thrombotic disorders

- Thrombocythaemia is a myeloproliferative disorder, associated with haemorrhagic and thrombotic complications, and is rare in pregnancy
- Due to the gestational fall in platelets, the count may normalise in pregnancy
- Women with platelet counts $> 500 \times 10^9/L$ should probably receive low dose aspirin. Other risks should also be considered and low molecular weight heparin (LMWH) prophylaxis may sometimes be appropriate
- Thrombophilic disorders affecting the clotting cascade are either inherited or acquired
- Inherited disorders and their associated risks of thrombosis in pregnancy are shown in **Table 35**. When considering anticoagulation during pregnancy and the puerperium, other risk factors such as age, parity and obesity should be considered on an individual basis (see Topic 104)

Table 35 Inherited thrombophilias and risk of thrombosis in pregnancy.			
Thrombophilia	% in population	% risk	Odds ratio
Antithrombin III	0.07	15–50	5–10
Compound heterozygote	-	1.8–15.8	9–107
Factor V Leiden heterozygote	3–5	2.1	5–8
Protein C deficiency	0.3	-	2–4.8
Protein S deficiency	0.2	-	3.2
Prothrombin gene heterozygote	1	2.3	3–10

- In previously asymptomatic women, those with lower risk thrombophilias such as factor V Leiden or prothrombin heterozygosity should be offered postnatal LMWH
- Protein C and protein S deficiency (protein S deficiency cannot be diagnosed in pregnancy as protein S falls physiologically) should be considered moderate risk factors, therefore may require LMWH
- Antithrombin III is associated with high thrombotic risk. These women are often resistant to heparin, so require high doses with monitoring within a multidisciplinary service. There is growing interest in covering these patients with antithrombin III replacement during times of particularly high risk of thrombosis, such as during delivery
- Acquired thrombophilia is usually antiphospholipid syndrome. The lupus anticoagulant is particularly associated with a high thrombotic risk. Management should involve rheumatologists and haematologists, but from a thrombosis perspective, postnatal LMWH as a minimum requirement. However, most will also receive antenatal treatment
- Women on antenatal LMWH should also receive it for 6 weeks postpartum
- It is important to remember general advice about long distance travel, hydration and compression stockings

Disseminated intravascular coagulation (DIC)

- DIC occurs secondary to a primary pathology such as haemorrhage, amniotic fluid embolism, prolonged retention of a dead fetus, sepsis, pre-eclampsia or HELLP syndrome. Stimulation of the clotting cascade and fibrinolysis cause massive consumption of platelets and clotting factors resulting in uncontrolled bleeding
- Diagnosis by finding increased fibrinogen degradation products (FDPs), increased fibrin, reduced platelet count and a low fibrinogen ($<2\,g/L$)
- Treatment is to manage the cause and intensive support with close involvement of haematologists and intensivists
- Supportive treatment may include factor replacement with fresh frozen plasma (FFP), blood transfusion to replace blood loss, platelet replacement and cryoprecipitate. Cryoprecipitate contains more fibrinogen than FFP and may be used if fibrinogen is less than $1\,g/L$

Diagnosis

Diagnosis of individual disorders is directed by history (especially family history) and tests of the coagulation system as outlined above.

Management

This should be multidisciplinary involving obstetricians, anaesthetists and specialist haematologists.

Further reading

James AH. Von Willebrand disease. Obstetrical & Gynecological Survey 2006; 61(2):136–145.

Thornton P, Douglas J. Coagulation in pregnancy Best practice & research clinical obstetrics and gynaecology 2010; 24:339–352.

RCOG Green-top Guideline No 37a. Reducing the risk of thrombosis and embolism during pregnancy and puerperium. London: RCOG, 2009.

Related topics of interest

Cord prolapse

Overview

Cord prolapse is defined as the presence of umbilical cord that has descended through the cervix to lie either beside the presenting part (occult) or below the presenting part (overt) in the presence of ruptured membranes. The incidence is between 0.1 and 0.6%. The incidence increases to >1% with breech presentation. Umbilical cord prolapse is a cause of stillbirth and neonatal deaths; a perinatal mortality rate of 91/1000 was determined by a large study. This is primarily attributed to prematurity, congenital malformations (which increase the incidence of cord prolapse) and birth asphyxia. Birth asphyxia occurs as a result of cord compression or cord vessels spasm due to the cold or handling.

Clinical features

Cord prolapse may occur without any clinical signs and in the presence of a normal fetal heart rate pattern. However, the presence of umbilical cord should be checked for at every vaginal examination and after artificial rupture of membranes. Vaginal examination should also be performed after spontaneous rupture of membranes if there are risk factors present or if fetal heart rate abnormalities begin to occur.

Risk factors

- The following risk factors predispose to the occurrence of cord prolapse:
  - Breech presentation
  - Prematurity (<37 weeks)
  - Transverse, oblique or unstable lie
  - Multiple pregnancy especially of the second twin
  - Low birth weight (<2.5 kg)
  - Fetal congenital malformations (particularly those which prevent engagement of the fetal head)
  - Polyhydramnios
  - Unengaged presenting part
  - Low-lying placenta

- The following obstetric procedures are also associated with an increased risk:
  - Artificial rupture of membranes
  - External cephalic version
  - Vaginal manipulation of the fetus in the presence of ruptured membranes including internal podalic version
  - Uterine pressure transducer insertion
  - Stabilising induction of labour

Approximately 50% of cord prolapse cases are preceded by obstetric procedures. These risk factors prevent the close approximation of the fetal head against the cervix and pelvic brim.

The following pre-emptive measures should be followed to avoid adverse effects following a cord prolapse. If there is transverse, oblique or unstable lie, elective admission after 37^{+6} weeks of gestation should be discussed and offered. If preterm rupture of membranes occurs in a fetus with a non-cephalic presentation, admission should be offered. If there is a high presenting part, artificial rupture of membranes should ideally not be performed. However, if required this should occur where facilities are available to proceed to emergency caesarean section if required. Rupture of membranes must be avoided if cord presentation is felt.

Diagnosis

If abnormal fetal heart rate occurs (bradycardia or variable decelerations), especially in the presence of risk factors and if they commence following spontaneous or artificial rupture of membranes, then cord prolapse should be suspected.

This must then be confirmed or excluded via prompt vaginal examination, with the use of speculum examination initially if preterm.

Every effort should be made to avoid handling the umbilical cord to prevent vasospasm.

Management

It is very important to firstly determine if the fetus is alive and the current stage of labour.

If the fetus is alive in the first stage of labour help should be called for immediately, and preparations made for immediate delivery in theatre.

To prevent cord compression the presenting part should be moved off the cord. This can be performed either digitally or via bladder filling via a urinary catheter.

Potential cord compression could be further reduced by advising the woman to adopt a knee–chest position or head down position in left lateral. Tocolysis should be considered if there are persistent fetal heart rate abnormalities despite reduction in cord compression. Delivery should not be delayed to achieve these manoeuvres or administer tocolysis.

A category I caesarean section is required, with delivery within 30 minutes if fetal heart rate abnormalities persist. A category II caesarean section (see Topic 62) is appropriate if the fetal heart trace is normal.

If cord prolapse occurs at full dilatation, in the second stage of labour, immediate delivery by forceps or ventouse can be performed. Breech extraction is a possibility after internal podalic version for the second twin.

A clinician with experience in neonatal resuscitation should be present at the birth and cord pH should be taken due to the increased risk of hypoxia/acidosis in the infant.

If cord prolapse occurs in the community, urgent hospital transfer via blue light (999) ambulance is required. During ambulance transfer the left lateral position should be adopted, whilst awaiting the ambulance the woman should adopt a knee–chest face down position. Manoeuvres for elevating the presenting part and avoiding cord vasospasm can be performed as before.

If the fetus is dead, diagnosed by lack of cord pulsations and verified by ultrasound scan finding no fetal heart beat then vaginal delivery should be prepared for.

If cord prolapse occurs at the limit of viability, then the woman should be counselled with regards her options, namely continuing with the pregnancy or termination. It may be possible to attempt replacement of the umbilical cord, although the effect on prognosis is uncertain.

Irrespective of the cause and location (home, midwifery-led unit or consultant-led unit) of the cord prolapse continuous explanation should be given to the woman and her partner, during their management, and full debriefing should occur postnatally.

Further reading

RCOG Green-top Guideline No. 50. Umbilical cord prolapse. London: RCOG, 2008.

Grady K, Howell C, Cox C. Managing Obstetric Emergencies and Trauma, 2nd edn. London: RCOG, 2007:233–237.

Related topics of interest

Diabetes in pregnancy

Overview

2–5% of pregnancies are affected by diabetes (pre-existing or gestational). Diabetes is a metabolic disorder characterised by chronic hyperglycaemia owing to a deficiency of or resistance to insulin. Pregnancy is a diabetogenic condition due to a number of factors: (i) human placental lactogen and human placental growth hormone have anti-insulin and lipolytic effects, (ii) corticosteroids and progesterone has an anti-insulin effect. A woman's antenatal, intrapartum and postnatal course are affected by diabetes, especially if poorly controlled. Maternal glucose crosses over the placenta into the fetal circulation by facilitated diffusion; therefore the fetal blood glucose closely mirrors that of the mother. Thus, the fetus may be adversely affected if the maternal condition is ignored.

Clinical features

Pre-existing diabetes mellitus puts women, the fetus and their babies at increased risk of a number of conditions listed in **Table 36**.

Risks associated with gestational diabetes mellitus (GDM) include: fetal macrosomia, birth trauma to mother and baby, operative delivery, transient neonatal morbidity, neonatal hypoglycaemia and diabetes developing later in the baby's life.

Aetiology

Type 1 diabetes is an absolute deficiency of insulin due to autoimmune destruction of the b cells of the pancreas. It typically presents before the age of 20 years.

Type 2 diabetes is associated with insulin resistance. Its incidence is increasing, typically presents over the age of 20 years and is associated with obesity.

GDM is a carbohydrate intolerance that begins or is first recognised during pregnancy and in most cases resolves after pregnancy. Women with GDM have an increased risk of GDM in future pregnancies and a > 50% chance of developing type 2 diabetes in later life. The incidence of both type 2 diabetes and GDM is increasing.

Diagnosis

Diagnosis of type 1 and type 2 diabetes has usually been made prior to pregnancy. However, occult diabetes should be suspected in patients who have elevated blood sugar readings prior to 20 weeks of gestation. There is much controversy regarding both screening and diagnosis of GDM. The Hyperglycaemia and Pregnancy Outcome (HAPO) study revealed a linear relationship between maternal plasma glucose and adverse outcomes. Results from the Australian Carbohydrate Intolerance Study

Table 36 Risks of pre-existing diabetes to mother, fetus and neonate		
Maternal risks	**Fetal risks**	**Neonatal risks**
	Miscarriage/stillbirth	Jaundice
	Congenital abnormalities (7%) Caudal regression syndrome is pathognomonic of a diabetic pregnancy with a prevalence of 1:1000 diabetic pregnancies	Hypoglycaemia – fetal hyperinsulinemia
Infection	Macrosomia	Hypocalcaemia/hypomagnesaemia
Pre-eclampsia	Fetal growth restriction	Polycythaemia
Operative delivery	Birth trauma	Respiratory distress syndrome
Birth trauma/shoulder dystocia	Preterm delivery	10-fold chance of developing diabetes in later life than infants of non-diabetic mothers (1% versus 0.1%)

in Pregnant Women (ACHOIS) have shown better pregnancy outcomes when gestational diabetes is treated. The International Association of Diabetes and Pregnancy Study Groups (IADPSG) recommend a one step screening for all women in pregnancy not known to be diabetic at 24–28 weeks of gestation. At present most UK obstetric departments adhere to the National Institute of Health and Clinical Excellence (NICE) guidelines. NICE recommend screening for gestational diabetes in women with any of the following risk factors.

- Body mass index above 30 kg/m^2
- Previous macrosomic baby weighing 4.5 kg or above
- Previous GDM
- First-degree relative with diabetes
- Family origin with a high prevalence of diabetes (South Asian, black Caribbean and Middle Eastern)

Many obstetricians will screen for GDM if glycosuria is present on more than one occasion, despite not being recommended by NICE.

In the UK screening for GDM uses the 2 hours 75 g oral glucose tolerance test (OGTT). It is performed between 26–28 weeks' gestation and 16–18 weeks' gestation in women with a previous history of GDM. NICE guidance states GDM is diagnosed with a fasting glucose of > 7 mmol/L and/or a 2-hour postprandial > 7.8 mmol/L. According to the IADSPG, if one or more of the following values are exceeded (fasting ≥ 5.1 mmol/L, 1-hour ≥ 10.0 mmol/L, 2-hour ≥ 8.5 mmol/L) using a 75 mg OGTT GDM should be diagnosed.

Management

To ensure improved outcome, care of the pregnant woman with diabetes is ideally provided by an obstetrician, a diabetic physician, a diabetes specialist midwife and a dietician.

Pre-existing diabetes

Preconception counselling

The importance of strict diabetic control prior to conception should be discussed. If it is safe to do so, aim for HbA1c < 6.1%,

(43.2 mmol/mol). Contraception should be used until adequate control is achieved. Current medication should be reviewed as many women with diabetes may be taking an angiotensin-coverting enzyme (ACE) inhibitor. Due to its fetotoxicity women should be advised to discontinue this. Calcium channel blockers are safe alternatives in those women with hypertension. Renal assessment should be offered and referral made to a nephrologist if serum creatinine is > 120 µmol/L. Retinal screening is advised if it has not been undertaken during the preceding 6 months. General measures include: checking rubella status, 5 mg folic acid daily preconception until 12 weeks of gestation to reduce the risk of neural tube defects, 75 mg aspirin daily to reduce the risk of pre-eclampsia and healthy diet and lifestyle advice.

Antenatal care

At the initial appointment advice is given regarding glycaemic control and monitoring. Blood glucose levels should be tested premeals and 1 hour postmeals, aiming for levels for fasting between 3.5–5.9 mmol/L and 1-hour postprandial < 7.8 mmol/L. Self-monitoring is vital, and some clinics now draw upon the technology of glucometers with a capacity to store the preceding 2 weeks' results, which can then be printed out in the clinic. Most insulin regimens use a mixture of short-acting and long-acting insulins. Insulin pumps can be used in pregnancy; they tend to be used by women using them preconception or in those having difficulty obtaining good glycaemic control with alternative regimens.

Women with type 2 diabetes may either continue taking metformin, or add insulin if required; other oral hypoglycaemics should be discontinued. Renal assessment is offered with consideration to the use of thromboprophylaxis if proteinuria > 5 g/day. Retinal assessment by digital imaging is recommended and general advice given regarding recognition of hypoglycaemia and the use of glucagon if required.

Anomaly and fetal size ultrasound (from 26–28 weeks) scanning should be performed to evaluate fetal growth. In uncomplicated pregnancies, induction of labour may be offered at 38–40 weeks' gestation. However, most centres have a caesarean section rate of at least 30% in pregnant women with diabetes. Continuous fetal monitoring is recommended during labour with hourly blood glucose assessments, and use of a sliding scale aiming for a blood glucose level of 4–6 mmol/L.

Pregnant women with diabetes are particularly prone to three complications, namely pre-eclampsia (14.4%), polyhydramnios (25%) and preterm labour (17%). If required, tocolysis and corticosteroids can be used in the diabetic patient. Corticosteroids will, however, have a deleterious effect on glycaemic control.

Postnatally, women with diabetes should be encouraged to breastfeed and contraception should be discussed prior to leaving hospital.

Gestational diabetes mellitus

Women with newly diagnosed GDM should be given advice on the risks of GDM. Review with a dietician should be offered and advice regarding glycaemic monitoring and control is similar to that of a woman with pre-existing diabetes. GDM can be managed by diet control alone or with the use of metformin and/or insulin depending on glycaemic control. Repeated ultrasound assessment should be offered for assessment of fetal growth.

NICE recommend offering delivery at 38 weeks' gestation and increased fetal surveillance if women opt to await spontaneous labour. The Royal College of Obstetricians and Gynaecologists (RCOG) recommend delivery between 38 and 40 weeks of gestation depending on clinical circumstances.

Postnatally the majority of women discontinue treatment. Women should be offered a postnatal GTT and informed regarding a > 50% chance of developing type 2 diabetes in later life. Yearly fasting glucose tests are recommended.

Further reading

NICE Clinical Guideline No. 63: Diabetes in pregnancy. Management of diabetes and its complications from pre-conception to the postnatal period. London: NICE, 2008.

Alwan N, Tuffnell DJ, West J. Treatments for gestational diabetes. Cochrane Database of Systematic Reviews, 2009; 3:CD003395. DOI: 10.1002/14651858.CD003395.pub2.

Royal College of Obstetricians and Gynaecologists. Scientific Impact, Opinion Paper 23. Diagnosis and treatment of gestational diabetes. London: RCOG, 2011.

Related topics of interest

Domestic abuse

Overview

Domestic abuse is defined as any incident of threatening behaviour, violence or abuse (psychological, physical, sexual, financial or emotional) between adults who are or have been intimate partners or family members, regardless of gender or sexuality. Domestic abuse occurs across all social classes and ethnic groups. It has an association with young age, marital separation, financial pressures, drug and alcohol abuse and disability and ill health.

In the UK, the annual prevalence of domestic violence is estimated to be 1:9–10. One in four women worldwide will suffer domestic abuse during their lifetime. It is thought that 5–11% of women presenting to accident and emergency departments do so as a consequence of domestic violence and it is estimated that women in abusive relationships will suffer more than 30 physical assaults before disclosing.

Domestic abuse also includes issues such as so-called 'honour' based violence, female genital mutilation (FGM) and forced marriage, and is clear that victims are not confined to one gender or ethnic group. The definition has recently been extended to include victims aged 16–18 years and controlling behaviour.

'Controlling behaviour' are acts designed to make a person subordinate and/or dependent by isolating them from sources of support, exploiting their resources for personal gain, depriving them of the means needed for independence, resistance and escape and regulating their everyday behaviour. This differs from 'coercive behaviour' which is an act or a pattern of acts of assault, threats, humiliation and intimidation or other abuse that is used to harm, punish or frighten their victim. Both are domestic abuse.

Impact on women's health

Gynaecology

Reproductive coercion can manifest as either pregnancy promoting behaviours or pressure to terminate a pregnancy. The provision of long-acting reversible contraception may be instrumental in interrupting a cycle of contraceptive sabotage, male decision making over pregnancy outcome and unwanted pregnancy or termination. Current domestic violence has been shown to be more prevalent among women seeking termination of pregnancy.

Canadian women seeking termination of pregnancy were found to be almost four times more likely to give a history of physical or sexual violence in the preceding 12 months than women continuing with their pregnancy (7.1% versus 1.8%). With repeated terminations of pregnancy the likelihood of the woman giving a history of domestic abuse increases. Physical and sexual violence is particularly common in women who do not disclose their pregnancy or termination of pregnancy to their partner (23.7% versus 12% in disclosers).

Obstetrics

Approximately 30% of domestic violence starts during pregnancy. Pregnancy may also exacerbate or lessen violent episodes. The pattern of violence may change with assaults being more likely to be directed to the abdomen, breasts or genitals. Domestic violence is strongly associated with psychiatric morbidity; antenatal and postnatal depressive symptoms may be the only presenting feature.

Late booking, threatened preterm labour, back pain, headaches and hyperemesis have all been associated with a history of domestic violence within the preceding 12 months. Physical abuse during pregnancy has been associated with fetal growth restriction, preterm labour, placental abruption, fetal fractures, miscarriage, stillbirth and maternal mortality – in addition to traumatic injuries to the mother. The incidence of preterm labour in women with a history of domestic abuse is 17%, four times higher than in women with no history of domestic abuse. A study looking at spousal violence in Sub-Saharan Africa suggested that the rate of stillbirth and miscarriage may be increased by 50% in women who suffer abuse during pregnancy.

Maternal mortality

Domestic homicide is a leading cause of maternal mortality. The Saving Mother's Lives Report from the triennium 2006–2008 reported that 12% of women who died during or after pregnancy (n = 39) had a history of domestic abuse, with eight women being murdered by their partner. 38% of these women had been late bookers or poor attendees for antenatal care. Many cases of maternal mortality were women who found it difficult to seek or maintain contact with maternity or other health services.

Child health

Children who witness domestic abuse are more likely to develop emotional, behavioural and learning problems. It is unclear if this is due to prenatal stress and adverse obstetric outcomes affecting fetal neurological development, the effects of abuse upon the bond between mother and baby or the coexistence of antenatal and postnatal psychiatric disorders in the mother.

Detection

The Royal College of Obstetricians and Gynaecologists and the recommendations of the triennial Centre for Maternal and Child Enquiries (CMACE) report advise routine enquiry as most women will not disclose abuse unless asked directly. All women attending for antenatal care must be 'asked the question' and be seen alone at least once during the course of the pregnancy. Sensitive questioning should take place if injuries are noted and all pregnant women should be given advice regarding domestic abuse. Local sources of help and emergency helpline telephone numbers should be displayed in suitable places in the antenatal clinic, e.g. the ladies' toilet. Indicators that domestic abuse may be occurring are show in **Table 37**.

Coercive relationships or forced marriage are closely linked to violence against women and clinicians should be alert to suspicious factors, such as patients who are:

- Quiet or display submissive behaviour

- Young with a history of multiple pregnancies
- Always accompanied to appointments/ have a controlling partner or carer
- Require translations because of cultural or language barriers

Family or partners should not be used for translation purposes. External interpretation services must be utilised. If coercive relationships are suspected clinicians should ensure documentation of next of kin, partner details and living arrangements. Concerns should be recorded in confidential notes, safeguarding teams should be notified, all injuries should be recorded and concerns should be shared with appropriate professionals such as the general practitioner (GP). The appropriate agencies should be contacted such as the Forced Marriage Unit.

Management

The role of health care professionals is key. Women want their experiences validated – they want to be believed and taken seriously. A negative or judgemental response from a health care professional may perpetuate the abusive power dynamics to which they are subject at home. The response must also be appropriate and effective. Women must be offered support, advice and thorough documentation of what they report. Documentation may provide key legal evidence in the event of a future court case.

Table 37　Indicators of domestic abuse in maternity care
Late booking and/or poor attendance at antenatal clinic
Unexplained admissions
Repeated attendances for seemingly trivial problems (e.g., at the general practitioner, antenatal clinic, emergency department)
Repeated presentations with psychological complaints
Self-discharging from hospital
Injuries of varying ages
Poor obstetric history (repeated miscarriage/ terminations, stillbirth, preterm labour)
Constant presence of partner
Patient reluctant to speak during consultations

Antenatal care

The NICE guideline on pregnant women with complex social factors addresses the needs of women who experience domestic abuse with specific recommendations to:

- Liaise with local support agencies to provide coordinated care for service users
- Develop a local protocol
- Offer a named midwife to provide the majority of antenatal care
- Offer women appropriate opportunity to disclose abuse in a secure environment
- Provide training for health care professionals
- Offer confidentiality, information and support

If domestic abuse is disclosed women should not be booked as 'low risk', and there must be an appropriate method of recording the disclosure on antenatal records but not in handheld records. Local strategies must be in place for referral to local multidisciplinary support networks. Inappropriate responses or advice from health care professionals can worsen the situation, e.g. confronting the partner. Appropriate referrals and advice should be given, e.g. Women's Aid Organisation (WAO), offer to contact the police, Multi-Agency Risk Assessment Conference (MARAC) notification.

The MARAC is part of a coordinated community response to domestic abuse, which aims to:

- Share information
- Determine whether the alleged perpetrator poses a significant risk
- Construct and implement a risk management plan
- Reduce repeat victimisation
- Improve agency accountability
- Improve support for staff involved in high risk domestic abuse cases

Women must understand the limits of confidentiality, as under the child protection act social services must be alerted if there are concerns about children within the home.

Further reading

NICE Clinical Guideline No. 110. Pregnancy and complex social factors. London: NICE, 2010.

Aston G, Bewley S. Abortion and domestic violence. The Obstetrician & Gynaecologist 2009; 11:163–168.

Bacchus L, Bewley S, Mezey G. Domestic violence and pregnancy. The Obstetrician & Gynaecologist 2001; 3:56–59.

Cantwell R, et al. Saving Mothers' Lives: Reviewing maternal deaths to make motherhood safer: 2006-2008. The Eighth Report of the Confidential Enquiries into Maternal Deaths in the United Kingdom. BJOG 2011; 118 (1):1–203.

Related topics of interest

- Preterm labour (p. 294)
- Maternal death (p. 255)
- Female genital mutilation (p. 41)

Dysfunctional labour

Overview

Dysfunctional labour describe a deviation away from the normal processes of labour. There are three main disorders contributing to dysfunctional labour:

- Prolonged latent phase of labour
- Primary dysfunctional labour
- Secondary arrest of labour

As progress in labour can be evaluated in terms of the 3 P's that is the passages (the bony pelvis and adjacent soft tissues), the passenger (the fetus) and the powers (the uterine contractions), dysfunctional labour can also be defined in relation to these, e.g. inadequate contractions.

Aetiology

Prolonged latent phase   This is the period of time during which cervical remodelling occurs to result in effacement and dilatation up to 3–4 cm. Women experience painful contractions and it can be lengthy, making it very distressing. Friedman described it as lasting up to 20 hours in nulliparous and 14 hours in multiparous women.

Management should be via reassurance and support, analgesia, and encourage adequate hydration, nutrition and mobilisation. Temptation to intervene by artificial rupture of membranes and augmentation with oxytocin should be resisted, as these do not increase the vaginal delivery rate, but instead cause a 10-fold increase in the rate of caesarean section.

Primary dysfunctional labour   This is defined as slow progress in the active first or second stage of labour. It affects up to 26% of nulliparous and 8% of multiparous women. While no single cause is responsible for all cases, the majority of cases will respond to augmentation with oxytocin. Other interventions include improvement of hydration and provision of one-to-one care. Ultimately, delivery may require caesarean section.

Secondary arrest   This is a cessation of cervical dilatation following a previously normal period of active first stage of labour. This is more likely to be associated with an underlying problem such as relative or absolute cephalopelvic disproportion (CPD). It can be described in terms of the 3 P's

- The passage
  There may be abnormalities in the shape of the pelvis, which do not allow normal progress through the pelvis. Congenital abnormalities of the pelvis such as Naegele's pelvis or acquired disorders such as pelvic fracture can contribute to CPD. Soft tissue abnormalities such as pelvic masses or vaginal septums can also impede passage of the fetus through the pelvis
- The passenger
  There are several potential causes of poor progress that can be attributed to the fetus. Malpresentation and malposition may contribute (see Topic 77 malpresentation and malposition). Macrosomia due to maternal diabetes or malformations such as hydrocephalus can cause CPD
- The powers
  This relates to the finding of inefficient uterine contractions, and augmentation of contractions with oxytocin is the only component that can be directly manipulated in dysfunctional labour, although there is evidence that administration of oxytocin has no effect on the incidence of obstetric intervention.

Diagnosis

Delay in the first stage of labour is defined as dilatation of < 2 cm in 4 hours in nulliparous women and cervical dilatation of < 2 cm in 4 hours or slowing of progress of labour in second or subsequent labours. The second stage is delayed if a nulliparous woman has not delivered within 2 hours of the onset of the active second stage of labour and if the multiparous woman has not delivered within 1 hour of the onset of the active second stage. This should prompt review by a health care professional trained in operative vaginal delivery.

Management

Delay in the first stage

Conservative measures should be adopted in the first instance. Rehydration may be all that is required to correct dysfunctional labour. Monitoring via a fluid balance chart and regular urinalysis looking for ketosis is important. Provision of one-to-one care by a caregiver other than the woman's birth partner has been shown to reduce the need for pain relief, reduce the likelihood of operative vaginal delivery and caesarean section and achieve a slight reduction in overall length of labour as well as improved Apgar scores. Pain may suppress uterine activity via the autonomic nervous system. Therefore, the provision of pain relief may have an impact in improving uterine contractions and progress in labour.

Before an intervention is considered, a careful abdominal and vaginal examination should be undertaken. Amniotomy should be performed if there is delay in the first stage of labour. The woman should be re-examined 2 hours later and if unsatisfactory progress has been made, consideration for intravenous oxytocin should be made. This can safely be used at any stage of dilatation in the nulliparous woman but caution should be applied before commencing it in multiparous women. This is especially true if they have made normal progress in the earlier stages of labour (i.e. have secondary arrest of labour). Multiparous women are at increased risk of uterine rupture following augmentation and if there is any suggestion of CPD, they should be delivered by caesarean section.

Oxytocin is given as an infusion of 10 IU in 500 mL of Hartmann's or 0.9% saline and commenced at a low rate. It should not be increased any more frequently that every 30 minutes in the first stage and titrated to achieve 4–5 contractions in 10 minutes. This helps to reduce the risk of hyperstimulation and if this occurs, the rate of oxytocin should be reduced. Vaginal examination should be repeated at 4 hourly intervals following initiation of oxytocin. The Royal College of Obstetricians and Gynaecologists (RCOG) recommends that caesarean section should not be considered in a nulliparous woman with dysfunctional labour without first trying augmentation with oxytocin.

Delay in the second stage

In nulliparous women, oxytocin can be commenced in the second stage if contractions are felt to be inadequate or malposition is present. If after 1 hour of pushing, the vertex is not visible, it would be appropriate to commence oxytocin. If delivery has not occurred in the presence of adequate contractions, a careful clinical assessment should be performed and if appropriate, operative vaginal delivery should be attempted. If operative vaginal delivery cannot be safely performed then the infant should be delivered by caesarean section.

In multiparous women with delay in the second stage, an experienced clinician should carry out a full clinical examination, with consideration as to whether an operative vaginal delivery is possible and safe. If it is not, caesarean section should be performed.

Further reading

National Collaborating Centre for Woman's and Children's Health. Intrapartum care: management and delivery of care to women in labour. NICE Clinical guideline no. 55. London: RCOG, 2008.

Luesley DM, Baker PN. Obstetrics and Gynaecology: an evidence-based text for MRCOG. 2nd edn. London: Hodder Arnold, 2010.

Friedman EA. Primagravid labor. Obstet Gynecol 1955; 6:567–589.

Hinshaw K, Simpson S, Cummings S, et al. A randomised controlled trial of early versus delayed oxytocin augmentation to treat primary dysfunctional labour in nulliparous women. BJOG 2008; 115(10):1289–1295.

Related topics of interest

Fetal growth restriction

Overview

Fetal growth restriction (FGR) (also referred to as intrauterine growth restriction) is an important condition affecting 5–8% of pregnancies; it is associated with increased perinatal mortality, iatrogenic preterm birth, intrapartum hypoxia, neurodevelopmental disorders and increased risk of diabetes and cardiovascular disease in later life.

FGR is not the same as being small for gestational age (SGA). SGA describes fetuses that are below a specific biometric measurement (e.g. estimated fetal weight). Various definitions of SGA exist including: < 10th centile, < 2 standard deviations below average. FGR describes fetuses that are failing to grow. The more severe the SGA, the greater the likelihood of FGR (20–30% of babies < 10th centile have FGR, 70% of babies < 3rd centile have FGR). However, not all FGR fetuses are SGA. For example, a fetus that was initially on the 80th centile, whose growth ceased and was on the 20th centile at delivery, would have FGR but not SGA.

Aetiology and epidemiology

SGA infants may be constitutionally small, have chromosomal abnormalities or have FGR. FGR is strongly associated with placental insufficiency.

Risk factors for FGR include: FGR in a previous pregnancy, previous stillbirth, teenage pregnancy, maternal age > 40 years, extremes of body mass index (underweight/obesity), cigarette smoking, alcohol or drug misuse, maternal medical disorders such as hypertension, renal disease, cardiac disease, diabetes and some thrombophilias, e.g. antiphospholipid syndrome, antithrombin III deficiency. FGR is increased in multiple pregnancies.

Diagnosis

Abdominal palpation alone has limited accuracy to predict a SGA/FGR fetus; it detects as few as 30% of small fetuses.

Similarly, symphysis-fundal height (SFH) measurement has limited accuracy to predict SGA infant (sensitivity 27–86%, specificity 80–93%). The sensitivity and specificity are improved by the use of customised growth charts that adjust for parity, ethnicity and maternal height and weight. However, measurement of SFH is a useful test to suspect SGA.

Ultrasound measurement of fetal biometry (usually abdominal circumference, head circumference and femur length, and the estimated fetal weight) is the gold standard investigation for suspected SGA. The individual components can be plotted to normal values, and estimated fetal weight plotted on a customised growth chart. The assessment of fetal growth should take into account growth velocity; hence serial ultrasound measurements have better prediction for FGR than one off evaluation. However, routine ultrasound measurement after 24 weeks of gestation does not improve pregnancy outcome.

More recently there has been significant interest in predicting pregnancies that will develop FGR before the onset of disease; these have focussed on tests which may indicate abnormal placental development. Pregnancies where alpha-fetoprotein is elevated > 2.5 multiples of the median (MoM) on the quadruple test (early second trimester) and there is no fetal anomaly have an increased risk of FGR (5–10x). Second-trimester uterine artery Doppler notching is a weak predictor of FGR (likelihood ratio = 3.6) as is isolated oligohydramnios (likelihood ratio = 2.3). Women who present with reduced fetal movements have a 2–3-fold increased risk of FGR. Other tests including placental growth factor (PlGF) and metabolomic analyses are still at the developmental stage, but may offer novel strategies to predict FGR.

Where there is severe early onset FGR (< 24 weeks) or there is also evidence of structural anomaly, chromosomal analysis by amniocentesis should be offered.

Management

Following the diagnosis of FGR the primary surveillance tool is umbilical artery Doppler; this reduces perinatal morbidity and mortality and is able to reliably predict poor perinatal outcomes in SGA fetuses. Umbilical artery Doppler assesses placental resistance which is increased in FGR due to altered placental vascular function, placental infarction and fibrin deposition.

Absent or reversed end-diastolic flow (EDF) is associated with increased perinatal morbidity and mortality [odds ratio = 4.0 (absent EDF) 10.6 (reversed EDF)]. Infants with abnormal EDF also have poorer neonatal outcome with increased risk of intraventricular haemorrhage, necrotising enterocolitis and hypoglycaemia.

The time interval between abnormal umbilical artery Doppler and changes in cardiotocograhpy (CTG)/biophysical profile indicating hypoxaemia ranges from 1–26 days. This makes determining the optimal time for delivery difficult, particularly in extremely preterm infants with FGR.

In addition to umbilical artery Doppler, liquor volume measured by amniotic fluid index or maximum pool depth may be used for fetal surveillance. Oligohydramnios (amniotic fluid index < 5 cm) is associated with increased perinatal morbidity in association with SGA/FGR.

Ultrasound biophysical profile is rarely abnormal when the umbilical artery Doppler is normal, but can add valuable information in preterm infants with absent EDF. The use of intermittent CTG has no positive effect on fetal outcome, but there is evidence that computerised analysis of the CTG using Dawes-Redman criteria may improve fetal outcome. The findings of the TRUFFLE study, which will compare timing of delivery based on short-term variability on CTG or on ductus venosus Doppler, are due to be reported in 2013.

The optimal frequency of ultrasound assessment is uncertain. When umbilical artery Doppler is abnormal this is usually every 2–3 days.

Several interventions have been used without success to improve the outcome of FGR after diagnosis, all attempted to increase uteroplacental perfusion. The following interventions should therefore not be used: hospitalisation for bed rest, beta-sympathomimetics, calcium channel blockers, oxygen, nutritional supplementation and aspirin. Currently there are studies to determine whether sildenafil (Viagra) can be used to increase uterine perfusion and treat severe early onset FGR.

Management of delivery

The optimal timing of delivery in FGR is uncertain, particularly in extremely preterm infants which have a high perinatal mortality and morbidity which is worsened in FGR and acidaemia. Therefore, parents should be carefully counselled and their wishes respected. Given the high incidence of neurodisability in extremely preterm FGR infants, conservative management is acceptable.

Draper et al. published tables of gestation and birthweight specific survival for different genders and ethnicities. These can be used to counsel parents about the likely survival rates.

The Growth Restriction Intervention Trial (GRIT) recruited women with FGR between 24–36 weeks when the clinician was uncertain whether to deliver. Women were randomised to immediate delivery or delivery when there was no uncertainty. There was no difference in perinatal mortality or long term disability between early or delayed delivery.

The DIGITAT study randomised 650 women with FGR over 36 weeks' gestation to induction of labour versus expectant management. There was no difference in perinatal mortality, caesarean section or instrumental delivery rate between the two groups. The induction group had lower birth weight (–130 g) and more immediate NICU admissions, but the expectant group had higher later NICU admissions and longer stays.

Current recommendations suggest that when umbilical EDF is normal then delivery is not indicated until 37 weeks. If expectant management is to be pursued, other methods of fetal surveillance should be used (although the evidence of value is weak): biophysical profile/ductus venosus Doppler, fetal movements, CTG.

When there is absent or reversed EDF < 34 weeks of gestation other methods of surveillance should be used including biophysical profile, ductus venosus Doppler, CTG, maternal hypertension. If any of these other surveillance methods also become abnormal then the infant should be delivered. When the infant is < 34 weeks and/or very small elective caesarean section should be considered.

If preterm delivery is planned corticosteroids should be administered to reduce the incidence of respiratory distress. Intravenous magnesium sulphate should be contemplated to reduce the risk of cerebral palsy in preterm infants.

Over 34 weeks' gestation, delivery should be considered even if other surveillance is normal. If induction of labour is planned, continuous fetal monitoring should be used in labour because of the increased risk of fetal acidaemia.

Delivery should occur where appropriate neonatal care is available and a skilled resuscitator should be present at the birth.

Further reading

Royal College of Obstetricians and Gynaecologists. The Investigation and Management of the Small for Gestational Age Fetus – Guideline 31. London: RCOG, 2013.

GRIT study group. A randomised trial of timed delivery for the compromised preterm fetus: short term outcomes and Bayesian interpretation. BJOG 2003; 110(1):27–32.

Thornton JG, Hornbuckle J, Vail A, et al. GRIT study group. Infant wellbeing at 2 years of age in the Growth Restriction Intervention Trial (GRIT): multicentre randomised controlled trial. Lancet 2004; 364(9433):513–520.

Boers KE, et al. Induction versus expectant monitoring for intrauterine growth restriction at term: randomised equivalence trial (DIGITAT). BMJ 2010; 341:c7087.

Alfirevic Z, Stampalija T, Gyte GM. Fetal and umbilical Doppler ultrasound in high-risk pregnancies. Cochrane Database of Systematic Reviews 2010; 1. CD007529.

Draper ES, et al. Prediction of survival for preterm births by weight and gestational age: retrospective population based study. BMJ 1999; 319:1093–1097.

Related topics of interest

Epilepsy in pregnancy

Overview

Approximately 0.5% of women of child-bearing age have epilepsy, making it the commonest neurological condition seen in pregnancy. Women with epilepsy have an increased risk of fetal anomaly and increased fit frequency in pregnancy (25–30%). In addition, pregnancy can alter the metabolism of antiepileptic drugs (AEDs). In the last Triennial report [Centre for Maternal and Child Enquiries (CMACE), 2011)], there were 14 maternal deaths from complications of epilepsy in pregnancy in the United Kingdom; of these cases 57% had not been reviewed by a neurologist. Consequently, multidisciplinary care is recommended in these patients.

Preconception counselling

In epilepsy, preconception counselling should: (i) establish the frequency and type of seizures, (ii) the current medication regimen, and (iii) if the patient has a regular review by a neurologist. In addition, women should be informed of an increased risk of congenital malformations, primarily neural tube defects, congenital heart defects and orofacial clefts. The risk of structural abnormalities is about 6–7% for one drug use, 15% for two drugs, against a background risk of 3%. There is a 5% risk of seizures in the child. To minimise the risk of neural tube defects 5 mg folic acid once a day should be after with cessation of contraceptive use. This should be continued throughout the pregnancy.

An attempt should be made to reduce the number of AEDs taken, and convert sodium valproate or phenytoin to AEDs with lower risks of fetal abnormalities, with advice from a neurologist. If medication is continued, increased seizure frequency is uncommon. In tonic-clonic seizures, the fetus may be at risk (of hypoxia) at the time of seizure, but this is low. In partial, absence or myoclonic seizures there is no risk to the fetus, other than as a consequence of a potential fall. However, there is a risk of sudden unexplained death in epilepsy (SUDEP), especially if medication is stopped suddenly. Women should be advised not to stop AEDs abruptly.

Antenatal management

- If preconception counselling has not occurred, then discussions about the risk of congenital anomaly and SUDEP should take place
- Folic acid 5 mg once a day should be prescribed for the whole duration of pregnancy
- Women should be made aware of the UK epilepsy and pregnancies register, and should be advised to register their pregnancy, or allow their clinician to do so
- The fetal anomaly scan, performed between 18 and 20^{+6} weeks should be offered to screen for congenital structural anomalies
- Women should have regular antenatal visits (24, 28, 32, 36 and weekly thereafter) on an individualised basis. This should include serial growth scans, as women with epilepsy are at increased risk of fetal growth restriction
- Routine monitoring of drug levels is not usually required. If seizure frequency is increased, drug levels should be checked and a neurologist consulted regarding ongoing AED therapy
- For women taking enzyme inducing AEDs (see specific section below), oral vitamin K 10 mg should be given once daily, from 36 weeks' gestation. Intramuscular administration of vitamin K should also be discussed, because of the increased risk of neonatal intracranial haemorrhage

AEDs in pregnancy

Enzyme inducing AEDs include: carbamazepine, oxcarbazepine, phenytoin, phenobarbitone, primidone and topiramate. Newer AEDs include: lamotrigine, gabapentin and tiagabine. All AEDs have a combined risk of major malformation of 4.6%. Sodium valproate alone has a risk of 8.7%, with a reduction in full scale IQ. Carbamazepine alone has a 2.9–3.3% risk, with no effect on IQ. Lamotrigine has a 2.7% risk. If the woman is currently taking sodium valproate, better control in pregnancy has been noted with slow release valproate medication, equally with slow release carbamazepine. Guidance from a neurologist prior to altering medication is essential.

Physiological changes in pregnancy [increased volume of distribution, altered metabolism, increased glomerular filtration rate (GFR)] lead to altered drug levels. Measurement of drug levels are not required if a woman is seizure-free; however, regular levels should be obtained in women with frequent seizures, and an increase in drug dosage may be required during pregnancy. Women should continue with their medication in labour, and repeat the dose if they vomit within an hour of taking their medicine.

Management of seizures

- In labour, 3.5% of women with epilepsy will have a seizure
- To reduce the risk of seizures, the woman should be well hydrated, have adequate pain relief and avoid sleep deprivation
- The initial management is the same as the management of maternal collapse. Secure the airway, breathing, circulation and intravenous access
- Treat seizures with IV lorazepam 4 mg or IV diazepam 10 mg. Lorazepam is preferable as it causes less sedation. Eclampsia should always be considered; however in a known epileptic with no hypertension, or

proteinuria treat as epilepsy. If uncertain, manage also as eclampsia

Postnatal management

- In the first 24 hours following delivery, 1–2% of women will have a seizure
- Women should be educated to minimise precipitating factors, including: sleep deprivation, excessive tiredness and dehydration
- Women should be encouraged to continue with their AEDs, and if doses have been increased in pregnancy, they may require reducing in the postnatal period
- Breastfeeding should be encouraged; most AEDs are excreted into breast milk but the dose is lower than in utero exposure
- General safety advice should be given to reduce potential risks of drowning, or injury to mother or baby. Advice includes to feed and change the baby on the floor, and not to bathe the baby or herself if alone
- Contraceptive advice should also be given. If the woman is taking enzyme-inducing AEDs, then the progesterone-only pill and progesterone implant should not be used. Depot progesterone injections should be given more frequently (every 10 weeks, as opposed to 12 weeks). If using the combined oral contraceptive pill, a higher dose of oestrogen is required. The minimum dose of ethinyl oestradiol is 50 µg, this can be increased to 75 or 100 µg if there is breakthrough bleeding.

Further reading

Cantwell R, et al. Saving Mothers' Lives: Reviewing maternal deaths to make motherhood safer: 2006-2008. The Eighth Report of the Confidential Enquiries into Maternal Deaths in the United Kingdom. BJOG 2011; 118 (1):1–203.
Nelson-Piercy C. Handbook of Obstetric Medicine, 2nd edn. Martin Dunitz Ltd, 2002:156–164.

NICE Clinical Guideline No. 137. Epilepsy. London: NICE, 2012.
Tomson T, Landmark CJ, Battino D. Antiepileptic drug treatment in pregnancy: changes in drug disposition and their clinical implications. Epilepsia 2013; 54(3):405–414.

Related topics of interest

- Teratogenic agents (p. 326)

Feticide and late termination of pregnancy

Overview

Termination of pregnancy (TOP) can be highly emotive for patients and medical professionals alike. Therefore, when discussing TOP it is important to be mindful of and sensitive to the perspective of others, whilst not prejudging a person's stance on TOP based on their ethnicity, age or religious background.

Under UK law, the 1967 Abortion Act (applicable in England, Scotland and Wales) states that a pregnancy can be legally terminated provided two registered medical practitioners are of the opinion the request satisfies one of the four clauses stipulated by the Act. The Abortion Act clauses are as follows:

a. That the pregnancy has not exceeded its 24th week and that the continuance of the pregnancy would involve risk, greater than if the pregnancy were terminated, of injury to the physical or mental health of the pregnant woman or any existing children of her family; or
b. That the termination is necessary to prevent grave permanent injury to the physical or mental health of the pregnant woman; or
c. That the continuance of the pregnancy would involve risk to the life of the pregnant woman, greater than if the pregnancy were terminated; or
d. That there is a substantial risk that if the child was born it would suffer from such physical or mental abnormalities as to be seriously handicapped

Indications

A request to terminate an unwanted pregnancy is usually covered by clause (a) provided two medical practitioners are in agreement and is not permissible once the pregnancy has completed 24 weeks.

Requests for TOP for unwanted pregnancies in the late second trimester are contentious and it may be difficult to obtain two medical practitioners willing to agree to such a request or indeed a National Health Service (NHS) facility that would offer such a service.

Where there is a risk of significant maternal morbidity or mortality by continuing the pregnancy, termination can be offered under clauses (b) and (c). At the limits of viability this can be a very difficult decision for the woman and her health care providers to make, and would ultimately require senior multidisciplinary involvement.

Department of Health statistics (Abortion Statistics, England and Wales, 2011) published in May 2012 state that approximately 98% (n = 185,973) terminations were carried out under clause (a) and 1% (n = 1,455) were undertaken to prevent serious maternal morbidity/mortality.

TOP can be offered at any gestation under clause (d) where there is a fetal abnormality leading to a significant risk of fetal disability. However, there is no legislation to define what constitutes 'significant risk' or 'handicap' and consequently this is a matter of judgement for clinicians and parents. When considering handicap and justification for termination of pregnancy, consideration should be given to the long term survival of a condition, the potential for treatment in utero or after delivery, the degree of suffering the individual would endure after birth and the ability for independent adult life.

Feticide

Some conditions for which late TOP may be offered will often result in the demise of the fetus during delivery or very shortly after birth (e.g. anencephaly, severe cardiac anomaly).

However, when TOP is performed for a condition such as ventriculomegaly or chromosomal abnormalities, there is a strong possibility that the fetus will survive delivery and be born alive, particularly at advanced gestations. This scenario is extremely difficult as neonatal staff are then legally obliged to deliver supportive medical care to the infant. In addition, the psychological impact of witnessing signs of life in a fetus delivered as a result of a termination can be devastating for parents and staff caring for the woman.

Therefore, the Royal College of Obstetricians and Gynaecologists (RCOG) recommend that any feticide is performed for any TOP taking place beyond 21weeks and 6 days of pregnancy to ensure fetal death prior to the delivery of the fetus.

The process of undergoing feticide is emotionally difficult and women who undergo this procedure require sympathetic counselling prior to the procedure.

Feticide should be performed in a specialised fetal medicine facility under aseptic conditions with continuous ultrasound guidance.

The procedure involves the administration of 15% potassium chloride (KCl) directly in the fetal heart or umbilical vein via a needle passed through the maternal abdomen. The volume of KCl administered to achieve asystole is in the range of 2–10 mL. Fetal asystole should be observed for 2 minutes and then confirmed by a repeat scan approximately 30 minutes later. Following the confirmation of fetal demise, the woman should then proceed with the process of medical management of the termination according to protocols appropriate for the gestation of the pregnancy.

Late TOP

There is currently no definition of the gestation which differentiates early from late TOP. However, medical and ethical difficulties increase with advancing gestation. Statham et al. (2006) described the varying attitudes and acceptability amongst specialists within UK fetal medicine centres with regards to when and for what conditions they would offer late TOP involving feticide.

Methods of TOP also vary with gestational age. Between 13 and 24 weeks, RCOG recommend mifepristone 200 mg orally, followed 36–48 hours later by misoprostol 800 μg vaginally, then misoprostol 400 μg orally or vaginally, 3-hourly, to a maximum of four further doses. Beyond 24 weeks, induction of labour would follow local policy.

Beyond 14 weeks of pregnancy, surgical TOP by vacuum aspiration is not recommended. Instead, dilation and evacuation of the uterus under continuous ultrasound guidance is performed. However, there are few operators within NHS facilities that are sufficiently experienced to provide this service. Women opting for this method should be reminded that this destructive method can limit postnatal investigations should they be desired.

Counselling and postdelivery care

Ideally, women should have been fully counselled about TOP prior to the procedure, particularly when performed for a fetal abnormality. Subjects such as seeing or holding the baby should be handled sensitively. When the TOP has been performed for a fetal abnormality, issues such as postmortem examination of the fetus, genetic assessment and chromosomal analysis should be discussed prior to discharge from hospital.

Routine postdelivery management should take place such as: anti-D prophylaxis in Rh negative women, offer cabergoline at advanced gestation to prevent the production of breast milk. It may also be appropriate to discuss contraception.

It is important to ensure that women undergoing TOP for fetal abnormalities have follow up arrangements made, ideally with the health care professional that cared for them during the pregnancy. At this meeting results of fetal investigations can be discussed and information given regarding recurrence risk and management of subsequent pregnancies.

Further reading

British Medical Association. The Law and Ethics of Abortion. BMA views. London: BMA, 2007.

Termination of Pregnancy for a Fetal Abnormality in England, Scotland and Wales, RCOG Working Party Report. London: RCOG, 2010.

Statham H, Solomou W, Green J. Late termination of pregnancy: law, policy and decision making in four English fetal medicine units. BJOG: An International Journal of Obstetrics & Gynaecology 2006; 113:1402–1411.

Related topics of interest

- Hydrops fetalis (p. 237)
- Invasive fetal testing (p. 250)

HIV in pregnancy

Overview

The incidence of HIV infection worldwide is increasing with two-thirds of those infected living in Sub-Saharan Africa. In the past 4 years, the numbers of new infections in adults have stabilised at about 2.5 million cases a year. At the end of 2010, there were about 95,000 HIV positive people in the UK with 24% of them undiagnosed. There were 6660 new diagnoses within the year; 32% were women and 50% were late diagnoses. The prevalence amongst pregnant women in the UK is 3.8 per 1000 in London and 1.1 per 1000 outside London.

In high-income countries HIV infection is now considered a chronic infection or carrier state because of early diagnosis and effective drug therapy. Appropriate drug treatment in pregnancy combined with appropriate mode of delivery, prophylaxis for the child and avoidance of breastfeeding can reduce the risk of vertical transmission from 15–25% to < 2%.

Screening

Screening for HIV should be offered to all pregnant women at booking and if negative, offered a repeat at 34–36 weeks for those at high risk. Those who decline testing at booking should be offered a test later and if they still refuse a third offer of testing should be offered at 36 weeks. A point of care test should be offered for women who first present to antenatal services in labour.

Screening is important both for maternal health and to prevent vertical transmission. About 20–30% of women who are found to be HIV positive on screening are not aware of their diagnosis, with significant risk of vertical transmission to their babies. The risk of vertical transmission could be significantly reduced if they are diagnosed and commenced on antiretroviral treatment and the babies receive postexposure prophylaxis at birth.

Management of HIV in pregnancy

The management of pregnant women with HIV should be multidisciplinary, involving: an obstetrician with a special interest in HIV, infectious disease/genitourinary medicine physicians, paediatricians that look after children with HIV, specialist midwives, counsellors and social workers.

The use of highly active antiretroviral therapy (HAART) can significantly reduce the risk of vertical transmission. Women who are currently on an effective HAART prior to conception should continue with this regimen. Those diagnosed in pregnancy should be offered sexual health and infectious disease screening including hepatitis B and C, herpes simplex virus, toxoplasma and herpes varicella zoster. Women should be commenced on HAART as early possible if they need it for maternal reasons, e.g. if CD4 count ≤ 350 cells/μL or ≤ 500 cells/μL if coinfected with hepatitis B or C.

All pregnant women should be on HAART by 24 weeks to prevent vertical transmission. Resistance testing should be done before commencing treatment. Liver function tests should be performed at initiation of HAART and at each visit as treatment could lead to deranged liver function. It is important to determine whether any derangement is secondary to treatment or caused by obstetric complications such as pre-eclampsia, HELLP syndrome, obstetric cholestasis or acute fatty liver of pregnancy. Adherence to medication especially with vomiting in early pregnancy and interaction with other medication should be reviewed.

Preventing vertical transmission

Vertical transmission can occur antepartum, intrapartum and postpartum with the greatest risk intrapartum and subsequently with breastfeeding. Risk factors for transmission include high viral load (VL), seroconversion in pregnancy, prolonged rupture of membranes, prematurity, vaginal delivery, concomitant sexually transmitted infections, chorioamnionitis and low birthweight.

The intrapartum risk can be reduced with antenatal treatment with HAART and the reduction of maternal VL. VL should be checked 2–4 weeks after commencing HAART, at least once every trimester, at 36 weeks and at delivery. If the VL is not < 50 HIV RNA copies/mL at 36 weeks, then check adherence and concomitant medication, resistance testing, therapeutic dose monitoring, consider optimising regimen or intensification.

Planning for delivery

The mode of delivery should be decided at 36 weeks based on VL and obstetric history. Vaginal delivery is suitable for women with VL < 50 HIV RNA copies/mL at 36 weeks if there are no other obstetric contraindications. They should have a point of care test at presentation in labour. Fetal blood sampling, the use of fetal scalp electrode and instrumental delivery except for low forceps delivery should be avoided. Labour should be induced immediately after prelabour spontaneous rupture of membranes at term, with antibiotics considered 4 hours postrupture if not delivered. No antiviral treatment is required in labour as long as the patient continues with her regular HAART medication. HIV is not a contraindication to vaginal birth after caesarean section.

If VL > 50 HIV RNA copies/mL at 36 weeks, then a planned caesarean section at 38–39 weeks should be organised. The patient should have intravenous zidovudine prior to delivery. If there is rupture of membranes then urgent caesarean section after intravenous zidovudine should be considered. Prelabour preterm rupture of membranes (PPROM) at < 34 weeks should be managed with intramuscular cortico steroids for fetal lung maturity and antibiotics in line with routine management of PPROM, HIV treatment optimised and a multidisciplinary decision made on the timing and mode of delivery.

There is no contraindication to external cephalic version in HIV patients.

Neonatal care

The aim of neonatal care is to assess whether vertical transmission has occurred and to reduce this risk postnatally. Infant postexposure prophylaxis should be initiated to reduce the incidence of transmission. Oral zidovudine monotherapy should be initiated within 4 hours of delivery if maternal VL < 50 HIV RNA copies/mL at 36 weeks or just before delivery. Triple drug therapy should be initiated if the mother was untreated or VL > 50 HIV RNA copies/mL at 36 weeks or at delivery.

All HIV positive mothers should be encouraged to exclusively formula feed from birth rather than breastfeed irrespective of whether they are on HAART or the baby is receiving postexposure prophylaxis. The mothers should receive cabergoline within 24 hours of delivery to prevent lactation. The babies should be washed prior to having injections such as vitamin K. They should have the regular national immunisation schedule.

The infant should be tested for HIV by DNA PCR (or HIV RNA) within 48 hours of birth and at 6 and 12 weeks of age. Seroconversion status is assessed at 18 months of life by HIV antibody testing. Maternal HIV antibody may persist in the child's blood for up to 18 months.

Further reading

Taylor GP, Clayden P, Dhar J, et al. British HIV Association guidelines for the management of HIV infection in pregnant women 2012. HIV Med 2012; 13(2):87–157.

Williams I, Churchill D, Anderson J, et al. British HIV Association guidelines for the treatment of HIV-1 positive adults with antiretroviral therapy 2012. HIV Med 2012; 13(2):1–85.

Nelson-Piercy C. Handbook of Obstetric Medicine, 4th edn. London: Informa Healthcare, 2010; 258–265.

Related topics of interest

- Antenatal care (p. 183)
- Infection in pregnancy (p. 243)
- Sexually transmitted infection (p. 135)

Hydrops fetalis

Overview

Hydrops fetalis describes accumulation of fluid in at least two serous cavities in the fetus. This can include subcutaneous skin oedema, pleural effusion (**Figure 21**), pericardial effusion or ascites. There may be associated polyhydramnios and/or placental oedema.

Hydrops fetalis is sub-divided into two categories: immune and non-immune hydrops.

Clinical features

In general, the diagnosis of hydrops fetalis is made following an ultrasound scan of the fetus and often is detected after routine first or second trimester scans. However, clinical features which may prompt an additional scan include reduced fetal movements or a clinical suspicion of polyhydramnios. Hydrops fetalis may be detected by ultrasound screening after parvovirus infection is known to have occurred during pregnancy. Hydrops may also be seen after an abnormal fetal heart rate (tachycardia or bradycardia) is heard on auscultation of the fetal heart during antenatal care.

Aetiology

Immune fetal hydrops occurs when there is incompatibility between maternal and fetal blood groups. When the mother is sensitised, circulating red cell antibodies are able to cross the placenta and destroy fetal red blood cells. The haemolysis of fetal blood cells leads to fetal anaemia and if severe enough, will result in hydrops. The most common and clinically significant alloantibodies are anti-D, anti-C, anti-Kell and anti-E. A multitude of atypical red cell antibodies have been described and have the potential to cause haemolytic disease of the fetus and newborn (HDFN) but these are rare and the effects are generally mild. Whilst anti-D remains the most common cause of immune fetal hydrops, the widespread introduction of routine prophylactic anti-D to Rhesus negative women has greatly reduced the incidence over the last 40 years.

Non-immune hydrops is a heterogenous disorder which has a wide variety of potential underlying causes, examples of which are shown in **Table 38**.

Diagnosis

The diagnosis of fetal hydrops is made on the basis of the ultrasonographic features of fluid accumulation in two serous cavities. Following the diagnosis, further investigation of both fetus and mother is necessary to help elicit whether the condition is immune or non-immune:

- Detailed ultrasound assessment of fetal anatomy to investigate for any underlying structure abnormality which could cause non-immune hydrops
- Fetal middle cerebral artery Doppler to investigate potential for fetal anaemia (raised peak systolic velocity)
- Maternal investigations should include an indirect Coombs antibody screen, maternal blood type, Kleihauer stain, TORCH and parvovirus B19 IgG and IgM levels
- Offer karyotyping (amniocentesis/chorionic villi sampling)

Management

The management of the remainder of the pregnancy and the treatment options

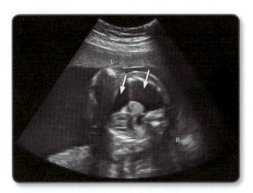

Figure 21 Fetal pleural effusion (marked with arrows)

Table 38 Underlying conditions causing non-immune fetal hydrops	
Cardiac abnormalities	Hypoplastic left heart syndrome, atrial septal defect (ASD), ventricular septal defect (VSD), tetralogy of Fallot, transposition of the great vessels, supraventricular tachycardia, heart block, atrial flutter, heart block
Aneuploidy	Trisomies 21, 18, 13, Turner's syndrome, triploidy
Haematological disorders	Alpha thalassemias, fetomaternal haemorrhage, fetal red cell enzyme deficiencies
Thoracic abnormality	Cystic adenomatous malformation of Lung (CAML) lung lesions, diaphragmatic hernia, intrathoracic mass, bronchogenic cysts
Genetic syndromes	Arthrogryposis, Noonan's syndrome, tuberous sclerosis, myotonic dystrophy
Infections	Parvovirus B19, cytomegalovirus, toxoplasmosis, syphilis, rubella
Skeletal dysplasias	Achondroplasia, osteogenesis imperfect a thanatophoric dwarfism
Gastrointestinal disorders	Oesophageal atresia, imperforate anus, meconium peritonitis, intestinal duplication, gut malrotation
Genitourinary conditions	Hypoplastic kidney, polycystic kidneys, bladder outlet obstruction
Neoplastic conditions	Neuroblastoma, teratoma, congenital leukaemia
Neurological disorders	Encephalocele, fetal intracranial haemorrhage
Vascular disorders	Arteriovenous malformation, sacrococcygeal teratoma
Placental/cord anomalies	Chorioangioma, umbilical vein torsion, angiomyxoma of cord
Maternal associations	Mirror syndrome, severe maternal anaemia, diabetes or hypoproteinaemia

available are dependent on the underlying condition causing hydrops. All cases should be managed by a consultant with a specialist interest in fetal medicine.

Immune hydrops has a well-established fetal intervention programme. Once the presence of maternal red cell antibodies has been confirmed, the peak systolic velocity within the middle cerebral artery is measured as a sensitive predictor of fetal anaemia. Once hydrops has developed the fetus is likely to be severely anaemic and on average has a haematocrit one-third below normal. Following full discussion of risks, the woman should be offered fetal blood sampling with a view to performing intrauterine blood transfusion via cordocentesis in a specialist fetal medicine unit.

Intrauterine blood transfusion should take place in sterile conditions under continuous ultrasound guidance. A 20 gauge needle is passed through the maternal abdomen and uterus. The preferred target is the umbilical vein, close to the placental insertion. Fetal blood is aspirated and equipment should be available to check fetal haemoglobin, haematocrit and platelet count. Blood should be available for transfusion; the

product should be group O, negative for the antibody to which the mother is immunised, cytomegalovirus negative and Kell negative. The volume of blood to be transfused is dependent on how anaemic the fetus is. However, care should be taken in the presence of hydrops as these fetuses are susceptible to volume overload. The fetus will require continued surveillance throughout pregnancy with many babies requiring repeat transfusions every 2–3 weeks. Generally when transfusion is performed between 24 and 34 weeks, corticosteroids for fetal lung maturity should be administered beforehand. Beyond 34 weeks, persistent fetal anaemia should prompt discussion with the woman regarding elective preterm delivery.

Because of the diverse aetiology of non-immune hydrops, the management is not as well defined. The fetal mortality for non-immune hydrops is 75–90% and termination of pregnancy could be offered in this scenario. If the woman wishes to continue the pregnancy, the management will depend on the underlying abnormality and may require input from fetal medicine specialists, neonatologists, neonatal surgeons and geneticists. The role for elective preterm delivery in non-immune fetal hydrops is less clear and each case should be judged individually. Some cases are amenable to treatment, e.g. fetal supraventricular tachycardia which can be controlled by oral digoxin or flecainide.

Mirror syndrome

Mirror syndrome (also known as Ballantyne's syndrome) is a rare condition characterised by the combination of fetal hydrops and maternal oedema, i.e. the mother 'mirrors' the hydropic fetus. Mirror syndrome is associated with both immune and non-immune causes of fetal hydrops. Mirror syndrome is related to pre-eclampsia, as clinical signs are common to both disorders including: hypertension, oedema, proteinuria, low haematocrit. Mirror syndrome is associated with a substantial increase in fetal mortality and maternal morbidity. However, the pathophysiology of mirror syndrome is poorly understood, but placental oedema and enlargement is often observed.

Further reading

Gajjar K, Spencer C. Diagnosis and management of non anti-D red cell antibodies in pregnancy. The Obstetrician and Gynaecologist 2009;11:89–95.

Sohan K, Carroll SG, De La Fuente S, et al. Analysis of outcome in hydrops fetalis in relation to gestational age at diagnosis, cause and treatment. Acta Obstet Gynecol Scand 2001; 80(8):726–730.

Soothill P. Intrauterine blood transfusion for non-immune hydrops fetalis due to parvovirus B19 infection. Lancet 1990; 336(8707):121–122.

Related topics of interest

- Feticide and late termination of pregnancy (p. 231)
- Infection in pregnancy (p. 243)
- Rhesus disease (p. 314)

Induction of labour

Overview

Induction of labour (IOL) describes the process of stimulating uterine contractions prior to the spontaneous onset of labour with the intention of causing progressive cervical effacement and dilatation. The ultimate aim of IOL is vaginal delivery of the baby.

IOL is common; according to the National Institute of Health and Clinical Excellence (NICE), between 2004 and 2005 one-fifth of all pregnancies in the UK were induced. As with normal labour, IOL is not without a risk of intervention: 15% of IOL ended with an instrumental delivery and 22% with a caesarean section. However, large scale retrospective studies suggest that women undergoing IOL have no significantly increased risk of intervention. Nevertheless, IOL should be clinically justified.

Women should be adequately counselled regarding the methods of IOL as many will find that it is more painful than spontaneous labour and increases the need for epidural analgesia. IOL also has an impact on the workload on the consultant-led delivery unit.

There are numerous reasons why IOL is considered as it occurs when it is thought that interrupting the pregnancy is more beneficial to mother, baby or both, than letting it continue.

If IOL is indicated at preterm gestations, the risks of prematurity and availability of a neonatal cot must be considered.

The majority of IOL are for prolonged pregnancy as it is known that the stillbirth rate increases from 1 in 1000 at 37 weeks to 6 in 1000 at 43 weeks. As a result, the majority of units will have a policy to offer IOL between 41 and 42 weeks.

Aetiology

The exact mechanisms underlying the onset of labour in humans are not fully understood. They have been studied in animal models where it is known to involve the hypothalamic-pituitary axis. Fetal cortisol is released which causes an increase in placental oestrogens and prostaglandins. These in turn sensitise the myometrium to circulating oxytocin which initiates labour. As prostaglandins have a central role in the onset of labour, synthetic prostaglandins are commonly used to induce labour.

Management

All women should be provided with information regarding why, when, where and how IOL will be carried out, and the risks involved, including the risk of failed IOL. It is good practice to provide information about labour and options for pain relief.

In the case of prolonged pregnancy they should also receive information about alternative arrangements should they not wish to proceed with IOL.

A vaginal examination should be performed to assess the cervix and documented using a modified Bishop's score (see **Table 39**). The higher the score, the more favourable for IOL the woman is. Women with a Bishop's score >4 should be suitable for artificial rupture of membranes (ARM) without the need for other methods of IOL. The following interventions should be discussed:

Table 39 Modified Bishop's score				
Score	0	1	2	3
Cervical dilatation	0	1–2	3–4	5
Cervical length	3	2	1	< 1
Consistency	Firm	Medium	Soft	–
Position	Posterior	Mid-position	Anterior	
Station of presenting part	−3	−2	−1 to 0	+1

Membrane sweep This can be performed at the same time as carrying out a vaginal examination to assess the cervix. Membrane sweeping aims to strip the chorion away from the decidua, which increases local production of prostaglandins.

A membrane sweep should be offered to nulliparous women between 40–41 weeks and to multiparous women after 41 weeks as it increases the chance of spontaneous labour, reducing the need for formal induction. There may be some benefit in repeated membrane sweep if the woman is agreeable. It can be uncomfortable and cause a small amount of vaginal bleeding so adequate counselling is important.

Pharmacological IOL Vaginal prostaglandin E2 is the preferred pharmacological method of induction. It can be given as either as gel, tablet or as a controlled-release pessary using the following regimens:

- One cycle of vaginal PGE2 in gel or tablet form, i.e. one dose which may be repeated if necessary 6 hours later if labour has not established
- One cycle of vaginal PGE2 in controlled-release pessary form left in place for 24 hours

Most obstetric units will conduct pharmacological IOL as an inpatient but some units carry out outpatient IOL. There should be robust policies in place and both practices should be continuously audited.

Pharmacological methods may cause uterine hyperstimulation (>5 contractions in 10 minutes), so a policy should be in place regarding the use of tocolysis. The aim is for established labour to occur after the administration of PGE2 or to achieve change in the Bishop's score so that amniotomy may then be performed. It is not recommended that amniotomy alone or in conjunction with intravenous oxytocin should be used as a primary method of induction unless there are clinical reasons such as specifically wanting to reduce the risk of hyperstimulation.

Intracervical balloon (Figure 22) Balloon is placed through cervical canal on vaginal examination; most devices have two balloons, one above the cervix and one in the vagina.

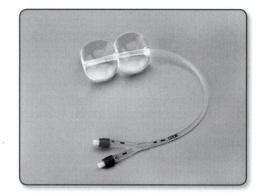

Figure 22 Intracervical balloon for induction of labour. (Permission for use granted by Cook Medical Incorporated, Bloomington, Indiana.)

The balloon in above the cervix is inflated with saline followed by the balloon in the vagina. The balloon is left in situ for 24 hours. This method is usually employed for IOL in women where there is a high risk of uterine rupture, e.g. previous caesarean section, grand multiparous women.

Intravenous oxytocin After artificial or spontaneous rupture of membranes, uterine contractions may be induced by administration of oxytocin according to a protocol. This should be followed to give 3–4 contractions in 10 minutes. Cervical dilatation should routinely be assessed at 4 hourly intervals. Women with previous uterine scars should be informed that there is a 2–3 fold increased risk of scar dehiscence/rupture with intravenous oxytocin (but this is less than with prostaglandins).

Expectant management If a woman decides she does not want to proceed with IOL following appropriate counselling her wishes should be respected and appropriate observation commenced. This will depend on the indication for IOL. After 42 weeks she should be seen twice weekly for cardiotocography (CTG) monitoring and ultrasound scans to assess fetal well-being and maximum amniotic pool depth.

Complications of IOL

Failed induction This has occurred if labour cannot be initiated via pharmacological or mechanical means. A further attempt at IOL may be considered at this point by repeating one of the cycles outlined above. This depends on the woman's wishes and the clinical situation. Mechanical procedures such as intracervical ripening balloons are not used routinely as a first attempt at IOL but they may have a place in this situation, after discussion with the woman. The alternative is to deliver the baby via caesarean section.

Cord prolapse   This may occur at the time of amniotomy or spontaneous rupture of membranes if the presenting part is high. Therefore, engagement of the presenting part should be assessed prior to undertaking IOL and amniotomy should be avoided if the head is high or if cord is present.

Uterine rupture   This is a rare obstetric emergency and should prompt urgent delivery by caesarean section once suspected. There is a 2–3-fold increased risk of uterine rupture in women undergoing pharmacological IOL who have previously had a caesarean section so antenatal counselling is particularly important in this group.

Special circumstances

Prelabour rupture of membranes (PROM)   If PROM occurs after 37 weeks, IOL with vaginal PGE2 or intravenous oxytocin should be offered 24 hours later to reduce the risk of infection. There are no data to favour one approach. If PROM occurs between 34 and 37 weeks, a discussion regarding IOL versus expectant management should take place regarding the increased chance of chorioamnionitis and the risks this poses to mother and baby. This should be weighed against the risks of prematurity and availability of a local neonatal cot.

Intrauterine fetal death   In the absence of complications, women may be offered expectant management or immediate IOL after the diagnosis of fetal death in utero. If there is evidence of ruptured membranes, infection or bleeding, IOL should be immediate. 200 mg mifepristone is given and reduces the length of time to induce labour but requires 24–48 hours to work. Misoprostol or PGE2 can be used to induce labour, they are equally safe, but misoprostol appears slightly more effective. Misoprostol should be administered vaginally (less side effects) and should be adjusted according to gestational age (100 µg 6-hourly before 26 weeks; 25–50 µg 4-hourly at 27 weeks or more). This is an unlicensed use of misoprostol but is recommended by the Royal College of Obstetricians and Gynaecologists (RCOG).

Suspected fetal macrosomia   In the absence of maternal diabetes, IOL should not be routinely offered.

Maternal request   IOL should not be offered routinely but if there are exceptional circumstances it may be considered after 40 weeks.

Further reading

NICE Clinical Guideline No. 70. Induction of labour. London: NICE, 2008.

Stock SJ, Ferguson E, Duffy A, et al. Outcomes of elective induction of labour compared with expectant management: population based study. BMJ 2012; 344:e2838.

RCOG Green-top Guideline No. 55. Late intrauterine fetal death and stillbirth. London: RCOG, 2010.

Related topics of interest

Infection in pregnancy

Overview

Infections in pregnancy can be broadly divided into those which predominantly have maternal effects and those which affect the fetus, either by transplacental transmission in utero or by direct infection via the lower genital tract during parturition.

Fever in early pregnancy can cause miscarriage and in later pregnancy may lead to premature labour. Therefore, any infection associated with significant pyrexia may carry a risk to the fetus. Maternal sepsis is an extremely serious condition which is associated with maternal mortality; this is covered separately in Topic 83.

Clinical features

Symptoms of sepsis in pregnancy may be less distinctive or absent compared to the non-pregnant population. Therefore, clinicians should be vigilant and consider infection as a differential diagnosis. Infections that have significant fetal/neonatal effects such as cytomegalovirus or Group B streptococcus may cause little, if any, maternal symptoms. Conversely, some viral infections that normally have a relatively benign course may be severe and even fatal in pregnancy (e.g. herpes varicella zoster and influenza esp. H1N1).

Aetiology/management

Maternal infection

Pregnancy predisposes to certain infections, notably of the urinary system and lower genital tract.

- Untreated urinary tract infection (UTI) predisposes to premature labour, and repeated infection may cause renal impairment
- The normal vaginal flora is affected by the hormonal changes in pregnancy, causing an increase in candidiasis (overall frequency 16%), particularly in women with gestational diabetes and/or after antibiotic use
- Potential pathogens may colonize the vagina and are related to the development of chorioamnionitis and puerperal sepsis including β-haemolytic and Group A streptococcus

Fetal infection

Certain infective agents cross the placenta and lead to fetal death, miscarriage or congenital anomalies.

- Maternal symptoms may be minor, leading to a delay in diagnosis. Direct transmission (from the maternal genital tract to the fetus) occurs at delivery. The increased severity of the illness in the neonate reflects an immature immune system

Transplacental infection

Rubella   Rubella causes few symptoms in pregnancy (flu like symptoms and mild rash). Fetal effects vary depending on gestation and may result in miscarriage (20%), stillbirth, congenital anomaly (typically patent ductus arteriosus, fetal growth restriction, deafness and blindness) and/or later handicap.

Diagnosis is on serology (rubella IgM) and termination is offered for proven infection before 17 weeks' gestation as greatest risk of fetal anomaly is the first trimester (50% transmission risk; minimal risk after 20 weeks).

All women should have rubella serology at booking. Women who are non-immune are offered vaccination postpartum.

Cytomegalovirus (CMV)   It is the commonest congenital infection in the UK (200–300 cases per annum), characterised by neurodevelopmental delay and sensorineural deafness.

Detection of CMV in amniotic fluid (culture or PCR) accurately identifies an infected fetus; see **Table 40**.

In the first half of pregnancy transplacental passage is about 40%. Disease manifestations [detected by ultrasound scan (USS)], include enlarged placenta, fetal growth restriction, microcephaly, ventriculomegaly, periventricular calcifications, serous effusions and echogenic bowel.

Table 40 Key tests for diagnosis of maternal CMV infection				
Type of infection	Serum PCR	Urine PCR	IgM	IgG
Acute	Positive	Positive	Positive	Absent on low avidity antibody
Recurrent or Reactivated	Usually negative	May be positive	Usually negative, but secondary response can occur	Positive for high avidity antibody

For those severely affected 30% die, with 80% of survivors having serious sequelae, although most (>90%) are asymptomatic at birth.

When primary maternal infection occurs in the third trimester the risk of transplacental transmission is higher – 75% to 80%. However, the risk of serious fetal injury is very low.

Therapy with hyperimmune globulin may be beneficial.

Immune mothers may suffer reinfection, causing difficulty in diagnosis and giving advice regarding prognosis.

Toxoplasmosis This occurs after ingestion of a protozoon found in inadequately cooked meat or contaminated cat faeces usually causing a non-specific infection characterised by lymphadenopathy and lethargy.

Fetal infection results in miscarriage or congenital cerebral, ocular and aural (deafness) anomalies.

In the UK about 2 in 1000 babies are infected, but only about 6 babies per year show signs of congenital infection at birth.

Spiramycin is an antibiotic used in pregnancy to prevent the infection of the child.

Screening is not recommended (RCOG 1992).

Listeria monocytogenes A Gram-positive rod, is widely prevalent in inadequately stored food. A rare disease, it is 20 times more common in pregnancy because of reduced cell-mediated immunity. Typically causing a non-specific maternal illness, fetal/neonatal infection is severe and frequently fatal (20-30%) – consequences include premature delivery of an infant with respiratory distress, liver impairment and neurological problems. Ampicillin is indicated if positive maternal blood cultures.

Preterm meconium staining of the liquor is suggestive of listeriosis.

Herpes Varicella Zoster (chickenpox) It is a virus that crosses the placenta. Fetal effects include congenital varicella syndrome (chorioretinitis, cerebral cortical atrophy, hydronephrosis, and cutaneous and partial limb reduction; rare – 0.4% <13 weeks, 2% between 13–20 weeks) or neonatal varicella (infection within the first 10 days of life, before maternal antibody transmission) with potential mortality (30%) due to pneumonia. Affected neonates are given varicella zoster immunoglobulin immediately to reduce risk/attenuate disease.

Maternal Varicella Zoster Secondary episodes of varicella infection (shingles) poses no risk to the fetus as IgG is already present. However, primary maternal varicella infection should be treated with oral antiviral agents. Intravenous acyclovir can be considered for severe complications (pneumonia/pneumonitis), liver disease and/or encephalitis

Parvovirus It is a common infection occurring in epidemics, and affecting 1 in 400 women at risk. Fetal transmission occurs in 30%, particularly in the second trimester, with a peak risk between 17–24 weeks' gestation. Fetal loss rate is approximately 10% before 20 weeks of gestation. It causes anaemia and/or hydrops in 15% of cases.

Direct transmission

Direct transmission occurs when organisms are transmitted to the fetus from the maternal genital tract.

Chlamydia trachomatis and *Neisseria gonorrhoea* These are both associated with ocular infection which may lead to neonatal blindness if appropriate treatment is delayed.

Herpes simplex virus It causes generalised neonatal infection, involving the central nervous system, liver, lungs and eyes.

Mortality is high. Almost all neonatal herpes occur from direct contact with infected maternal secretions, when it usually causes a generalised, severe infection. Transmission is greater with primary rather than secondary infection, in the third trimester and within 6 weeks of delivery (approximately 40%). Type-specific HSV antibody testing (IgG to HSV-1 and HSV-2) confirms primary infection when caesarean section should be offered unless the membranes have been ruptured for ≥ 4 hours. Acyclovir reduces both the duration/severity of symptoms and viral shedding. Its use in labour to reduce transmission risk [along with avoidance of amniotomy (ARM), fetal blood sampling (FBS) and fetal scalp electrode (FSE)] is assumed but not proven.

Limited evidence to support prophylaxis (RCOG, 2007) as recurrent lesions do not require elective caesarean but avoidance of internal procedures unless necessary, e.g. (artificial rupture of membranes, fetal blood sampling, and/or fetal scalp electrode).

Other infections

The neonate is at particular risk in certain situations because of the immaturity of its immune system.

Mothers who have a chronic infection may transmit this to the neonate. The most important examples of this type of infection are hepatitis B and HIV infection.

Hepatitis B virus   This can induce a carrier state; prevalence of about 200 million worldwide. The presence of hepatitis E antigen carries a greater risk of vertical transmission (90% versus 10%); this is limited by avoiding FSE and FBS in labour, and possibly maternal lamivudine from 36 weeks.

Spread is via infected blood and the perinatal period is of particularly high risk. Although maternal antibody may also be transmitted to the fetus, this disappears and persistence beyond 9 months suggests an infected baby.

At-risk babies are given active and passive immunisation at birth.

Infected mothers can breastfeed as there is no additional risk of transmission

HIV infection   see (HIV and Pregnancy Topic 75)

Influenza – RNA retrovirus   Influenza activity in the UK is declining. Influenza B is now being reported more frequently than H1N1.

Pregnant women are recognised as being at significantly increased risk of complications, particularly in the second/third trimester, including death (maternal mortality rate three times greater than non-pregnant population) from chest infection, because of the flu itself, or secondary bacterial infection.

Hospitalisation with H1N1 is associated with three times risk of preterm birth, and five times risk of stillbirth/early neonatal death.

The seasonal influenza vaccine (2010–2011) contains three flu virus strains, including H1N1 (2009). All pregnant women should be vaccinated, also providing passive immunisation to the newborn (first 6 months of life).

Antivirals are effective in treating flu, and appear safe. Oral oseltamivir capsules or inhaled zanamivir can be given.

Breastfeeding is not contraindicated, and can be continued whilst the mother is receiving antiviral treatment/prophylaxis.

Further reading

Jangu EB. Viral Infections in pregnancy. In: De Swiet M (Ed.). Medical Disorders in Obstetric Practice, 4th edn. Oxford: Blackwell Scientific Publications, 2002; 513–531.

Byrne BMP, Crowley PA, Carrington. D. Chickenpox in pregnancy. RCOG Guidelines No. 13. London: RCOG, 2007.

Low-Beer NM, Kinghorn GR. Management of genital herpes in pregnancy. RCOG Guidelines No. 30. London: RCOG, 2007.

Royal College of Obstetricians and Gynaecologists. Prenatal screening for toxoplasmosis in the UK. Report of a multidisciplinary working group. London: RCOG, 1992.

Yates L, Pierce M, Stephens S, et al. Influenza A/ H1N1v in pregnancy: an investigation of the characteristics and management of affected women and the relationship to pregnancy outcomes for mother and infant. Health Technol Assess 2010; 14(34):109–182.

Related topics of interest

- HIV in pregnancy (p. 234)
- Hydrops fetalis (p. 237)

- Maternal sepsis (p. 259)

Instrumental delivery

Operative vaginal delivery can be achieved with either forceps (rotational or non-rotational) or ventouse. Forceps may also be used to facilitate delivery of the aftercoming head during a vaginal breech delivery or to deliver the head at caesarean section. An operator should use the appropriate instrument for the clinical situation taking into account their experience and competence.

Types of forceps

Outlet forceps   Non-rotational used more at caesarean section; rarely used for vaginal delivery. Wrigley's forceps have a fixed pivot lock and short handles, with a pelvic and a cephalic curve to the blades.
Non-rotational forceps   There are many types of such forceps with Simpson's and Neville-Barnes being the commonest in use. These also have a pelvic and cephalic curve but with longer handles so that more traction can be applied.
Rotational forceps   Kielland's forceps have a sliding lock, a cephalic curve, but only a minimal pelvic curve to enable rotation of the head.

Types of ventouse

Rigid cup   Including the metal vacuum cups of Malstrom (vacuum tubing and traction chain coming off the centre of the cup) and Bird (vacuum hose and traction chain on the rim of the cup – this modified cup was intended to be used for posterior or lateral positions of the occiput as it allows easier placement over the flexion point).
Soft/flexible cup   Cone shaped silastic or disposable plastic.
Disposable vacuum cup   This is a disposable device with an integral handpump vacuum delivery system.

Significant caput on the fetal head may inhibit achievement of a good vacuum seal and forceps may be a more appropriate choice of instrument if this is present. Successful vacuum delivery also requires good maternal effort. Vacuum extraction should not be used at gestations of $< 34^{+0}$ weeks and caution and careful consideration is required if the ventouse is used between $34–36^{+0}$ weeks.

Classification of operative vaginal delivery

Outlet   Fetal head is at or on the perineum
Low   Leading point of the skull is a station +2 cm or lower
Mid-cavity   Leading point of the skull is higher than +2 cm but not above the level of the ischial spines
High   The presenting part of the head is above the level of the ischial spines – this is not recommended in modern obstetrics; caesarean section would be the recommended mode of delivery

Additionally, a delivery may require fetal head rotation prior to applying traction. Rotation of the fetal head can be achieved by manual rotation, rotational vacuum extraction or Kielland's forceps depending on the experience of the operator.

Indications

- Delay in second stage: Depending on parity, clinical circumstances and use of regional anaesthesia, delay in the second stage may be diagnosed between 1 and 3 hours (total of active and passive second stage). If a patient has an epidural in situ pushing should be delayed for 1–2 hours or until there is a strong urge to push as this reduces the need for mid-cavity and rotational operative vaginal delivery
- Maternal exhaustion
- Maternal compromise requiring limitation of active second stage, e.g. eclampsia/severe pre-eclampsia, cardiac or pulmonary disease
- Presumed fetal compromise (e.g. pathological fetal heart rate trace/fetal bradycardia)

Prerequisites for an instrumental delivery

- Maternal consent should have been obtained (either verbal or written)
- The fetal head should be ≤ 1/5 palpable per abdomen
- The bladder should have been catheterised
- The fetal head position and station should have been identified on vaginal examination. Should the position not be determined with the use of sutures and fontanelle lines, feeling for the location of the ear and assessing its position and which direction it faces can help diagnose fetal position
- The cervix should be fully dilated and the membranes ruptured
- There should be no apparent cephalo-pelvic disproportion – an assessment of caput and moulding should be made on vaginal examination
- Appropriate analgesia should be used. For a rotational delivery, regional anaesthesia should be employed. For a mid-cavity delivery, especially if the patient is in pain/distress regional analgesia should also be considered. For low cavity/outlet deliveries perineal infiltration ± a pudendal nerve block should be utilised
- Personnel trained in neonatal resuscitation should be present prior to delivery
- Cases which have a higher chance of a failed instrumental delivery, e.g. malposition (occipito-transverse or posterior), maternal increased body mass index, mid-cavity delivery should be considered a trial of instrumental delivery. Appropriate personnel should be in place in case of a failed instrumental delivery, that is anaesthetists and theatre team so a caesarean section can be facilitated without delay. Many obstetricians will choose to conduct such trials of instrumental delivery in an operating theatre.

When should an operative vaginal delivery be abandoned?

Traction to the instrument is applied during a uterine contraction. Delivery should be abandoned in favour of caesarean section if there is no evidence of progressive descent over each contraction or when delivery is not imminent following three contractions.

The use of sequential instruments should be minimised as there is an increased risk of neonatal trauma – however, after a failed ventouse the relative merits of proceeding with a forceps or abandoning the vaginal delivery for a caesarean section should be considered.

Complications

Maternal   The perineum, vagina and cervix can be damaged, with extension of the episiotomy to a third/fourth degree tear often with associated postpartum haemorrhage. Damage to both the bladder and urethra can occur which may result in fistula formation. Urinary complications such as retention and infection can occur. The patient can also be prone to back strain and nerve root or sciatic plexus damage by poor positioning during delivery and also if excessive movement occurs. Ventouse delivery is more likely to lead to a failed instrumental delivery but is less likely to be associated with significant perineal or vaginal trauma. Care must be taken to ensure there is no entrapment of maternal tissue between the cup edge and the fetal head. Depending on maternal complications it should be considered whether the administration of antibiotics or thromboprophylaxis is required.

Fetal   If a ventouse has been utilised then a baby's head will show a chignon – this resolves rapidly, usually within hours/days. A cephalhaematoma can occur which is haemorrhage between the skull and the periosteum secondary to rupture of blood vessels. A more severe haemorrhage is a subgaleal bleed, which has a high associated rate of head trauma. This swelling typically develops 12–72 hours after delivery and can cause haemorrhagic shock. These complications are more common with the use of the ventouse. Skull fractures and facial nerve palsy are associated more with forceps delivery. Jaundice postdelivery is also common (more often with the ventouse). Retinal haemorrhages (unknown significance) seem to be more common with the ventouse.

Further reading

RCOG Green-top Guideline No. 26. Operative vaginal delivery. London: RCOG, 2011.

Johanson RB, Menon V. Vacuum extraction versus forceps for assisted vaginal delivery. Cochrane Database Syst Rev 2007:CD000224.

RCOG. Operative vaginal delivery RCOG consent advice number 11 London: RCOG, 2010.

Doumouchtsis SK, Arulkumaran S. Head injuries after instrumental vaginal deliveries. Curr Opin Obstet Gynecol 2006; 18(2):129–134.

Murphy DJ, et al. A cohort study of maternal and neonatal morbidity in relation to use of sequential instruments at operative vaginal delivery. Eur J Obstet Gynecol Reprod Biol 2011; 156(1):41–45.

Murphy DJ, Koh DK. Cohort study of the decision to delivery interval and neonatal outcome for emergency operative vaginal delivery. Am J Obstet Gynecol 2007; 196(2):145.

Related topics of interest

Invasive fetal testing

Overview

Invasive procedures performed within pregnancy are generally carried out for the purpose of providing prenatal diagnosis, fetal treatment or to terminate a fetus (singleton/multiple). These procedures are deemed as invasive as they involve the passage of a 20–22 gauge needle through the maternal abdomen and uterus to enter the amniotic sac and possibly cord/fetus. Due to the invasive nature of such procedures they carry a risk of miscarriage/preterm labour and fetal death. The procedures considered here include amniocentesis, chorionic villus biopsy and fetal therapy. Feticide is described in Topic 74.

Amniocentesis

Amniocentesis describes sampling the amniotic fluid around the fetus for the purposes of prenatal diagnosis. Amniocentesis was originally used to measure bilirubin levels in Rhesus disease, but this has been superseded by fetal middle cerebral artery Doppler. Current indications for amniocentesis include:
- To determine fetal karyotype (either following a high risk screening result or for a high risk known familial condition)
- To test for a known genetic or biochemical disorder
- To assess amniotic fluid for infection

Amniocentesis is performed under aseptic conditions with continuous ultrasound guidance. The procedure is performed from 15 weeks of gestation. Early pregnancy amniocentesis has been abandoned due to high culture failure rates, increased need for more than one needle puncture, a significantly higher pregnancy loss rate than when performed early in the second trimester and an association with fetal talipes. Patients should be counselled about the risks of the procedure and sign a written consent form. The risks that should be discussed include:

- 1% risk of miscarriage (or preterm delivery if being performed after 24 weeks)
- Failure to obtain a sample
- Failure to culture fetal cells in the laboratory (may need to undergo a second procedure)
- Maternal cell contamination
- Blood staining of liquor may mean that rapid qfPCR (for trisomies 21, 18, 13) may not be possible

Women should be informed to expect mild abdominal cramps for 1–2 hours following the procedure and that they may feel tender over the puncture site for 1–2 days. They should, be advised that if this does not settle with simple analgesia or is associated with watery or a bloody loss per vagina that they should seek medical advice.

It is also important that women are aware of how the results will be communicated to them and in what time frame to expect their results. For fetal karyotype, the laboratory aim to produce a rapid result (by qfPCR) for the most common chromosome abnormalities (trisomy 21, 18 and 13) within 2–3 working days. The remainder of the fetal karyotype will usually be available with 10–14 working days. Tests for rarer genetic conditions may take longer and often require the sample to be transported to a specialised laboratory.

Chorionic villus biopsy

This technique involves aspiration of the chorionic villi as a means of analysing the fetal karyotype or looking for a genetic syndrome. This technique can be performed from 11 weeks of gestation and thus provides women with the opportunity to receive prenatal diagnosis earlier in pregnancy. This allows them the option of earlier medical and surgical termination of pregnancy (TOP). This is desirable as many women find the prospect of TOP more difficult the longer the pregnancy progresses.

Chorionic villus biopsy (CVB) should only be performed after an ultrasound scan has been performed by the operator to confirm fetal viability; a crown–rump measurement confirms gestation and the accessibility of the placenta.

The procedure is then performed with aseptic technique, under continuous ultrasound guidance and generally performed after administration of local anaesthetic to the maternal skin and subcutaneous tissue. Most operators in the UK perform CVB by a transabdominal approach using a double lumen CVB needle (or a 20 gauge spinal needle) which is passed through maternal tissues directly into the placenta. The double lumen CVB needle has an inner stylet (see **Figure 23**) which is removed following correct placement, allowing the assistant to place the aspirating needle down into the placenta with a 20 mL syringe attached to create negative pressure. Analysis requires approximately 30 mg of villous material for analysis thus it is advisable to visually inspect the aspirate to ensure the sample appears adequate prior to the removal of the needle from the maternal uterus.

The procedure can also be performed by the transcervical route. A speculum is inserted into the vagina and a catheter is then passed through the cervical os until the tip is seen (by ultrasound) entering the placenta.

Women should be counselled about what to expect during and after the procedure and to sign a written consent form. The risks of CVB are similar to amniocentesis but the following should be discussed:
- The fetal loss rate following CVB is 2–3%; this higher rate seems to reflect the fact that the test is performed at an earlier gestation than amniocentesis where the background loss rate is higher. Studies suggest that the procedure related loss is around 1%

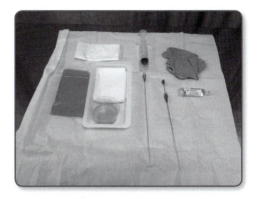

Figure 23 Equipment used in chorionic villus biopsy

- The presence of placental mosaicism (~1%) may make results difficult to interpret and women may require a further amniocentesis to help interpretation
- CVB should not be performed under 10 weeks of gestation due to an association with severe limb defects
- Both amniocentesis and CVB can be performed in multiple pregnancies but it is recommended that such procedures are performed by an experienced operator

Invasive fetal therapy

Invasive procedures can be performed for the purpose of fetal therapy. Such procedures should be carried out by trained fetal medicine specialists.

Invasive antenatal procedures include intrauterine blood transfusion (also discussed in Topic 76 Hydrops fetalis), laser ablation of anastomotic placental vessels in twin-to-twin transfusion syndrome and the insertion of vesicoamniotic shunts in bladder outlet obstruction.

Some centres are beginning to publish the results of prenatal surgery for conditions such as congenital diaphragmatic hernia and spina bifida. Such procedures have not been established in UK practice.

Further reading

RCOG Green-top Guideline No. 8. Amniocentesis and chorionic villus sampling. London: RCOG, 2010.

Johnson A, Wapner RJ. Mosaicism: implications for postnatal outcome. Curr Opin Obstet Gynecol 1997; 9(2):126–135.

Ruano R, Yoshisaki CT, da Silva MM, et al. Randomized controlled trial of fetal endoscopic tracheal occlusion versus postnatal management of severe isolated congenital diaphragmatic hernia. Ultrasound Obstet Gynecol 2012; 39(1):20–27.

Related topics of interest

- Hydrops fetalis (p. 237)
- Feticide and late termination of pregnancy (p. 231)

Malpresentation and malposition

Overview

The presentation refers to the part of the fetus overlying the internal cervical os. By term, the vertex will present in 95% of cases. This is a diamond shaped area defined by the parietal eminences laterally, and the anterior and posterior fontanelles to the front and back. A malpresentation occurs when the presenting part is not cephalic.

The denominator is a term used to describe the bony landmark on the presenting part that is used to define the position. Due to the shape of the pelvic floor, in a normal labour the vertex will present in the occipitoanterior (OA) position and the occiput is then said to be the denominator. Flexion of the head is encouraged and this presents the smallest anteroposterior (AP) and lateral diameters of the head to the pelvis, meaning spontaneous vaginal delivery is much more likely. Deviation away from this is termed malposition.

Aetiology

The aetiology of malpresentation and malposition are varied. They can be thought of as related to the 3 P's:

Passenger (related to malpresentation)
- Multiple pregnancy
- Polyhydramnios
- Anatomical abnormalities such as sacrococcygeal tumour or hydrocephalus

Passage (related to malpresentation or malposition)
- Pelvic abnormalities
- Pelvic tumours
- Uterine abnormalities

Powers (related to malposition)
- Inadequate uterine contractions (which are insufficient to rotate the fetal head to an OA position)

Management

The management of malpresentation or malposition is dependent on the problem and its cause.

Fetal abnormalities will mostly be detected in the antenatal period, e.g. the presence of hydrocephalus or sacrococcygeal teratoma. Some malpresentations (e.g. breech presentation or transverse lie) can also be picked up antenatally. This allows planning to take place regarding whether to attempt external cephalic version to facilitate a normal delivery or to proceed to caesarean section. Any discussions should involve the woman and her partner and take into account the safety of the proposed method of delivery for both woman and baby.

Malpositions are detected during vaginal examinations during labour. This may be the first time a malpresentation such as undiagnosed breech is detected. Further management will then depend on other issues such as fetal well-being, parity, maternal wishes and progress during labour if it is deemed safe to have a vaginal birth.

Malpositions

Occipitoposterior (OP)   This position is necessarily associated with a degree of extension of the head. Thus, the larger anteroposterior diameter presents. It is possible to deliver spontaneously, particularly in multiparae but labours tend to be slower and more painful. OP may correct spontaneously to a more favourable OA position. To achieve sufficient uterine contractions to rotate to an OA position intravenous oxytocin may be required, particularly in nulliparous women.

If delay in the second stage occurs due to persistent OP, an instrumental delivery may be possible, utilising either manual rotation to OA and direct application of forceps or rotational ventouse or forceps delivery depending on the skill of the operator.

Occipitotransverse (OT)   In OT position the sagittal suture is palpable in the transverse diameter (as opposed to AP). The fetus may be right OT, where the occiput is on the maternal right or left OT, where the occiput is on the maternal left. As the transverse diameter of the pelvis is largest in the mid-cavity, persistent OT positions tend to have a higher station than OP or OA. Like OP positions, OT may correct to OA, which may require labour to be augmented with intravenous oxytocin. An instrumental delivery may also be possible by manual rotation or rotational ventouse or Kielland's forceps.

Brow   This occurs in about 1 in 1500–3000 deliveries and is commoner in preterm gestations. The largest possible diameter (mentovertical) presents. Spontaneous delivery may be possible if flexion occurs to a vertex presentation or if further extension occurs resulting in face presentation. In early labour, it is appropriate to observe whether either of these corrections occur, as a brow presentation is inherently unstable. If correction does not occur, vaginal delivery is not a possibility and caesarean section will be required.

Face   This occurs in around 1 in 500–1000 deliveries. It is more common in fetal goitre or anencephaly. It is detected in labour if the eye sockets, nose and gum margins are palpable, but even this may be difficult due to swelling of the face. A vaginal delivery is possible in the mentoanterior position but not in the mentoposterior position, where a caesarean section will be required.

Asynclitism   This is usually associated with OT positions when the fetal head is tilted more to one side than the other, i.e one parietal bone is felt closer to the pelvic outlet than the other. It will usually correct itself with flexion and rotation of the head.

Malpresentations

Breech   See Topic 61: Breech presentation.
Transverse and oblique lie   This may occur due to uterine abnormalities but may also occur in multiparas with no other risk factors due to increased laxity of the uterus. The incidence at term is around 1 in 400. It may correct itself spontaneously to a longitudinal lie at the onset of uterine contractions. Prior to the onset of established labour, external cephalic version can be considered, with or without induction of labour, if appropriate. In the presence of ruptured membranes, there is a significant risk of cord prolapse and an emergency caesarean section should be performed if this occurs (see Topic 68). If transverse lie persists and cannot be corrected, delivery should be by caesarean section. This may pose technical difficulties, especially if the back is inferior; it should be performed by an experienced operator and may require a classical incision on the uterus.
Compound   This refers to the presentation of a fetal extremity, usually the hand, alongside the head. It may correct spontaneously, proving no barrier to a normal vaginal delivery. Occasionally, an entire limb can present below the head and in these cases, it is much less likely to resolve and a caesarean section will be required.

Further reading

Edmonds, DK. Malpresentation, malposition, cephalopelvic disproportion and obstetric procedures. In: Dewhurst's Textbook of Obstetrics & Gynaecology, 7th edn (DK Edmonds). Oxford: Blackwell Publishing, 2008.

Related topics of interest

Maternal death

Overview

Maternal death is one of the most significant challenges to obstetrics. There are more than 350,000 maternal deaths worldwide per year; the majority (99%) of which occur in low-income countries. The majority of maternal deaths are avoidable. This is reflected in the United Nations Millennium Development Goal 5, which aims to reduce the maternal mortality ratio by three-quarters.

In the UK there is an established confidential enquiry into maternal deaths. The most recent mortality report 'Saving Mother's Lives' covers the triennium 2006–8 and was published in March 2011. This was the 8th Report on Confidential Enquiries into Maternal Deaths in the UK and investigated 261 maternal deaths, giving a maternal mortality ratio of 11.39 per 100,000 births which represents a slight decrease from the previous triennium (2003–2005).

Definitions

Maternal death is defined as a woman who dies while pregnant or in the 42 days following the end of the pregnancy. The cause must be related to, or exacerbated by, the pregnancy or its management. Deaths from accidental or incidental causes are not included in this definition.

Direct deaths result directly from pregnancy complications, e.g. postpartum haemorrhage, eclampsia and puerperal sepsis.

Indirect deaths result from a pre-existing disease or a disease that developed during pregnancy. The disease is exacerbated by the physiological effects of pregnancy but is not a direct result of obstetric causes.

Maternal deaths are most commonly a result of indirect causes.

Aetiology/epidemiology

In 2006–2008 there were 4.27 direct deaths per 100,000 births, down from 6.24 per 100,000 births in 2003–2005. The most common causes of direct maternal deaths are shown in **Table 41**. Although the order changes in each triennium, the most frequent causes of direct death are venous thromboembolism (VTE), preeclampsia/eclampsia, sepsis, haemorrhage and amniotic fluid embolism.

The two single most important causes of indirect maternal deaths were pre-existing cardiac disease and psychiatric conditions (**Table 42**).

Table 41 Direct causes of maternal deaths in the UK broken down by triennium			
Cause	2006–2008	2003–2005	2000–2002
Venous thromboembolism	18	41	30
Eclampsia/pre-eclampsia	19	18	14
Haemorrhage	9	14	17
Amniotic fluid embolism	13	17	5
Early pregnancy deaths	11	14	15
Sepsis	26	18	13
Anaesthetic	7	6	6
Other	4	4	6
TOTAL	107	132	106

Data from Centre for Maternal and Child Enquiries (CMACE). Saving Mothers' Lives: reviewing maternal deaths to make motherhood safer: 2006–2008. The Eighth Report on Confidential Enquiries into Maternal Deaths in the United Kingdom. BJOG 2011; 118 (Suppl 1):1–203.

Table 42 Indirect causes of maternal deaths in the UK broken down by triennium			
Cause	2006–2008	2003–2005	2000–2002
Cardiac	53	48	44
Indirect psychiatric	13	18	16
Other indirect	85	87	90
Indirect malignancies	3	10	5
TOTAL	154	163	155
Coincidental deaths	50	55	36

Data from Centre for Maternal and Child Enquiries (CMACE). Saving Mothers' Lives: reviewing maternal deaths to make motherhood safer: 2006–2008. The Eighth Report on Confidential Enquiries into Maternal Deaths in the United Kingdom. BJOG, 2011; 118 (Suppl 1):1–203.

In the UK, maternal mortality is strongly related to poor health status (e.g. cigarette smoking and obesity). 50% of deaths occurred in obese women and 6% of deaths in morbidly obese women. The most significant causes of death in obese women were VTE and cardiac causes. In addition, 11% of women who died had history of substance abuse.

Social exclusion is also an important risk factor for maternal mortality as maternal death is five times more common in women from deprived areas compared to affluent areas and women from Black African origin or asylum seekers are six times more likely to die than women from White British origin. This may reflect less engagement with antenatal care. 17% of maternal deaths occurred in women who booked after 22 weeks gestation, 14% of women who died declared they were subject to domestic abuse and 10% were known to child protection services.

Avoidable factors

In total, suboptimal care was evident in 70% of direct maternal deaths and was felt to be major when it contributed significantly to the death (44% of direct deaths). Major suboptimal care was most common in preeclampsia and related disorders. Of concern, is that the proportion of cases of suboptimal care has not fallen significantly from 50% in 1997–99. The 2006–08 Confidential Enquiry identified several important avoidable factors relating to the provision of care in cases of maternal death

including inadequate resuscitation skills and a failure to identify and recognise common non-obstetric medical emergencies, e.g. sepsis, pulmonary embolism. There was also a need to better recognise the needs of vulnerable women, e.g. those who are socially excluded, ethnic minorities, lack of spoken English. A significant proportion of avoidable factors focussed on communication between professionals and their ability to function as a team with tasks delegated inappropriately, short consultations by phone rather than in person, or a lack of sharing information between health professionals.

Recommendations

The 8th report of the Confidential Enquiries into Maternal Deaths in the UK made a Top 10 recommendation to reduce the number of maternal deaths. The key points of these recommendations are summarised below:

Pre-pregnancy care All women with a significant pre-existing medical illness which requires a change of medication or is likely to deteriorate in pregnancy should be informed of the risks of pregnancy at every opportunity to increase the proportion of planned vs. unplanned pregnancies in this group. A management plan should be made for such women by clinicians with knowledge of that condition in pregnancy. Conditions which need pre-pregnancy counselling include: asthma, cardiac disease, diabetes, epilepsy, HIV, liver disease, obesity, renal disease and severe psychiatric illness.

Professional interpretation services   To ensure that women from non-English speaking groups can adequately access care and actively participate in their management, professional interpreters should be used. Use of family members should be discouraged as this may reduce discussion of personal problems (e.g. domestic violence) or sensitive previous history (e.g. termination of pregnancy), and the quality of the translation cannot be ensured.

Communications and referrals   All referrals to specialist services (e.g. specialist physicians or mental-health services) regarding pregnant patients should be prioritised as urgent. Complex patients should be seen by senior members of the obstetric team and referrals should be made at a senior level, e.g. consultant to consultant. Remember to include communication to/from primary care.

Women with potentially serious medical conditions require specialist care   When a potentially serious medical problem is identified at booking or during pregnancy, women should be referred to specialist centres with experience of caring for obstetric and medical conditions. Such referrals should be made promptly and with an explanation that urgent review is required. In conditions which present before pregnancy this should be a consultant review in early pregnancy. However, women who develop complications during their pregnancy should be referred immediately to a centre with expertise in caring for that obstetric and medical condition. Referrals should be made between clinicians of appropriate seniority.

Clinical skills and training   To address the reported deficiencies in the identification and management of serious medical conditions, and in the provision of maternal resuscitation, it was recommended that all clinical staff must have training in the identification and initial management of serious obstetric conditions, and common medical and mental health emergencies. This training should also include advanced life support skills. Although focussed on maternity professionals, this training should also be offered for general practitioners and staff in emergency departments who may also see women who are seriously ill in pregnancy.

Identifying and managing very sick women   Although the modified early warning score (MEOWS) was recommended in the 7th Confidential Enquiry into maternal deaths (2003–05) this has not been universally adopted. Consequently, this report repeated the recommendation that a MEOWS chart should be used for all pregnant or postpartum women who become unwell and require maternity (or gynaecology) services. In other clinical settings early warning score charts help identify patients with developing critical illness and facilitate prompt referral and treatment. Several reports have identified cases of maternal death where severe pain was not evaluated appropriately. Therefore, this report recommended that women with unexplained pain severe enough to require opiate analgesia should have an urgent review. Importantly, the management of women who are unwell in pregnancy or postpartum requires a multidisciplinary approach using the right seniority of staff from the right specialities.

Systolic hypertension requires treatment   The most frequently identified instance of suboptimal care in the 8th report was inadequate control of hypertension resulting in intracranial haemorrhage. Women with a systolic blood pressure of ≥150 mmHg need urgent and effective antihypertensive treatment to control systolic blood pressure <150 mmHg. Due to the variation in clinical presentation of preeclampsia consideration should be given to antihypertensives at lower levels of blood pressure if there is a rapid deterioration in the patient's condition.

Genital tract sepsis   Sepsis is an increasing cause of maternal death which needs to be urgently addressed. Prevention of sepsis is essential, to this end all maternity professionals should adhere to infection control protocols (e.g. aseptic non-touch technique) when performing invasive procedures (including cannulation and catheterisation). Women should also be informed how to prevent transmission of infection. To facilitate early identification of sepsis all women should be informed of the signs and symptoms of genital tract infection. Any suspected severe infection should be referred back to obstetric services immediately. Where sepsis is suspected, broad spectrum antibiotics should be started as soon as possible (within first hour of signs of sepsis).

Serious Incident Reporting   Incident reviews were not undertaken in 20% of cases of maternal deaths between 2006 and 2008, and when incident reviews were carried out these were not always of high-quality. This deprives maternity services of an opportunity to identify and learn from suboptimal care. A high-quality, multidisciplinary local review is recommended for all maternal deaths, this should involve representatives from all relevant fields and the results disseminated to the same clinical environment. As with any critical incident review, it is important for recommendations to be implemented and their impact audited regularly.

Pathology   In 2006–8 autopsies performed in 85% of maternal deaths, although the quality of autopsies was questioned in some cases. Maternal death can be complex and needs additional specialist involvement as specific causes of death or signs at autopsy may need to be sought. Maternal deaths should be reported to the coroner when appropriate. Due to changes in the law, there is likely to be reduction in autopsies ordered by coroners, consequently there should be an attempt to obtain more consented hospital autopsies to ensure that there is as much information as possible to determine the cause of maternal death.

Further reading

Centre for Maternal and Child Enquiries (CMACE). Saving Mothers' Lives: reviewing maternal deaths to make motherhood safer: 2006–2008. The Eighth Report on Confidential Enquiries into Maternal Deaths in the United Kingdom. BJOG 2011; 118 (Suppl 1):1–203.

Investigation into 10 maternal deaths at, or following delivery at, Northwick Park Hospital, North West London Hospitals NHS Trust, between April 2002 and April 2005. London: Healthcare Commission, 2006.

Related topics of interest

- Amniotic fluid embolism (p. 174)
- Cardiac disease (p. 204)
- Infection in pregnancy (p. 243)
- Postpartum haemorrhage (p. 287)
- Pre-eclampsia and eclampsia (p. 290)
- Puerperal psychosis and postnatal depression (p. 303)
- Venous thromboembolism (p. 335)

Maternal sepsis

Overview

Historically, puerperal sepsis was a major cause of maternal mortality until the introduction of basic hygienic practice on the labour ward (after the observations of Semmelweis in the 1840s), coupled with the introduction of antibiotics in the middle of the 20th century.

One concerning finding is that the proportion of maternal deaths because of sepsis has increased, making sepsis the most common cause of direct maternal death in 8th Report of the Confidential Enquiries into Maternal Deaths. Genital tract sepsis caused 26 direct maternal deaths (out of a total 261 maternal deaths). In addition there were three late maternal deaths associated with sepsis occurring more than 6 weeks postnatally.

Clinical features

- Factors predisposing to sepsis include:
  - Black or ethnic minority
  - Preterm and/or prolonged rupture of membranes
  - Obesity
  - Retained products of conception
  - History of pelvic inflammatory disease/ vaginal discharge
  - Amniocentesis or similar invasive procedure
  - Group A streptococcus infection in close contacts
  - History of Group B streptococcus infection
  - Cervical cerclage
  - Prolonged use of catheters/wound drain/ intravenous cannula
  - Caesarean section
  - Underlying disease that may compromise immune system, e.g. diabetes, sickle cell disease/trait, anaemia
- Resistance to infection is lowered by malnutrition, exhaustion, anaemia or intercurrent disease
- Patients are usually febrile. Genital tract sepsis presents with pelvic discomfort, offensive lochia, which may be increased in amount and associated with an increased blood loss
- Established infection in the pelvis may be painful
- Abscess formation is associated with swinging pyrexia and signs of shock may supervene
- Onset of sepsis may be insidious at first but may deteriorate into septic shock, disseminated intravascular coagulopathy and multi-organ failure
- Group A streptococcus infection can progress very rapidly, with a median of 2 hours between first signs of infection to severe sepsis

Aetiology

Causative organisms may be exogenous or endogenous to the lower gastrointestinal tract or more rarely the vagina.

- Infective organisms ascend via the lower genital tract under the favourable conditions after delivery and colonize the uterine cavity
- Once infection is established it can spread directly through the pelvis and via the bloodstream to cause pelvic sepsis with abscess formation, septic thrombosis of pelvic veins and septicaemia. The end result is septic shock, which carries a high mortality
- There has been an increase over the last decade in community-acquired Lancefield Group A streptococcus (GAS), i.e. *Streptococcus pyogenes*. This is carried asymptomatically in 5–30% of the population with transmission via direct contact or droplets
- Other microbes implicated in genital tract sepsis include *Escherichia Coli, Enterococcus faecalis, Staphylococcus, Streptococcus pneumoniae, Morganella morganii* and *Clostridium septicum*

Diagnosis

Sepsis may be defined as infection plus systemic manifestations of infection, whilst severe sepsis may be defined as infection plus sepsis-induced organ dysfunction or tissue hypoperfusion. Septic shock is defined as the persistence of hypoperfusion despite adequate aggressive management with intravenous fluid replacement. Common symptoms include: productive cough, fever, urinary symptoms, diarrhoea, vomiting, pelvic pain, offensive vaginal discharge, rash or general non-specific symptoms such as lethargy or reduced appetite. However, clinical signs including pyrexia are not always related to the severity of the sepsis. Wound infection may be evident.

Diagnosis of sepsis is by a combination of infection (documented or suspected) and any of the following:

- Tachycardia (>90 beats per minute)
- Tachypnoea (>20 breaths per minute)
- Ileus (absent bowel sounds)
- Decreased capillary refill or mottling
- Impaired mental state, altered conscious level
- Fever (>38°C) or hypothermia (core temperature <36°C)
- Oliguria or oedema
- Arterial hypotension
- Coagulation abnormalities including thrombocytopenia (platelet count $<100 \times 10^9$/L)
- Hyperbilirubinemia (total bilirubin >70 µmol/L)
- Serum lactate >4 mmol/L (indicative of tissue hypoperfusion)
- Hyperglycaemia (plasma glucose >7.7 mmol/L) in the absence of diabetes
- White blood cell (WBC) count $>12 \times 10^9$/L or leucopenia (WBC count $<4 \times 10^9$/L)
- Plasma C-reactive protein >7 mg/L (usually significantly higher in bacterial sepsis)
- Creatinine rise of >44.2 µmol/L; sepsis is severe if creatinine level >176 µmol/L

If sepsis is suspected, the following investigations should be performed:
- Blood culture prior to any antibiotic administration
- Other samples to screen for infection should be guided by clinical suspicion: throat swab, midstream specimen of urine, high vaginal swab, cerebrospinal fluid, rapid MRSA screening (if status unknown)
- Relevant imaging studies including: chest X-ray, ultrasound and computed tomography (CT) scans should be performed promptly in an attempt to confirm the source of infection and identify abscess formation
- Full blood count, coagulation profile, C-reactive protein, urea and electrolytes, liver function tests. Arterial blood gas should be performed for pH, base excess and lactate

Management

Early recognition and initiation of treatment is the mainstay of sepsis management. Broad-spectrum antibiotic should be given within 1 hour of recognition of severe sepsis. Treatment should be promptly instituted whilst awaiting antibiotic sensitivities. Severe sepsis with acute organ dysfunction has a mortality rate of 20–40%, which increases to 60% if septic shock develops.

Diagnosis is on clinical grounds, confirmed by appropriate bacteriological investigation. It is important to cover the more virulent organisms such as streptococci, E coli and anaerobic bacteria. The decision to change antibiotic therapy is taken on clinical grounds, due to a lack of improvement in clinical condition. Antibiotic therapy is recommended as initial empirical treatment for presumed genital tract infection (**Table 43**).

Table 43 Initial empirical antibiotic treatment for maternal sepsis	
Sepsis degree	**Antibiotic therapy**
Non-severe sepsis	IV cefuroxime 750 mg 8-hourly + IV metronidazole 500 mg 8-hourly Penicillin allergy (anaphylaxis): IV clindamycin 900 mg 8-hourly + IV gentamicin once-daily (see local antibiotic guidelines for dosage - usually 3-5 mg/kg)
Severe sepsis or septic shock	Seek urgent microbiology advice/access local guidelines: IV meropenem 1 g 8-hourly + IV clindamycin 900 mg 8-hourly

- Genital tract sepsis may also occur after early pregnancy loss and first-trimester termination of pregnancy, hence antibiotics of metronidazole and azithromycin at the time of procedure or a course of doxycycline should be offered in accordance with Royal College of Obstetricians and Gynaecologists (RCOG) guidelines
- It is important to remember rare but potentially serious pathogens such as *Clostridium welchii* in situations where there is no clinical response to a broad-spectrum antibiotic therapy
- Surgical treatment options should always be considered, such as evacuation of the uterus or drainage of perineal or pelvic abscesses. Abscess may be drained under radiological guidance
- Record Modified Obstetric Early Warning Score (MOEWS) on an obstetric high-dependency chart (including documentation of fluid input/output)
- Involvement of senior multidisplinary team of consultant microbiologist, obstetrician, anaesthetist and critical care team
- Delivery if antenatal and likely to be beneficial to mother or baby
- If preterm and delivery is planned, cautious consideration should be given to use of antenatal steroids to improve fetal lung maturity
- Epidural/spinal anaesthesia should be avoided in women with sepsis and a general anaesthetic will usually be required for operative procedures

In conclusion, maternal sepsis should be regarded as an obstetric emergency, which requires prompt diagnosis and treatment with expertise from microbiologists. Consideration should be given to antibiotic prophylaxis in high risk situations to keep mortality and morbidity to a minimum.

Further reading

RCOG Green-top Guideline No. 64a. Bacterial sepsis in pregnancy. London: RCOG, 2012.
RCOG Green-top Guideline No. 7. The care of women requesting induced abortion. London: RCOG, 2004.

Centre for Maternal and Child Enquiries (CMACE). Saving Mothers' Lives: reviewing maternal deaths to make motherhood safer: 2006–2008. The Eighth Report on Confidential Enquiries into Maternal Deaths in the United Kingdom. BJOG 2011; 118 (Suppl 1):1–203.

Related topics of interest

Monitoring in labour

Low and high risk labours

Prior to commencing monitoring in labour it needs to be ascertained whether the labour is low or high risk dependent on maternal and/or fetal conditions. Illustrated below are factors for which a labour would be considered high risk for mother, fetus or both (this should not be regarded as an exhaustive list).

- **Pre-existing maternal medical conditions** Essential hypertension, bleeding/clotting disorders, cardiac disease, renal disease, diabetes, systemic lupus erythematosus, body mass index (BMI) > 35
- **Prior obstetric history** Previous postpartum haemorrhage, retained placenta, prior delivery by caesarean section, shoulder dystocia
- **Development of increased risk during current pregnancy** Pre-eclampsia, pregnancy induced hypertension, multiple pregnancy, gestational diabetes, preterm labour, recurrent reduced fetal movements, polyhydramnios
- **Fetal indications** Fetal growth restriction, some congenital abnormalities, e.g. gastroschisis/exomphalos, oligohydramnios
- **Development of increased risk during labour** Meconium stained liquor, pyrexia, new onset hypertension, use of oxytocin, delay in the first or second stage of labour, antepartum haemorrhage, epidural analgesia, prolonged rupture of membranes

Low risk labour

Maternal monitoring

Maternal observations should be performed on admission with established labour to confirm low risk status including: blood pressure, pulse and temperature. Once in established labour, management of labour should be with the aid of a partogram and minimum care should include 4-hourly blood pressure and temperature, hourly pulse, documentation of the strength and frequency of the contractions and vaginal examination 4-hourly in the first stage of labour. If monitoring detects slow progress in labour then interventions should be recommended, e.g. artificial rupture of membranes, intravenous oxytocin. If blood pressure, pulse and temperature are outside normal ranges then a change in maternal risk status should be noted and appropriate action taken; this may include transfer of care from a midwifery-led to a consultant-led unit.

Fetal monitoring

Fetal monitoring aims to detect fetal compromise to allow timely obstetric intervention to prevent fetal morbidity but to minimise unnecessary intervention. Continuous electronic fetal monitoring was introduced with the aim of reducing perinatal mortality and cerebral palsy. However, this reduction has not been demonstrated in systematic reviews but an increase in maternal intervention has been shown. Therefore, continuous electronic fetal monitoring is not advocated for low risk women. Intermittent auscultation with a handheld instrument (e.g. Doppler ultrasound or Pinard stethoscope) is the recommended method of monitoring for fetal well-being in low risk women. Intermittent auscultation of the fetal heart is recommended after a contraction, for at least 1 minute, at a minimum of 15 minute intervals during the first stage of labour. During the second stage of labour the frequency of intermittent auscultation should be increased to a minimum of 5 minute intervals.

If the risk status of the labour changes or there are any concerns detected by intermittent auscultation then continuous electronic fetal monitoring should be commenced.

High risk labour

Maternal monitoring

The close monitoring of patients, physiological parameters is the cornerstone of early detection of critical illness. However, it has been widely demonstrated that early changes in patient observations are often not detected or communicated to the appropriate personnel leading to a delay in intervention. The Early Warning Scoring System (EWS) was developed with the aim of providing a simple scoring system which could be readily applied by nurses and doctors to help identify patients developing critical illness. The EWS can be described as an aggregate weighted scoring system with six physiological parameters:

- Respiratory rate
- Oxygen saturations
- Pulse rate
- Blood pressure
- Temperature
- Neurological status

These parameters are scored between 0 and 3 with a score of ≥ 3 initiating the protocol. The Confidential Enquiry into Maternal Deaths in 2007 highlighted, as one of its top ten recommendations, an urgent need for the routine use of a national obstetric early warning chart. The report had highlighted that in many cases the early warning signs of impending maternal collapse went unrecognised. Obstetric early warning scores should now routinely form the basic monitoring in high risk mothers. The frequency of the individual observations and early warning score calculations are based on the clinical risks, e.g. a patient who has pre-eclampsia will need more frequent blood pressure monitoring than a mother who is high risk because she has renal disease with no additional complications.

Other monitoring of the progress of labour such as frequency of contractions and vaginal examinations is often the same as in a low risk labour – potentially with a lower threshold for an increased frequency to ensure adequate progress.

Fetal monitoring

Continuous electronic fetal monitoring should be utilised in all cases deemed high risk. This makes use of a cardiotocograph (CTG) which continuously depicts the fetal heart rate and the contraction pattern. Interpretation of the fetal heart rate needs to take into account which risk factors are present, the gestation, the prior tracing and the stage of labour. Since 2001, interpretation of CTGs has become more consistent with national published guidance. Classifications of the fetal heart rate tracings should now fall into three categories:

- Normal – when all four fetal heart features are reassuring
- Suspicious – when one feature is classified as non-reassuring
- Pathological – when two or more features are classified as non-reassuring or when one of more features are classified as abnormal

The above classification is illustrated in **Table 44**.

Table 44 Classification of fetal heart rate patterns				
Features	Baseline rate (bpm)	Variability (bpm)	Decelerations	Accelerations
Reassuring	110–160	≥ 5	none	Present
Non-reassuring	100–109 161–180	< 5 for 40–90	Typical variable decelerations with > 50% contractions for > 90 minutes Or Single prolonged deceleration up to 3 minutes duration	The absence of accelerations with an otherwise normal fetal heart rate trace is of uncertain significance – when in established labour
Abnormal	< 100 > 180	< 5 for 90	Atypical variable decelerations with > 50% contractions for > 30 minutes Or Late decelerations for > 30 minutes Or Single prolonged deceleration for > 3 minutes	

Table 45 Classification of fetal blood sample result with appropriate action plan		
pH Value	Classification	Recommended action
≥7.25	Normal FBS result	Repeat after no more than 1 hour if the FHR trace remains pathological, or sooner if there are further abnormalities
7.21–7.24	Borderline FBS result	Repeat after no more than 30 minutes if the FHR trace remains pathological, or sooner if there are further abnormalities
≤7.20	Abnormal FBS result	Inform senior obstetrician; delivery by the most appropriate method in the majority of cases.

It is recommended that the fetal heart rate pattern should be assessed at a minimum of hourly intervals. It is good practice to have a 'buddy' review of the fetal heart tracing with the main caregiver. Alternatively at regular intervals another midwife/obstetrician should review the fetal heart rate tracing – the fresh eyes approach.

Suspicious CTGs can be treated with conservative measures, e.g. change in maternal position, intravenous fluids, reduction in oxytocin dosage (in the presence of excessive contractions). If the fetal heart rate tracing is classified as pathological then fetal status should be ascertained by a fetal blood sample (FBS) taken from the fetal scalp.

If this is not possible (e.g. contraindicated, not technically possible because of minimal dilatation of the cervix) then delivery should be expedited by caesarean section. If a prolonged bradycardia occurs (> 3 minutes) then a plan should be made to expedite delivery of the baby should this not recover. If FBS is performed, appropriate action should depend upon the result (**Table 45**). If the fetal heart rate trace remains unchanged and the FBS result is stable after the second test, a further sample may be deferred unless additional abnormalities develop. Where a third FBS is considered necessary, consultant obstetric opinion should be sought.

Further reading

NICE clinical guideline no. 55. Intrapartum care. London: NICE, 2007.

Devane D, Lalor JG, Daly S, et al. Cardiotocography versus intermittent auscultation of fetal heart on admission to labour ward for assessment of fetal well-being. Cochrane Database Syst Rev 2012 Feb 15;2:CD005122.

Alfirevic Z, Devane D, Gyte GM. Continuous cardiotocography (CTG) as a form of electronic fetal monitoring (EFM) for fetal assessment during labour. Cochrane Database Syst Rev 2006; 19;(3):CD006066.

Centre for Maternal and Child Enquiries (CMACE). Saving Mothers' Lives: reviewing maternal deaths to make motherhood safer: 2006–2008. The Eighth Report on Confidential Enquiries into Maternal Deaths in the United Kingdom. BJOG 2011; 118 (Suppl 1):1–203.

Related topics of interest

Multiple pregnancy

Overview

Twin pregnancy occurs in about 1 in 80 spontaneous conceptions in the UK. Higher multiples follow Hellin's law. The incidence of higher multiples is reduced by a higher spontaneous miscarriage rate but is increased as a result of assisted conception techniques.

The incidence of multiple pregnancy increases with advancing maternal age and a family history of multiple pregnancy. The rate of monozygotic twins is fairly constant at 3–5 per 1000 maternities worldwide whereas dizygotic twin rates vary geographically being highest in the Yoruba tribe of Nigeria at 49/1000 maternities.

Clinical features

Multiple pregnancies can be classified either by zygosity (number of zygotes) or more importantly clinically by chorionicity (number of placenta) and amnionicity (number of amniotic sacs). 80% of all twin pregnancies are dizygotic and 20% monozygotic and thus identical. Depending on the timing of division of the zygote into two embryos, monozygotic twins could be dichorionic (splitting into two embryos < 4 days after fertilisation, 30%) or monochorionic (70%). Furthermore monochorionic twins could be diamniotic (splitting 4–8 days postfertilisation), monoamniotic (splitting 8–13 days) or conjoined (> 13 days).

Aetiology

The physiological changes of pregnancy are exaggerated in multiple pregnancy, notably an increase in plasma volume, a lesser increase in red cell mass, with a consequent tendency to anaemia. There is increased glomerular filtration rate and an increase in pregnancy-related hormones and placental proteins. There is a decreased tolerance to a blood glucose load, tending to the development of gestational diabetes.

Diagnosis

Chorionicity and amnionicity should be determined at the dating scan in the first trimester with the lambda sign confirming the presence of multiple placentas. Determining chorionicity and amnionicity is more difficult later in the second trimester especially if there is one placenta and the fetuses are same gender. Inter-twin membrane thickness < 2 mm is predictive of monochorionic twins. Screening for risk of Down's syndrome using the combined screening and specific nuchal translucency to calculate individual risks for the twins can be offered. The anomaly scan is at 18–20 weeks.

Chorionic villus sampling and amniocentesis for one or all fetuses for raised screening risk, genetic disorders and structural abnormalities are offered by fetal medicine specialists.

Twin-to-twin transfusion syndrome (TTTS) and is suspected, diagnosed and severity determined by difference in size, oligohydramnios/polyhydramnios, absent bladder and abnormal umbilical artery Dopplers in the donor and recipient twins. TTTS occurs in 5–15% of monochorionic twins. Therefore, fortnightly scans should be performed from 16–24 weeks and thereafter 3–4 weekly whereas dichorionic twins have growth scans every 3–4 weeks from 24 weeks.

Management
Complications

Most pregnancy-related problems are more frequent and more severe in multiple pregnancy. The diagnosis may be suspected by exaggerated symptoms of early pregnancy, particularly nausea and vomiting.

- Anaemia is more common, as is gestational diabetes, pre-eclampsia, preterm labour, fetal growth restriction and polyhydramnios. Recent studies suggest no significant increase in the incidence of antepartum haemorrhage. In higher order multiple pregnancies selective fetal reduction could reduce the risk of these complications

- TTTS occurs in 5–15% of monochorionic twins. If acute, the syndrome has a high mortality of 79–100% at 18–26 weeks. The effective treatment for severe forms of this is laser ablation of the communicating placental vessels. This requires expert input from a fetal medicine unit
- There is increased risk of chromosomal and structural abnormalities with the possibility of twins discordant for anomaly and the difficulty of subsequent management. This is particularly difficult in monochorionic pregnancy where one fetus has a lethal condition which carries an attendant risk of death and neurological damage to the normal fetus if the affected fetus dies. This dilemma also occurs with severe selective growth restriction in previable monochorionic twins. In monochorionic twins laser ablation of the placenta to separate the circulations or cord occlusion for the affected twin could save the normal fetus from the effects of the demise of the affected twin
- Cord entanglement can occur in monoamniotic pregnancies
- Other pregnancy-related symptoms may be more exaggerated in multiple pregnancy and cause significant distress, e.g. heartburn, constipation, backache, tiredness and discomfort from haemorrhoids

Antenatal care

Patients should be managed by consultant-led care, and seen regularly in the antenatal clinic; iron and folate supplements are routinely prescribed. Blood pressure and fetal growth are regularly monitored, with ultrasound scans at least at 4-weekly intervals in later pregnancy.

Management of labour

In the absence of complications dichorionic twins are usually delivered at 38–40 weeks, monochorionic diamniotic twins at 36–37 weeks and monoamniotic twins at 32–34 weeks. Twins may deliver vaginally if the presenting twin is cephalic and there are no other complications. The labour should be supervised by an experienced obstetrician with an anaesthetist present and facilities for emergency caesarean section and expert neonatal care readily available.

Elective caesarean section may be considered if there is a malpresentation of the first twin; or if maternal or fetal circumstances warrant. Elective caesarean section is the preferred mode of delivery for monoamniotic twins, and higher multiples.

Perinatal mortality

For twins and triplets the perinatal mortality rate is about five times that of singleton births. The main aetiological factor is prematurity.

Rare causes of twin mortality include locked and conjoined twins. The second and third triplets are at greater risk, with a delay in delivery of 5 minutes after the birth of the first triplet being significant. The maturity of the triplets is of greater prognostic significance than their size.

Further reading

Twining P. Abnormalities of twin pregnancy. In: Twining P, McHugo JM, Pilling DW (Eds). Textbook of Fetal Abnormalities. Edinburgh: Churchill Livingstone, 2007:405–426.

Engineer N, Fisk N. Multiple pregnancy. In: Rodeck CH, Whittle MJ (Eds). Fetal Medicine: Basic Science and Clinical Practice. Edinburgh: Churchill Livingstone, 2009:649–677.

Crowther CA. Multiple pregnancy including delivery. In: James DK, et al (Eds). High Risk Pregnancy Management Options. London: WB Saunders, 1994: 137–149.

Daw E. Triplet pregnancy. In: Studd J (Ed.). Progress in Obstetrics and Gynaecology, Vol. 6. Edinburgh: Churchill Livingstone, 1987:119–131.

MacGillivray I. Multiple pregnancy. In: Turnbull Sir AC, Chamberlain GC (Eds). Obstetrics. Edinburgh: Churchill Livingstone, 1989:493–502.

Related topics of interest

- Antenatal care (p. 183)
- Changes to maternal physiology in pregnancy (p. 210)

- Feticide and late termination of pregnancy (p. 231)

Neonatal resuscitation

Overview

Labour and birth are stressful events for the neonate. Contractions lead to periods of hypoxia as the retroplacental pool of oxygenated maternal blood is expelled from the uterus. The majority of infants tolerate this period of hypoxia–reperfusion well. However, approximately 6% of term infants require some bag and mask ventilation, but only 0.4% of term infants require intubation.

Unlike adults, the primary event leading to cardiorespiratory collapse is respiratory not cardiac.

Prolonged intrauterine hypoxia leads to an attempt to breathe. If this hypoxia persists then the fetus will lose consciousness and the neurons in the respiratory centre will fail to stimulate breathing; this is termed primary apnoea. The heart rate then reduces as the myocardium switches to anaerobic metabolism and blood is shunted away from the peripheries to vital organs. The anaerobic metabolism leads to a lactic acidosis. If the hypoxic stimulus persists, the fetus will gasp (at a rate of ~12/min). If these gasps don't aerate the lungs, then a period of secondary or terminal apnoea will occur. Without intervention the infant will die.

75% of babies who died in the neonatal period in the UK in 2008 had absent or ineffective respiratory activity at 5 minutes and 31% had a heart rate that was persistently < 100.

As the primary event is respiratory, intervention focuses on aerating the lungs and delivering oxygen to the heart and brain to enable the myocardium and respiratory centre to recover and resume control of breathing and circulation. Rarely, chest compressions are needed to move oxygenated blood from the lungs to the myocardium.

Aetiology

Fetal hypoxia may result from a variety of intrauterine causes including placental insufficiency, cord compression, placental abruption and fetomaternal haemorrhage.

Where fetal hypoxia is anticipated, appropriate staff should be present at delivery to manage neonatal resuscitation.

Clinical management

Advanced Neonatal Life Support should be provided by expert neonatologists/nurses.

This chapter discusses basic newborn life support as recommended by the Resuscitation Council, UK.

This is simplified in the algorithm shown in **Figure 24**.

After birth of uncompromised infants, clamping of the umbilical cord should be delayed for 60 seconds. Where an infant is severely compromised (or severe compromise is anticipated), there should be no delay in cord clamping.

Infants that are pale, floppy with no respiratory effort and heart rate < 100 require resuscitation.

At birth all babies should be handled gently, wrapped and kept warm after the cord is clamped.

If a baby does not have good tone, colour, respiratory effort and heart rate it should be transferred to a flat surface which should ideally have good lighting and a source of radiant heat. In the hospital setting, this is usually a Resuscitaire. The baby's condition should be reassessed every 30 seconds – key features include: tone, colour, respiratory rate and heart rate. The heart rate should be listened to using a stethoscope. The easiest way to assess oxygenation and heart rate is to use a pulse oximeter.

If the baby is gasping or not breathing at 30 seconds of age then the airway should be opened by placing the head in a neutral position, then five inflation breaths should be delivered.

Inflation breaths are best delivered using air. Each breath should last about 2–3 seconds. As oxygenated blood reaches the myocardium the heart rate may improve. If the chest does not move after five breaths or there is no improvement in the heart rate then the lungs are not being aerated.

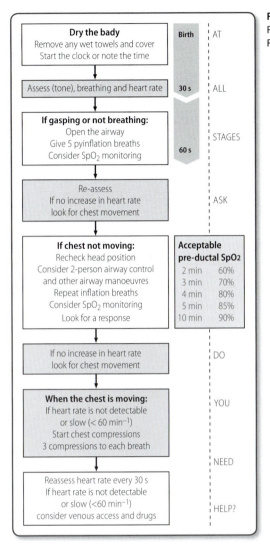

Figure 24 Algorithm for Newborn Life Support. Reproduced with the kind permission of the Resuscitation Council (UK).

If this is the case, the airway should be checked and further inflation breaths given. If the heart rate is < 100 beats per minute despite good chest movements, cardiac compressions should be started. The airway should be inspected using a laryngoscope and any solid matter removed by suctioning.

Chest compressions should be delivered by grasping the infant's chest so that both thumbs press down upon the lower third of the sternum. The chest should be compressed quickly and briskly to a depth of one-third of the chest. The ratio of compressions is three compressions to one breath.

The job of the chest compressions is to move oxygen from the lungs to the myocardium. Good ventilation of the lungs should not be compromised to facilitate rapid chest compressions.

Very few term infants (< 1:1000) require drugs for resuscitation. Drugs used in this setting include adrenaline, sodium bicarbonate and dextrose. If hypovolaemia is suspected then saline may be given intravenously.

In a term newborn with no cardiac activity, and with cardiac activity that remains undetectable for 10 minutes, it is appropriate to consider stopping resuscitation. The decision to continue resuscitation efforts beyond 10 minutes with no cardiac activity is often complex and may be influenced by issues such as the presumed aetiology of the arrest, the gestation of the baby, the presence or absence of complications, and the parents' previous expressed feelings about acceptable risk of morbidity. Hence, the decision to cease resuscitation must be taken by the most senior member of the neonatal team present.

Further reading

Resuscitation Council UK. Resuscitation Guidelines, Chapter 11 Newborn Life Support. London: Resuscitation Council UK, 2010.

Chan LC, Hey E. Can all neonatal resuscitation be managed by nurse practitioners? Arch Dis Child Fetal Neonatal 2006; 91(1):F52–F55.

Owen CJ, Wyllie JP. Determination of heart rate in the baby at birth. Resuscitation 2004; 60(2):213–217.

Related topics of interest

- Caesarean section (p. 198)
- Instrumental delivery (p. 247)
- Monitoring in labour (p. 262)
- Shoulder dystocia (p. 319)

Normal labour

Overview

Normal labour is defined as the onset of regular, painful uterine contractions which cause progressive effacement and dilatation of the cervix. There is accompanied descent and rotation of the fetal head until full dilatation is reached. At this point, contractions become expulsive and with the aid of maternal effort, the baby is delivered. Labour is complete when the placenta and membranes are delivered.

Labour is divided into three stages:
- First stage: onset of labour to full dilatation.
- Second stage: from full dilatation to delivery of the baby.
- Third stage: the period following delivery of the baby until expulsion of the placenta and membranes is complete

Aetiology

The process by which the cervix must transform from a rigid, tubular structure to a soft structure capable of effacement and dilatation is known as cervical ripening. The cervix is composed of connective tissue, mainly collagen, and a key aspect to cervical ripening is the rearrangement and realignment of collagen fibres. It also involves an inflammatory reaction and cervical tissue at term has an inflammatory cell infiltrate. The uterine smooth muscle, responds to stimuli to cause the cells to contract.

The main triggers for the initiation of labour are still uncertain in humans. Both aspects of cervical ripening and uterine contraction seem to involve prostaglandins, making this the key pharmacological target for inducing labour.

The first stage

The latent phase is the period of time, which is not necessarily continuous, where painful contractions and cervical effacement occur. Dilatation up to 4 cm should also occur. After this point, the established first stage of labour is said to have started and there should be progressive cervical dilatation.

The duration of labour is variable, depending on many factors such as parity, gestation and the size of the baby. The rate of expected dilatation was originally described by Friedman in the 1950s using observational data (Friedman's curve). This data has been updated over time and now the National Institute for Health and Clinical Excellence (NICE) suggests that first labours should last on average 8 hours and usually no longer than 18 hours. Second and subsequent labours should last on average 5 hours and usually no longer than 12 hours.

Progress in established labour is monitored by repeated vaginal examinations every 4 hours and is traditionally plotted on a partogram, with a 4-hour action line as recommended by the World Health Organization (WHO) (**Figure 25**). All aspects of progress in labour should be taken into consideration, including cervical dilatation, descent and rotation of the fetal head and the duration, strength and frequency of contractions.

Observations in the first stage should include:
- Four-hourly temperature and blood pressure measurements
- Hourly pulse
- Half hourly documentation of frequency of contractions
- Four-hourly vaginal examination. Vaginal examination should take into account colour of the amniotic fluid (e.g. blood-stained, meconium-stained) if membranes are ruptured; dilatation of the cervix; station of the presenting part in relation to the ischial spines; position of the vertex, and the presence or absence of caput and moulding
- Frequency of bladder emptying
- The fetal heart rate should be checked every 15 minutes and be recorded for at least 1 minute.

The package known as 'active management of labour' as adopted by O'Driscoll et al. should not be routinely offered in a normally progressing labour.

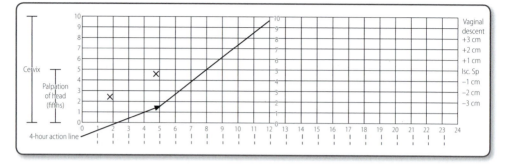

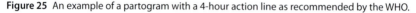

Figure 25 An example of a partogram with a 4-hour action line as recommended by the WHO.

The second stage

This is divided into the passive stage, which is when full dilatation is diagnosed but there are no expulsive contractions. The active second stage is defined as either when the baby is visible; expulsive contractions occur and full dilatation is detected; or when active maternal effort is encouraged in the absence of expulsive contraction, full dilatation having previously been diagnosed. If full dilatation is detected in a woman who does not have an epidural and who has no urges to push, she should be reassessed after 1 hour. This allows further time for rotation and descent of the head to occur.

In nulliparous women delivery should be expected to have occurred within 3 hours of the onset of active second stage. In multiparous women, delivery should have occurred within 2 hours of the onset of active second stage. If delivery has not occurred after 2 hours of active second stage in nulliparous women and 1 hour in multiparous women, the woman should be assessed by a health care professional with consideration to undertaking an operative vaginal delivery.

Observations in the second stage should include:
- Hourly blood pressure and pulse
- 4-hourly temperature
- Vaginal examination hourly
- Half hourly documentation of frequency of contractions
- Frequency of bladder emptying
- Assessment of effectiveness of maternal pushing

- Intermittent auscultation of the fetal heart after a contraction. This should occur every 5 minutes and be recorded for at least 1 minute.

The mechanism of normal birth

The fetus has to pass through the maternal pelvis. Normally the head enters the pelvic brim in the occipitolateral position. The fetal neck flexes which presents the smallest diameter of the head – the suboccipito-bregmatic. Uterine contractions encourage descent of the fetal head through the pelvis and once it reaches the pelvic floor, it rotates through 90° to the most favourable occipitoanterior position. It continues to descend until it reaches the perineum when the head delivers via extension.

Simultaneously, the shoulders enter the pelvis in the transverse position. They also rotate to an anteroposterior position once they reach the pelvic floor. Once the head has delivered, it rotates back to the transverse position via a process called restitution. The shoulders are then delivered by gentle downward traction to release the anterior shoulder from under the pelvic brim. Delivery is completed by upward traction to release the posterior shoulder and the remainder of the body.

The third stage

This can either be active or physiological. Active management involves the routine use of uterotonic drugs; early clamping and cutting of the umbilical cord, and controlled cord traction. This is recommended as it reduces the risk of postpartum haemorrhage. It is also associated with an increased rate of side effects such as nausea, vomiting and hypertension when ergometrine is used. Physiological management involves not using uterotonic drugs; avoidance of clamping the cord until pulsation has ceased, and delivery of the placenta by maternal effort.

Active management should be complete within 30 minutes following delivery of the baby and physiological management within 60 minutes. If physiological management is not complete within this time or if there are complications such as bleeding, active management should be initiated or if the woman requests it at any point during the third stage.

Observations in the third stage should include:

- Documentation of maternal general physical condition and observations
- Vaginal blood loss

Further reading

National Collaborating Centre for Woman's and Children's Health. Intrapartum care: management and delivery of care to women in labour. NICE Clinical guideline no. 55. London: RCOG, 2008.

O'Driscoll K, Jackson JA, Gallagher JT. Prevention of prolonged labour. BMJ 1969; 2:447–480.

Friedman EA. Primagravid labor. Obstet Gynecol 1955; 6:567–589.

Friedman EA. Labor in multiparas. Obstet Gynecol 1956; 8:691–703.

WHO, World Health Organization partograph in the management of labour. World Health Organization Maternal Health and Safe Motherhood Programme. Lancet 1994; 343:1399–1404.

Related topics of interest

Obstetric cholestasis and acute fatty liver of pregnancy

Overview

Obstetric cholestasis (OC) describes a condition with pruritus in the absence of a skin rash, and abnormal liver function tests (LFTs) which have no other cause, and resolve after birth. OC affects 0.7% of pregnancies in the UK; the incidence rises to 1.2–1.5% in Indian or Pakistani women. OC is more common in multiple pregnancies and in 35% there is a family history.

The potential risks to the fetus are:
- Spontaneous preterm delivery (4–12%)
- Iatrogenic preterm delivery (7–25%)
- Meconium-stained liquor (25% in preterm OC and 12% in term OC)
- Intrapartum fetal distress
- Caesarean section delivery rate (up to 36%)
- Stillbirth – in treated OC the perinatal death rate is 9.1–10.6 per 1000 which compares with the rate for the general population (8.3–13.4 per 1000).

Acute fatty liver of pregnancy (AFLP) is a rare condition, with an incidence of 1 in 9–13,000 pregnancies. It is more common in nulliparous women, obese women, male fetuses and multiple pregnancies. AFLP has an approximately 10–20% risk of maternal mortality and a 20–30% risk of perinatal mortality.

Aetiology

Obstetric cholestasis is hypothesised to be associated with increased circulating oestrogens having a cholestatic effect, as the increased oestrogens lead to a reduced sulphation of bile acids. There is also a reduction in the fluidity of the liver cells. Genetic factors imply an autosomal dominant sex-limited inheritance.

The pathophysiology of AFLP is poorly understood. There is microvesicular fatty infiltration of hepatocytes. Some patients with AFLP have defects in fatty acid oxidation.

Clinical features

OC is characterised by intense pruritus, especially affecting palms and soles, which usually occurs in the third trimester. The pruritus may result in insomnia and distress. There is no rash visible, but sometimes excoriations are evident from the pruritus. Abnormal LFTs including elevated bilirubin and alanine transaminase (ALT) may occur. Pale stools, dark urine and anorexia may also occur.

AFLP classically presents after 34 weeks' gestation. Significant vomiting and abdominal pain can occur. Marked hypoglycaemia and raised urate levels can be a feature. There is a risk of disseminated intravascular coagulation (DIC), and fulminant liver failure including hepatic encephalopathy.

Diagnosis

OC The diagnosis is made if there is pruritus without a rash, in the presence of raised bile acids when other causes have been excluded. Other causes of pruritus include eczema or polymorphic eruption of pregnancy, although a rash should be evident in both these conditions. Other causes of abnormal LFTs include pre-eclampsia, AFLP, viral infection, gallstones and autoimmune causes.

The diagnosis of OC can be confirmed postnatally when symptoms of pruritus resolve and the elevated bile acids and LFTs return to normal.

Investigations taken if OC is suspected include full blood count (FBC), clotting screen, LFTs and bile acids. Bile acids are raised, and may be the only abnormal parameter; > 14 mmol/L is abnormal. ALT shows a moderate rise, a mild rise in bilirubin is less common (pregnancy reference ranges: ALT 5–40 U/L and bilirubin 0–22 U/L).

If initial blood results are normal but the patient's symptoms continue, then tests should be repeated weekly, as the symptoms can predate the abnormalities. If the diagnosis is unclear, consider further investigations depending on maternal history including: viral screen for hepatitis A, B, C, cytomegalovirus and Epstein–Barr virus, liver autoimmune screen, (comprising of antismooth muscle and antimitochondrial antibodies for chronic active hepatitis and primary biliary cirrhosis). Ultrasound scan (USS) of the liver and biliary tree, to exclude gallstones, hepatitis and cirrhosis.

AFLP   This may be confused with liver damage from pre-eclampsia (PE) or HELLP syndrome. However, in PE/HELLP blood pressure will be raised and proteinuria present. Intravascular haemolysis is a late feature of AFLP but is evident in HELLP syndrome. USS and computed tomography (CT) scan of the liver have been used to differentiate between AFLP and other causes of liver dysfunction. In AFLP, ammonia, LFTs and urates are raised, with hypoglycaemia. Imaging may demonstrate fatty infiltration of the liver. A comparison of OC and AFLP diagnosis can be seen in **Table 46**.

Table 46 Comparison of OC and AFLP for diagnosis . –, not present; +, present; ++, strongly present for each condition.		
Findings	OC	AFLP
Pruritus	++	–
Vomiting + abdominal pain	–	++
Hypertension	–	+
Proteinuria	–	+
Raised LFTs	+	++
Hypoglycaemia	–	++
Raised urates	–	++
Disseminated intravascular coagulation	–	++
Liver USS	Normal	Fatty infiltration
Ratio of male: female fetus	M:F 1:1	M:F 3:1

Management

OC   After diagnosis women must be counselled with regards the potential risks of the condition. Treatment is offered for relief of pruritus and to improve levels of LFTs and bile acids. Currently, there is no evidence that present treatment improves perinatal outcomes. There are no biochemical or ultrasound investigations that predict poor pregnancy outcome.

Emollients, for example aqueous cream, can help with the pruritus. Ursodeoxycholic acid (UDCA) reduces pruritus and normalises LFTs in women with OC. The starting dose is 300 mg 8-hourly and this can be increased to 1800 mg per day. It is not licensed for use in pregnancy, but has been used widely with no reports of adverse effects.

There is a theoretical risk that absorption of vitamin K is reduced in OC. If prothrombin time is prolonged 5–10 mg per day aqueous vitamin K should be prescribed. When prothrombin time is normal, women should be carefully counselled about potential benefits and risks of vitamin K. Dexamethasone 10 mg per day for 7 days, followed by 3 days off, should not be given outside randomised controlled trials without careful consultation between the woman and her consultant obstetrician.

As stillbirth in OC cannot be predicted, delivery should be offered between 37 and 38 weeks. However, a discussion should include information of the increased risk of perinatal and maternal morbidity from early intervention (after 37 weeks of gestation). The case for induction of labour may be stronger in those with more severe biochemical abnormality (ALT and bile acids).

In the postpartum period advice should be given to avoid oestrogen-containing contraceptives and that there is a 60% recurrence risk of OC. LFTs should be rechecked 48 hours after delivery and 2 weeks later to ensure a return to normal.

Management of AFLP involves correcting the hypoglycaemia with intravenous dextrose, treating the coagulopathy with fresh frozen plasma and/or cryoprecipitate. Red cell transfusions may be required to replace blood loss. After maternal condition has been stabilised, delivery should be expedited.

Further reading

Nelson-Piercy C. Handbook of Obstetric Medicine, 2nd edn. London: Martin Dunitz 2002: 204–212.

RCOG Green-top Guideline No. 43. Obstetric cholestasis. London: RCOG, 2011.

Related topics of interest

Oligohydramnios and polyhydramnios

Overview

The assessment of reduced (oligohydramnios) or excessive (polyhydramnios) volumes of liquor are clinically highly subjective. The use of ultrasound has enabled a semiquantitative method of fluid volume determination. The largest pocket of liquor is identified and measured. Fluid volume is defined as normal when the largest pocket measures > 2 cm and < 8 cm in its maximal vertical diameter.

Polyhydramnios is therefore defined as a pool depth of > 8 cm, with a pool depth < 2 cm (in some reports 1 cm) defined as oligohydramnios. Semiquantative four-quadrant assessment of liquor volume measurement known as Amniotic Fluid Index (AFI) is also widely used. AFI is known to varying according to gestation, but a general definition of polyhydramnios is an AFI > 24 cm and oligohydramnios when the AFI is < 8 cm (see **Figure 26**)

Clinical features

Polyhydramnios

The diagnosis of polyhydramnios is often suspected clinically when examination reveals a greater than expected symphysis fundal height measurement for gestational age. This should be confirmed by ultrasound scan. Polyhydramnios, particularly if acute, can cause significant maternal discomfort and even respiratory compromise. Polyhydramnios is associated with a 17-fold increase in major fetal abnormalities and a 7-fold increase in perinatal mortality. Other fetal risks associated with polyhydramnios include:

- Unstable lie
- Cord prolapse
- Premature labour
- Preterm rupture of membranes
- Placental abruption

Tapping of amniotic fluid in severe cases is possible, but only causes brief respite from symptoms and can be associated with premature labour and introduction of infection into the amniotic cavity.

Oligohydramnios

Oligohydramnios is suspected clinically when a smaller than expected symphysis fundal height is measured and fetal parts are particularly easy to palpate. The clinical impact of oligohydramnios is dependent on

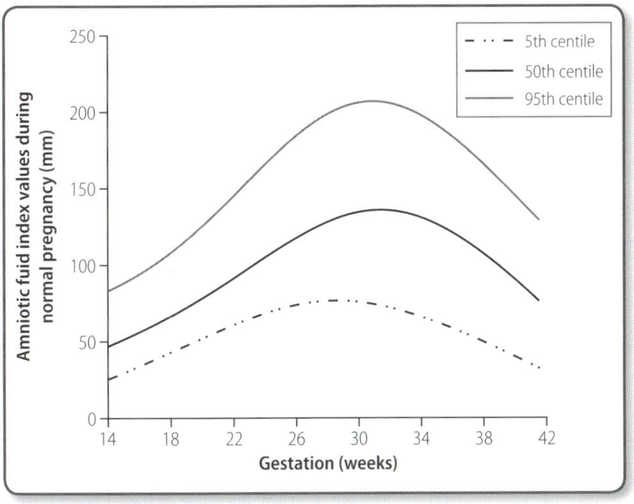

Figure 26 Change in amniotic fluid index over gestation.

the gestation at which it is discovered. There is an increase in major fetal abnormalities in oligohydramnios compared to pregnancies with normal liquor volume. Other fetal risks associated with oligohydramnios are: fetal growth restriction (FGR), chronic intrauterine asphyxia and stillbirth.

The importance of oligohydramnios as a parameter in the biophysical profile has been established. The decrease in amniotic fluid in chronic fetal compromise is that fetal blood flow away from fetal lungs and kidneys, which are the two main areas of amniotic fluid production.

Aetiology

Amniotic fluid volume is the result of flow into and out of the amniotic sac. In the early stages of pregnancy the amniotic fluid is produced by active transport of sodium and chloride ions across the amniotic membrane and fetal skin, with water moving according to osmotic gradients. In the second half of pregnancy, the amniotic fluid volume is the balance of fluid production by the fetal kidneys and respiratory secretions and that are swallowed by the fetus.

Polyhydramnios can have a maternal or fetal origin:

- 50% idiopathic
- Increased production by fetus, e.g. hydrops
- Impaired fetal swallowing, e.g. oesophageal atresia
- 15% are associated with maternal diabetes
- Twin-to-twin transfusion syndrome in multiple pregnancies

The underlying causes of oligohydramnios are as follows:

- Premature rupture of membranes
- Placental insufficiency (reduced perfusion of the fetal kidneys as blood is preferentially shunted to the brain, resulting in reduced urine output); this may be associated with FGR or pre-eclampsia
- Fetal abnormalities (e.g. bladder outlet obstruction, if early anhydramnios consider bilateral renal agenesis)
- Prolonged pregnancy
- Maternal use of angiotensin-converting enzyme inhibitors

- Is associated with raised alpha-fetoprotein (AFP) in maternal serum

Diagnosis

Ultrasound assessment of liquor volume, using the parameters described above, is used to diagnose oligohydramnios and polyhydramnios. A detailed ultrasound assessment of fetal anatomy should then take place to look for fetal structural anomalies, assess fetal growth and if appropriate Doppler assessment of umbilical artery blood flow. In advanced gestation detailed assessment of fetal anatomy can be difficult.

In the presence of oligohydramnios, a careful maternal history should be obtained to elicit the possibility of premature rupture of membranes and speculum examination is advised to observe liquor.

Additional maternal investigations advisable upon the detection of polyhydramnios include serum screen for toxoplasmosis, rubella, cytomegalovirus and herpes simplex virus (TORCH) and screening for gestational diabetes in the form of a glucose tolerance test (GTT).

Management

Polyhydramnios

The management of polyhydramnios is dependent on the underlying cause, if one is found. If an underlying structural fetal abnormality or maternal infection is detected a referral should be made to a tertiary level fetal medicine unit for further management. If screening for maternal diabetes is positive, blood glucose monitoring should be instituted and arrangements made for further management in a joint multidisciplinary diabetic antenatal clinic.

Oligohydramnios

The management of oligohydramnios is dependent on the suspected underlying aetiology, but also the gestational age at which it occurs. Oligohydramnios detected before 22 weeks of gestation is a particularly serious finding because (i) there may be a lethal fetal abnormality, e.g. renal agenesis or

(ii) the incidence of pulmonary hypoplasia is very high as liquor plays an important role in lung development. This can be compounded further by premature delivery, which may be spontaneous or iatrogenic. Thus, when oligohydramnios is detected under 22 weeks women need to be counselled about the potential impact on fetal lung development and termination of pregnancy should be offered.

The management of other conditions are briefly outlined below:

- Preterm prelabour rupture of membranes: treat with antibiotics (as per local guidelines), corticosteroids after 24 weeks of gestation, monitor for signs of maternal sepsis, initiate preterm delivery if signs of maternal sepsis. Consider elective delivery between 34–36 weeks (see Topic 95 for more detail)
- Oligohydramnios with/without FGR: regular fetal surveillance in form of growth scans, umbilical artery Doppler, Ductus Venosus Doppler if umbilical artery Doppler is abnormal, consider elective induction of labour before term or earlier if static growth/abnormal Doppler waveform, may need steroid cover
- Fetal abnormality: referral to regional fetal medicine unit

Further reading

Golan A, et al. Oligohydramnios: maternal complications and fetal outcome in 145 cases. Gynecol Obstet Invest 1994; 37:91–94.

RCOG Green-top Guideline No. 31. The investigation and management of the small-for-gestational-age fetus. London: RCOG, 2013.

Harman CR. Amniotic fluid abnormalities. Semin Perinatol 2008; 32(4):288–294.

Related topics of interest

Perineal repair

Overview

Over 85% of women will experience some degree of perineal trauma at the time of a vaginal delivery. Trauma can result from an episiotomy or from tears. Tears can occur anteriorly, involving the labia, clitoris or urethra or posteriorly, involving the perineal skin, muscle or the anal sphincter.

Clinical features

Risk factors for perineal trauma:
- First vaginal delivery
- Fetal macrosomia
- Mode of delivery – instrumental > spontaneous vaginal delivery
- Malpresentation and malposition of the fetus
- Ethnicity – white women at greater risk than black women
- Age – older women at greater risk
- Poor nutritional status

Perineal trauma is associated with both short term and long term physical and psychological sequelae.
- Pain
  - Perineal pain is present in up to 42% of women 10–12 days postnatally
  - Perineal pain is present in up to 10% of women 3–18 months postnatally
  - Superficial dyspareunia occurs in up to 23% of women 3 months postnatally
- Incontinence
  - Urinary incontinence – present in up to 24% of women
  - Faecal incontinence – present in 3–10% of women

Classification

Since 2001 the classification of anal sphincter injury, described by Sultan, has been accepted by the Royal College of Obstetricians and Gynaecologists (RCOG) and the International Consultation on Incontinence (**Table 47**).

The incidence of third-degree tears is approximately 0.5–0.7% of vaginal deliveries.

Management

Prevention

The use of antenatal perineal massage has been advocated in reducing the incidence of perineal tears and/or episiotomies. Meta-analysis from four trials concluded:
- A significant reduction in the incidence in episiotomy rates in women without a previous vaginal birth only
- A reduction in the incidence of trauma requiring suturing
- No differences in the incidence of first- or second-degree perineal tears or third- or fourth-degree tears
- No significant differences in the incidence of instrumental deliveries, sexual satisfaction, or incontinence of urine, faeces or flatus for any women who practiced perineal massage compared with those who did not

Table 47 Classification of perineal trauma: external anal sphincter (EAS); and internal anal sphincter (IAS)		
Type of tear		**Nature of injury**
First-degree		Injury to perineal skin only
Second-degree		Injury to perineum involving perineal muscles but not involving the anal sphincter
Third-degree	3A	Less than 50% of EAS thickness torn
	3B	More than 50% of EAS thickness torn
	3C	Both EAS and IAS torn
Fourth-degree		Injury to perineum involving the anal sphincter complex (EAS and IAS) and anal epithelium

Restrictive episiotomy (a surgical incision only when there is a clear maternal or fetal indication) reduces the risk of posterior perineal trauma. A review of randomised trials comparing restrictive use of episiotomy with routine episiotomy reports less suturing, fewer healing complications and no difference in most pain measures with the use of restrictive episiotomy. There is no increased risk of third-degree tear with restrictive episiotomy.

If an episiotomy is required the mediolateral technique is recommended, as midline incisions are more likely to result in severe tears.

Labour/delivery

Continuous support in labour has been shown to reduce the need for assisted vaginal delivery, thereby reducing perineal trauma. A systematic review in 2012 reported a significant reduction in the incidence of third- and fourth-degree tears following the use of warm compresses compared with hands-off or no warm compress on.

Following delivery, women should be examined systematically by an experienced medical professional to assess the extent of trauma prior to repair.

Repair and surgical technique

All tears should be repaired by an appropriately trained professional and a clear description of the extent of perineal injury and repair method should be documented in all cases. A digital rectal examination should be performed in posterior vaginal and perineal trauma to exclude damage to the anal sphincters or mucosa.

Episiotomy and first/second-degree tear repairs

A review of eight randomised control trials report that the use of absorbable polyglycolic sutures (Vicryl/Dexon) result in less pain than catgut sutures. Incidence of short term pain, analgesia use and resuturing is reduced in the absorbable suture groups, but no difference is seen in the incidence of long term pain. There is evidence that the use of a continuous suturing technique compared with an interrupted technique is associated with less

immediate pain, but no significant difference in long term pain. Continuous subcutaneous skin closure appears to reduce short term pain up to 10 days postpartum, but evidence is limited.

There is some controversy regarding whether to suture first-degree perineal tears. It has been reported that not suturing reduces pain both immediately postpartum and up to 3 months postpartum; however, it may be associated with reduced healing. More research is needed to provide recommendations in clinical practice.

Repair of third/fourth-degree tears

All third/fourth-degree tears should be repaired in the operating theatre under regional or general anaesthesia, by adequately trained professionals.

Two techniques are described for repair of the external anal sphincter – end-to-end or overlapping method. Both have an equivalent outcome. Monofilament sutures or modern braided sutures are recommended for use in external anal sphincter (EAS) repair. An interrupted method is recommended for internal anal sphincter repair. A fine suture is recommended for internal anal sphincter (IAS) repair, as it may cause less discomfort. To prevent surgical knot migration, it is recommended that knots are buried beneath the superficial perineal muscles

Postnatal care

All women should be counselled regarding the extent of their perineal tears. Advice should be given regarding perineal hygiene, the use of analgesia and pelvic floor exercises.

Third/fourth-degree perineal tears

In addition to the above advice, women who have sustained third/fourth-degree tears should be advised regarding the use of laxatives to reduce the incidence of wound dehiscence secondary to straining on defaecation. A course of broad spectrum antibiotics to reduce infection and wound dehiscence should also be given. All women should be offered physiotherapy and pelvic floor exercises for 6–12 weeks postnatally and followed up 6–12 weeks postpartum by a consultant obstetrician and gynaecologist.

Symptoms of incontinence and dyspareunia are embarrassing; therefore the long term morbidity of third/fourth degree tears is often underreported by women. The prognosis following EAS repair is good, with 60–80% asymptomatic at 12 months. Mode of delivery in a subsequent pregnancy should be discussed with women with a history of third/fourth degree tears. They should be aware of the risk of developing incontinence or worsening symptoms with a subsequent vaginal delivery. Any woman with ongoing symptoms should be given the option of elective caesarean section.

Further reading

Aasheim V, Nilsen ABV, et al. Perineal techniques during the second stage of labour for reducing perineal trauma. Cochrane Database of Systematic Reviews 2011; (12) Art. No.: CD006672. doi: 10.1002/14651858.CD006672.pub2.

Kettle C, Dowswell T, Ismail KMK. Continuous and interrupted suturing techniques for repair of episiotomy or second-degree tears. Cochrane Database of Systematic Reviews, 2012, (11). Art. No.: CD000947. doi: 10.1002/14651858. CD000947.pub3.

Carroli G, Mignini L. Episiotomy for vaginal birth. Cochrane Database of Systematic Reviews 2009; (1). Art. No.: CD000081. doi: 10.1002/14651858. CD000081.pub2.

Beckmann MM, Garrett AJ. Antenatal perineal massage for reducing perineal trauma. Cochrane Database of Systematic Reviews 2006; (1). Art. No.: CD005123. DOI: 10.1002/14651858. CD005123.pub2.

Sultan AH. Obstetric perineal injury and anal incontinence. Clin Risk 1999; 5:193–196.

Related topics of interest

• Instrumental delivery (p. 247)

Placenta praevia and morbidly adherent placenta

Overview

Placenta praevia and morbidly adherent placenta (MAP) are associated with high rates of maternal mortality and morbidity including: massive blood product transfusion, peripartum hysterectomy, cystotomy and need for critical care.

Placenta praevia occurs when the placenta is inserted wholly or partly in the lower segment of the uterus. Using ultrasound; if the placenta lies over the internal cervical os it is a major praevia; if the leading placental edge is in the lower uterine segment but not covering the os a partial or minor placenta praevia exists.

A MAP develops when placental implantation is abnormal as a result of defect(s) in the decidua basalis which normally separates the myometrium from the anchoring placental villi. The precise pathogenesis is unclear. Hypotheses include (1) biological factors, e.g. abnormal maternal response to trophoblast invasion (2) mechanical factors, e.g. deficiency of the decidua as a result of uterine wall trauma (3) a combination. MAP has traditionally been divided into placenta accreta, placenta increta (placenta invades into the myometrium) and placenta percreta (placental invasion extends to the peritoneum). These are histological diagnoses and therefore more recently the term morbidly adherent placenta has been adopted.

The reported incidence of MAP varies widely, due to differences in diagnostic criteria, i.e. histological diagnosis versus diagnosis based on clinical criteria. In a recent study in the UK (2010–2011) the incidence of MAP was reported as 1.7 per 10,000 maternities. However, the incidence in women with both a previous caesarean delivery and placenta praevia was 577 per 10,000. Numerous studies worldwide have attributed the increase in MAP to the increase in known risk factors, particularly caesarean section. A multicentre observational study on women with multiple caesarean sections demonstrated a prevalence of placenta accreta of 0.24%, 0.31%, 0.57%, 2.13% and 6.7% after the first, second, third, fourth and fifth or more repeated caesarean sections. Of those who also had placenta praevia rates of MAP were 3%, 11%, 40%, 61% and 67% respectively.

Vasa praevia occurs when fetal vessels pass through the membranes over the internal cervical os unprotected by either placental tissue or umbilical cord. Vasa praevia is a significant risk to the fetus. A comparison of women diagnosed either antenatally or in the intrapartum period demonstrated neonatal survival rates of 97% and 44% respectively. Neonatal blood transfusion rates were 3.4% and 58.5% in the two groups.

Clinical features

Classically placenta praevia presents a painless or provoked antepartum haemorrhage in which the presenting part is high and the fetal lie is abnormal. CTG abnormalities are rare.

In the antenatal period there may be no clinical evidence of MAP. Historically, the diagnosis of MAP was made at the time of the third stage of labour when difficulty was encountered in delivery of the placenta with a failure of, or incomplete placental separation often associated with massive haemorrhage. With the advent of increased suspicion, in particular in the setting of an anterior placenta over a previous caesarean section scar a much higher proportion of patients with MAP are being diagnosed in the antenatal period.

Classically, vasa praevia presents as bleeding at the time of rupture of the membranes. This bleeding is secondary to vessel rupture and results in fetal exsanguination. It is associated with CTG abnormalities which progress rapidly to a sinusoidal fetal heart rate pattern and fetal death in utero. Occasionally, the fetal vessels can be felt in the membranes at the time of vaginal examination in labour.

Aetiology

Risk factors are outlined in **Table 48**.

Diagnosis

Placenta praevia

The Royal College of Obstetricians and Gynaecologists (RCOG) and National Institute for Health and Clinical Excellence (NICE) support placental localisation at the routine transabdominal 20-week ultrasound scan. If placenta praevia is suspected this should be confirmed by transvaginal scan. Follow up imaging should then be performed. This should be done:

- On an individualised basis in the case of women who bleed
- At 36 weeks' gestation if the woman is asymptomatic and the suspected praevia is minor
- At around 32 weeks in asymptomatic cases with suspected major praevia +/– MAP. This allows time for clarification of the diagnosis, further imaging if needed and also planning for delivery.

MAP

Any woman with placenta praevia or an anterior placenta positioned underneath an old caesarean section scar should have an ultrasound scan looking for signs of MAP. A variety of ultrasound imaging techniques has been described including greyscale, colour and/or three-D power Doppler.

Ultrasound findings suggestive of MAP include:

1. Obliteration of the bladder–uterine interface including loss of the normal hypoechogenic retroplacental myometrial zone
2. Adjacent sonolucent spaces
3. Increased vascularity of the bladder wall demonstrated on colour Doppler

Any one of these findings is consistent with abnormal placental invasion (sensitivity 0.77, specificity 0.96, positive predictive value 0.65 and negative predictive value 0.98). However, some authors suggest the loss of the hypoechogenicity zone between the retroplacental area and the myometrium can be seen in a normal placenta.

The role of magnetic resonance imaging (MRI) in diagnosing MAP is still under

Table 48 Risk factors for placenta praevia, morbidly adherent placenta and vasa praevia		
Placenta praevia	**Morbidly adherent placenta (risk factors present in 95% of cases)**	**Vasa praevia**
Previous caesarean section	Independent risk factors: • Previous caesarean section • Advanced maternal age • Coexistent placenta praevia	Placental abnormalities, e.g. succenturiate lobe or bilobar placenta
Advanced maternal age	Possible risk factors: • Multiparity • Previous uterine curettage • IVF • Previous uterine surgery	Multiple pregnancy
History of two or more induced abortions or spontaneous miscarriages	Known associations: • Abnormally elevated second-trimester free β subunit human chorionic gonadotropin and α-fetoprotein levels in maternal serum obtained during trisomy 21 screening programme	History of low-lying placenta in the second trimester
Previous placenta praevia		IVF (a number of theories have been expounded including vanishing embryos and disturbed orientation of the blastocyst at implantation)
Multiple pregnancy		
IVF, in vitro fertilisation.		

debate. A number of comparative studies have suggested that MRI and sonography are comparable with one study suggesting that MRI is better at detecting the depth of invasion in cases of placenta accreta ($p < 0.001$). Many units therefore utilise MRI, especially in cases when ultrasound findings are inconclusive. The main MRI features of MAP are:

- Uterine bulging
- The presence of dark intraplacental bands on T2-weighted imaging
- Heterogenous signal intensity within the placenta

In the US and Europe there is widespread experience in this clinical setting in the use of Gadolinium (to enhance imaging) which is not licensed for use in pregnancy in the UK. Therefore, its use should be considered on an individual patient basis following a risk–benefits analysis if the images are inconclusive.

Vasa praevia

This is rarely confirmed in the antenatal period but may be suspected if ultrasound reveals vessels crossing the membranes over the internal cervical os. Whilst there are those who advocate screening for vasa praevia using cord insertion identification +/- TV colour Doppler in women at high risk, e.g. those with a low-lying placenta, in vitro fertilisation (IVF) conceptions, multiple pregnancies, the UK national screening committee does not recommend this.

Management
Placenta praevia

- If the placental edge is ≥ 2 cm away from the internal os in the third trimester then vaginal delivery can be contemplated if the fetal head engages
- Transvaginal scanning should be considered if the head engages prior to an elective caesarean section
- There is no evidence to recommend the use of cervical cerclage or prophylactic tocolytics
- Tocolysis for treatment of bleeding may be useful in selected cases
- In the late third trimester women must be counselled on an individual basis

about their risks of preterm delivery and haemorrhage. Any home-based care requires close proximity to the maternity unit, a constant companion and informed consent

- In the case of antenatal admission decisions regarding blood availability should be based on blood bank services, antibody findings and the clinical picture

Major placenta praevia and/or antenatally suspected MAP

(e.g. women who have had a previous caesarean section and who have an anterior placenta underlying the previous scar.) Following a scan confirming major placenta praevia or MAP the woman should see a consultant obstetrician. The placenta accreta care bundle should be applied to all cases where there is a placenta praevia and for a suspected MAP. It was designed by a multidisciplinary expert group to highlight an approach to clinical care, which would reasonably be expected to reduce risks in a simple, practical and achievable way. The care bundle comprises six elements (highlighted below) which all need to be applied in order for the care bundle to be complied with.

- A consultant obstetrician should plan and directly supervise the delivery (using the care bundle). The need for caesarean section, the different surgical options and the risk of hysterectomy should all be discussed with the patient antenatally by a consultant obstetrician along with the use of blood transfusion, cell salvage (if available) and interventional radiology (see care bundle)
- The maternal and neonatal risks should be weighed up to determine the optimal timing of delivery, but this should not be done electively before 37 weeks
- 40% of women will present as an emergency therefore any plan should include anticipated skin and uterine incisions and whether proceeding straight to hysterectomy or conservative management is the preferred option in the situation where MAP is confirmed
- Any treatment refusals should be

discussed antenatally and effectively documented

- Plans may need to be made for patient to be transferred to a tertiary unit for delivery depending upon the expertise available and the degree of invasion, e.g. through into bladder or bowel
- Preoperative planning must be multidisciplinary (care bundle)
- At a minimum a level two critical care bed must be available (care bundle)
- A consultant anaesthetist should review the patient in the antenatal period, make a plan with regards to anaesthetic technique and directly supervise the anaesthetic (care bundle)
- Blood and blood products must be available on site (care bundle)
- If possible the surgeon should perform an ultrasound scan to plot out the position of the placenta before starting. The uterine incision should avoid the placenta if possible, as incising through the placenta to achieve delivery is associated with more bleeding and a higher chance of hysterectomy
- If the placenta fails to separate with standard measures and there is no bleeding both leaving it in place and closing and leaving it in place and proceeding to hysterectomy are associated with less blood loss than trying to separate it. The decision will obviously be influenced by antenatal discussion and past obstetric history
- If the placenta partially separates it needs

to be delivered and any haemorrhage should be dealt with using standard management protocols. Adherent portions can be left but in such circumstances blood loss can be high and massive haemorrhage management must be aggressive

- In all cases the woman must be debriefed by a senior member of the team. If part or all of the placenta is left in situ the woman must be warned of the risks of bleeding and infection
- Prophylactic antibiotics should be used as they may be helpful in reducing infection rates
- There is no evidence to recommend the use of methotrexate or arterial embolisation

Vasa praevia

If vasa praevia is suspected, transvaginal ultrasound using colour Doppler should be used to confirm the diagnosis. This modality has good specificity but the sensitivity is unclear. If the diagnosis is made in the second trimester this should be confirmed again in the third trimester as vasa praevia is reported to resolve in 15% of cases. Once the diagnosis is confirmed delivery should be by elective caesarean section ideally at term, prior to the onset of labour. Admission to a unit with appropriate neonatal facilities should be offered from 28–32 weeks of gestation and the use of prophylactic corticosteroids discussed. A grade 1 caesarean section should be carried out if an antepartum haemorrhage occurs.

In the future some cases of vasa praevia may be managed using laser ablation in utero.

Further reading

Grobman WA, Gersnoviez R, Landon MB, et al. Pregnancy outcomes for women with placenta previa in relation to the number of prior cesarean deliveries. Obstet Gynecol 2007; 110:1249–1255.

RCOG Green-top Guideline No. 27. Placenta praevia, placenta praevia accreta and vasa praevia:

diagnosis and management. London: RCOG, 2011.

Gagnon R, et al. Guidelines for the management of vasa previa. SOGC clinical practice guideline. Int J Gynecol and Obstetrics 2010; 108:85–89.

Related topics of interest

- Antepartum haemorrhage (p. 186)
- Blood transfusion (p. 192)
- Postpartum haemorrhage (p. 287)

Postpartum haemorrhage

Overview

Haemorrhage remains a major cause of maternal morbidity and mortality in high and low-income countries. In the last report on maternal mortality in the UK covering the period 2006–2008, nine women died of haemorrhage. This was the sixth highest cause of direct maternal death and although this number is decreasing, representing 0.39 per 100,000 maternities, it is still a concern as two-thirds of these women had substandard care implicated in their deaths.

Postpartum haemorrhage (PPH) is divided into:

- Primary PPH – defined by the World Health Organization (WHO) as > 500 mL blood loss from the genital tract in the first 24 hours following delivery. Even if the blood loss is < 500 mL, it can be classified as PPH if it causes hypovolaemic shock.
- Primary PPH may be further subdivided into:
    - Minor – 500–1000 mL
    - Moderate – > 1000 mL
    - Severe – > 2000 mL
- Secondary PPH – abnormal bleeding from the genital tract occurring more than 24 hours following delivery and up until 12 weeks.

Estimated blood loss is frequently inaccurate, which is compounded by the fact that young, fit women may compensate for large blood losses; they may not become hypotensive or tachycardic until they have lost > 20% of their blood volume. Pictorial charts may help improve clinicians estimate the amount of blood loss; where possible, all blood loss should be weighed to improve the accuracy of estimated blood loss.

Aetiology

The major causes of primary PPH are usually classified as 'the 4 T's':

Tone Uterine atony accounts for 79% of PPH
Trauma There may be substantial bleeding due to tears involving the vagina, cervix or episiotomy/perineum

Tissue Retained placental tissue can cause significant bleeding.
Thrombin Women may have an inherent coagulation disorder or be on anticoagulants, making PPH more likely. These women should have been identified antenatally. However, certain conditions developing in labour such as pre-eclampsia and amniotic fluid embolism can predispose to coagulopathy. Massive haemorrhage and subsequent transfusion itself can cause disseminated intravascular coagulation

Management

Consideration should be given to preventing and ameliorating the risks of PPH antenatally. Haemoglobin should be optimised with oral or intravenous iron to treat anaemia. Careful history of risk factors such as previous PPH should be taken into account and a discussion regarding the active management of the third stage should take place. Women at high risk of PPH should have intravenous access secured on admission in labour. Any woman on antenatal thromboprophylaxis should have a detailed care plan made regarding when to stop their medication.

Once PPH has occurred, women should be transferred to the consultant-led delivery unit (if not already managed there) and the Royal College of Obstetricians and Gynaecologists (RCOG) recommends a four-pronged approach. Each of these components should be considered simultaneously.

Communication

The person identifying the PPH should call for help. The management of PPH requires multidisciplinary input, initially the obstetric and anaesthetic registrars and senior midwife. Consideration should be given to involving the consultant obstetrician and anaesthetist at an early stage. Most units will have a major haemorrhage protocol which, when initiated (usually ≥ 2000 mL blood loss), will involve liaising with laboratory staff and haematologists to ensure prompt access to blood and blood products, as well as portering staff who are essential in ensuring blood products are delivered in a timely fashion.

Resuscitation

This should initially use Advanced Life Support approach i.e. Airway, Breathing, Circulation. High-flow oxygen via a facemask should be commenced and two large intravenous cannulae inserted. Blood tests should also be taken at this time for four units cross-matched red cells, full blood count (FBC) and clotting screen. Crystalloid or colloid may be rapidly infused although the best fluid replacement is compatible blood. Up to two units of type O-negative blood can be given in an emergency and this will be instantly accessible in many units. Group specific blood can be made available quicker than full cross match if necessary. The main therapeutic goals are to maintain: haemoglobin > 80 g/L, platelets > 75×10^9/L, prothrombin time < 1.5x mean control, activated prothrombin time < 1.5 x mean control, fibrinogen > 1.0 g/L.

Monitoring and investigation

Monitoring and documentation of observations on a Modified Obstetric Early Warnings score (MOEWs) chart should take place, and a person should be nominated to act as scribe. An indwelling catheter should be inserted with an hourly measurement recorded. An arterial and/or central line may be considered.

An investigation should determine which of the 4 T's is the most likely cause.

Arresting the bleeding

This will depend upon the cause. As uterine atony is the most common cause, this will be discussed further here. Initial assessment should involve bimanual examination to stimulate uterine contraction. This has the added benefit of allowing removal of clots from the cervix, which may be a factor in causing atony. If the bladder is not already catheterised, this should be done now. Pharmacological measures should then be initiated (**Table 49**). If these fail to control the bleeding, there should be quick recourse to transferring to theatre and initiating surgical interventions.

Surgical interventions

Examination under anaesthesia will enable repair of tears and removal of retained products.

If bleeding persists, the following treatments may be used:
- Intrauterine balloon tamponade. This is inserted into the uterus and inflated with up to 500 mL of saline until the bleeding is controlled. The balloon is then secured with a vaginal pack
- Haemostatic uterine brace suture. This is particularly useful if the PPH occurs at the time of caesarean section. It is recommended that a laminated diagram of the technique should be kept in theatre. This can be used in combination with an intrauterine balloon
- Internal iliac artery ligation may be considered but is thought to be less

Table 49 Pharmacological agents for treating PPH	
Pharmacological intervention	**Dose**
Syntocinon	5 IU by slow IV injection. This may be repeated
Ergometrine	0.5 mg by slow IV or IM injection (avoid if hypertensive)
Syntocinon infusion	40 IU in 500 mL Hartmann's solution/0.9% saline, administered at 125 mL per hour
Carboprost	0.25 mg by IM injection. Can be repeated at 15 minute intervals up to a maximum of 8 doses
	0.25 mg direct intramyometrial injection. It is not licensed via this route
Misoprostol	1000 µg rectally
Recombinant factor VIIa	May be given after discussion with a haematologist at a suggested dose of 90 µg/kg. Fibrinogen should be above 1 g/L and platelets above 20×10^9/L. In the absence of a clinical response, it can be repeated in 15–30 minutes

effective than balloon tamponade or brace suturing and is more difficult to perform
- Interventional radiology may be considered but has limited availability and the logistics are such that it may not be possible in an emergency. It may be used electively prior to surgery for known cases of placenta praevia or placenta accreta

Early resort to hysterectomy should be considered sooner rather than later and may be life-saving.

Secondary PPH

10% of cases will present with massive haemorrhage and initial management will be the same as that for primary PPH while establishing a cause. The main causes are:

- Endometritis
- Retained placental tissue

Investigation should involve taking vaginal swabs, blood tests for inflammatory markers (FBC, C-reactive protein) as well as blood tests for PPH described above +/- blood cultures if there are signs of sepsis. An ultrasound scan may be useful in detecting retained placental tissue but may also be non-specific. Treatment should be with broad spectrum antibiotics in cases of endometritis. If a surgical evacuation is necessary, this should be done with senior involvement because of the high risk of uterine perforation. Consideration should be given to sending histological samples to detect rare cases of choriocarcinoma.

Further reading

Centre for Maternal and Child Enquiries (CMACE). Saving Mothers' Lives: reviewing maternal deaths to make motherhood safer: 2006–2008. The Eighth Report on Confidential Enquiries into Maternal Deaths in the United Kingdom. BJOG 2011;118(1):1–203.

Royston E, Armstrong S. Preventing Maternal Deaths. Geneva: World Health Organization, 1989.
RCOG Green-top Guideline No. 52. Prevention and management of postpartum haemorrhage. London; RCOG, 2009.
RCOG Green-top Guideline No. 47. Blood transfusion in obstetrics. London; RCOG Press, 2008.

Related topics of interest

Pre-eclampsia and eclampsia

Overview

Pre-eclampsia (PE) and eclampsia are associated with increased maternal and fetal mortality and morbidity.

PE is associated with reduced depth of spiral artery conversion in early pregnancy, which is thought to expose the placenta to hypoxic or oxidative stress. In response the placenta releases vasoactive factor(s) into the maternal circulation which alter endothelial permeability and vascular reactivity. This results in the multisystem disorder of PE identified by maternal hypertension and proteinuria.

Definitions and clinical features

Blood pressure (BP) should be measured on accurate, calibrated equipment using Korotkoff V (disappearance of heart sounds) to measure diastolic BP.

PE is defined as a BP ≥ 140/90 mmHg with significant proteinuria (≥ 2 + on urine dipstick/> 0.3 g/24 hours per protein:creatinine ratio ≥ 30 mg/mmol) occurring for the first time after 20 weeks of gestation. Severe PE describes PE where BP is ≥ 160/110 mmHg.

- Pre-existing hypertension is BP ≥ 140/90 mmHg prior to pregnancy or before 20 weeks of gestation.
- Gestational hypertension (GH) is BP ≥ 140/90 mmHg after 20 weeks of gestation with no significant proteinuria.
- Superimposed PE describes the development of features of PE in a woman with pre-existing hypertension.
- Eclampsia is the occurrence of fits, convulsions or coma without another neurological cause after 20 weeks of pregnancy.
- HELLP syndrome describes a manifestation of severe PE when there is haemolysis, elevated liver function tests and low platelets (HELLP).

Symptoms include headache and visual disturbances (particularly severe pounding frontal headache and bright flashing visual disturbances) and epigastric pain which may be severe and associated with vomiting. Oedema is evident in the majority of women in late pregnancy; oedema in PE may involve hands and face and worsen rapidly.

Aetiology and epidemiology

In the UK, PE has an incidence of between 3 and 5%, with severe PE complicating 0.5% of pregnancies. Eclampsia affects 0.05% of pregnancies in the UK.

There are a number of risk factors which predispose women to developing PE, including: primiparity, obesity, previous pre-eclampsia/eclampsia, age < 20 or > 40, family history of first-degree relative with PE or eclampsia, essential hypertension, renal disease, multiple pregnancy.

In severe early-onset cases PE may coexist with fetal growth restriction (FGR). Very rarely, PE may be associated with fetal hydrops in Mirror or Ballantyne's syndrome.

Antenatal care and prevention of pre-eclampsia

Women at increased risk of PE should be offered 75 mg of aspirin once a day which reduces the risk of developing PE by approximately 30%. Women who should be offered aspirin include: women with hypertensive disease during a previous pregnancy, chronic kidney disease, autoimmune disease including systemic lupus erythematosus or antiphospholipid syndrome, pre-existing diabetes and chronic hypertension/renal disease.

Women who are calcium-deplete should be offered calcium supplementation. Women with pre-existing hypertension need to be on therapeutic agents suitable for pregnancy. Ideally, these women should be seen prior to conception. Antihypertensive agents unsuitable for use in pregnancy include angiotensin converting enzyme inhibitors, angiotensin receptor blockers and chlorothiazide diuretics.

- The target BP for women with pre-existing hypertension is < 150/100 mmHg. In women with end-organ damage (e.g. renal disease) aim for < 140/90 mmHg.
- Women with pre-existing hypertension or renal disease should be managed in specialist antenatal clinics with appointment schedule dependent on maternal and fetal condition.

Management of gestational hypertension

If BP is ≥ 160/110 mmHg admit to hospital, and give antihypertensive (e.g. Labetalol 200 mg orally). Measure BP at least four times a day, test for proteinuria using protein:creatinine ratio or automated strip reader. Blood tests for full blood count (FBC), renal and liver function, then monitor weekly.

If BP ≥ 150/100 mmHg and ≤ 160/110 mmHg patients do not require admission but should commence antihypertensive (e.g. labetalol 200 mg three times a day) to keep BP < 150/100 mmHg. The woman should be seen twice a week to assess BP and proteinuria. Blood tests for FBC, renal and liver function at presentation which don't need repeating unless proteinuria develops.

If BP < 150/100 mmHg – BP and proteinuria assessed no more than twice a week. If < 32 weeks or at high risk of PE then measure BP and test for proteinuria twice a week.

Fetal well-being should be assessed by ultrasound biometry with liquor volume and umbilical artery Doppler. In the absence of an abnormality, this should be performed at 2-week intervals. Cardiotocography (CTG) should be performed if there is a reduction in fetal movements or if BP ≥ 160/110 mmHg.

If BP > 160/110 mmHg and refractory to treatment the woman may need preterm delivery, otherwise consider delivery after 37 weeks of gestation following discussion with the mother (based on the HYPITAT trial).

Women with GH are at increased risk of developing PE (42–50% of cases).

Management of pre-eclampsia

All women with PE should be admitted to hospital. Do not reassess proteinuria.

If BP < 150/100 mmHg measure BP four times a day, check FBC, liver and renal function tests twice a week.

If BP is ≥ 150/100 mmHg and ≤ 160/110 mmHg, treat with first line antihypertensive (e.g. labetalol 200 mg three times a day or nifedipine LA 20 mg) to keep blood pressure < 150/80–100 mmHg. Measure BP at least four times a day and check FBC, liver and renal function tests three times a week.

If BP > 160/110 mmHg treat with first line oral antihypertensive (e.g. labetalol 200 mg three times a day or nifedipine LA 20 mg) to keep BP < 150/80–100 mmHg. Measure BP more than four times a day depending on clinical condition; daily FBC, liver and renal function tests.

Fetal well-being should be assessed by ultrasound biometry with liquor volume and umbilical artery Doppler. In the absence of an abnormality this should be performed at 2-week intervals. CTG should be performed if there is a reduction in fetal movements or if BP ≥ 160/110 mmHg.

If severe PE or HELLP syndrome, consider the need for high-dependency care. BP should be controlled with labetalol (oral or intravenous), hydralazine (intravenous) or nifedipine (oral, do not give sublingually). Consider need for seizure prophylaxis with magnesium sulphate (see section on management of eclampsia for dose).

Offer delivery to all women with PE after 37 weeks of gestation. Between 34–37 weeks of gestation: plan delivery if severe hypertension that is resistant to treatment, worsening maternal condition or fetal indication (e.g. FGR). Before 34 weeks, aim to manage condition conservatively, senior obstetric staff should document maternal (biochemical, haematological and clinical) and fetal indications for elective birth before 34 weeks.

Before 37 weeks corticosteroids should be given for fetal lung maturity and delivery should take place where there are suitable neonatal facilities.

Management of eclampsia

Eclamptic fits may present antepartum (30%), intrapartum (30%) and postpartum (40%). Eclampsia is one clinical manifestation of severe PE, and fits may precede signs and symptoms of PE; the severity of hypertension does not correlate with the incidence of fits. Signs and symptoms of impending eclampsia include clonus, visual disturbances and severe headache.

Eclamptic fits are thought to result from cerebral vasospasm or hypertensive encephalopathy.

Important differential diagnoses include cerebrovascular accident, intracranial tumour, drug withdrawal (alcohol, cocaine) and epilepsy.

Eclamptic fits are generalised, self-limiting and usually last ≤ 2 minutes, but approximately 1–2% of women will have persistent neurological symptoms following an eclamptic fit. Women with focal neurological signs or persistent seizures require neuroimaging [computed tomograghy (CT) or magnetic resonance imaging (MRI)].

- Initial management should focus on: Airway, Breathing and Circulation (remembering left lateral tilt). Get help – a senior anaesthetist and obstetrician should be involved
- Intravenous access should be obtained. Blood should be taken for FBC, clotting profile, urea and electrolytes, liver function tests and urate
- Magnesium sulphate 4 g is used to control the seizure given intravenously over 10 minutes. If intravenous access cannot be obtained, this dose can be given intramuscularly
- For recurrent seizures another 2 g bolus of magnesium is given and the maintenance increased to 20 mL/hour (2 g/hour), alternatively 5–10 mg diazepam (although this will lead to sedation)

- If antepartum or intrapartum, eclamptic seizures are often accompanied by a fetal bradycardia (due to maternal hypoxia) the primary concern is maternal well-being. Delivery should be planned when the mother's condition is stabilised.

Postnatal management of severe pre-eclampsia or eclampsia

In the majority of cases, severe PE and eclampsia will resolve spontaneously following delivery of the infant and placenta. However, care is needed to prevent postnatal complications including fluid overload and venous thromboembolism.

- Patients should be managed in a 1:1 environment (ideally in a high dependency area on the delivery suite) with continuous monitoring of pulse and oxygen saturation
- Maternal observations should be recorded on a maternity early warning score (MEOWS) chart together with hourly fluid balance
- BP should be recorded regularly, initially every 15–30 minutes. If BP is unstable, intra-arterial monitoring may be appropriate
- Fluid restrict to 2 L in 24 hours (e.g. 83 mL/hour). This means all fluids intravenous and oral
- FBC, urea and electrolytes, liver function test and clotting studies every 6–12 hours dependent on maternal condition
- Magnesium sulphate infusion should be continued for 24 hours after the last seizure or 24 hours after birth whichever is the longest. Deep tendon reflexes should be checked every 4 hours while patients are on intravenous magnesium. If tendon reflexes are absent, the rate of magnesium infusion should be reduced by half. If respiratory rate is < 12 minutes the infusion should be stopped and magnesium levels checked. If there is respiratory depression 10 mL of 10% calcium gluconate should be given intravenously

- Prior to discharge from hospital women should be debriefed to ensure they understood events. This should include counselling about the risk of recurrence of PE/gestational hypertension which affects 13–53% of future pregnancies. The risk of PE is 16% in future pregnancies, but increases to 25% if they had severe pre-eclampsia, HELLP syndrome or eclampsia before 34 weeks and to 55% if it led to birth before 28 weeks.
- Women with severe pre-eclampsia/ eclampsia/HELLP syndrome should be offered medical review 6–8 weeks postnatally.

Further reading

NICE Clinical Guideline No. 107. Hypertension in pregnancy. NICE: London, 2010.

NICE Clinical Guideline No. 62. Antenatal care. NICE: London, 2008.

Koopmans CM, Bijlenga D, Groen H, et al. HYPITAT study group. Induction of labour versus expectant monitoring for gestational hypertension or mild pre-eclampsia after 36 weeks' gestation (HYPITAT): a multicentre, open-label randomised controlled trial. Lancet 2009; 374(9694):979–988.

Milne F, Redman C, Walker J, et al. The pre-eclampsia community guideline (PRECOG): how to screen for and detect onset of pre-eclampsia in the community. BMJ 2005; 330(7491):576–580.

Milne F, Redman C, Walker J, et al. PRECOG II Group. Assessing the onset of pre-eclampsia in the hospital day unit: summary of the pre-eclampsia guideline (PRECOG II). BMJ 2009; 339:b3129.

Related topics of interest

Premature labour

Overview

Premature labour (PTL) is the occurrence of regular painful uterine contractions which result in cervical change prior to 37 weeks of gestation. In high-income countries the incidence of PTL varies between 5–12%. In the UK in 2009, infant mortality amongst babies born between 24 and 36 weeks was 27.5 per 1000 live births, compared with 4.2 per 1000 live births overall. For extremely preterm infants (< 24 weeks) infant mortality was 864 per 1000 live births. Those infants who survive are at increased risk of repeated admission to hospital and adverse outcomes including cerebral palsy and long term disability. These risks increase with decreasing gestational age at delivery.

Clinical features

Women may present with regular painful uterine contractions, non-specific abdominal pain, change in vaginal discharge or vaginal pressure. Some women with cervical weakness present with a sensation of vaginal fullness or an urge to push.

Aetiology and predisposing factors

Maternal   Primigravidae, maternal age < 20 years or > 35 years, pre-pregnancy weight < 50 kg, non-caucasian ethnicity, stress, having been a preterm infant, previous cone biopsy, cervical trachelectomy, large loop excision of the transformation zone (LLETZ) and cigarette smoking.

Socio-economic factors   Lower social class, a heavy or stressful work load, suboptimal antenatal care and single women.

Past reproductive history   Previous PTL [at least 2.5-fold increase in risk, up to 70% recurrence risk if two or more preterm births (PTBs)], spontaneous second-trimester miscarriage, uterine abnormalities (congenital, fibroids, trauma), cervical weakness and previous bleeding in pregnancy.

Present pregnancy   Uterine over-distension (e.g. polyhydramnios), multiple pregnancy, antepartum haemorrhage, fetal congenital anomalies, maternal illness and retained intrauterine contraceptive device (IUCD).

Infection   Inflammation of the intrauterine tissues occurs in both term and PTL. A causal link between infection and prematurity has been established and at least 40% of all PTBs are associated with infection. Bacterial vaginosis (BV), a bacterial imbalance of normal vaginal flora, is associated with a risk of preterm prelabour rupture of membranes (PPROM), prematurity and chorioamnionitis. A recent meta-analysis demonstrated that pregnant women with BV have an over 2-fold increase in risk of PTB Odds Ratio (OR) 2.16 (95% CI: 1.56–3.00). However, there are no benefits to screening for BV in the low risk population and arguments in favour of screening and treatment of BV in women at high risk of PTB remain insufficient.

PPROM   This occurs in 2–3% of pregnancies and one-third of PTBs.

Diagnosis

Often difficult, but evidence of cervical change must be present. Approximately 90% of women presenting with signs and symptoms of spontaneous PTL will not deliver within 7 days indeed almost 75% will deliver at term. Risk scoring has a low positive predictive value and poor reproducibility.

- Examination of the cervix with ultrasound is superior to digital cervical assessment. Transvaginal ultrasound is a reliable method to measure cervical length (CL) and a better predictor of PTB than obstetric history. The risk of spontaneous PTB is almost 50% at ≤ 32 weeks if the CL is ≤ 15 mm. Overall the sensitivity and positive predictive value of CL measurements are too low to justify it as a population based screening tool
- Randomised controlled trials have indicated that ambulatory uterine contraction frequency monitoring is not useful in reducing PTB rates

- Fetal fibronectin (fFN) is an extracellular matrix glycoprotein produced by amniocytes and by cytotrophoblast; there are very high levels in amniotic fluid in the second trimester. fFN can be detected in cervicovaginal secretions using a bedside test (10–15 minutes). Positive results have been associated with an increased risk of spontaneous PTB but may occur if there has been sexual intercourse in the preceding 24 hours or vaginal bleeding. In patients presenting in PTL, the positive predictive value of fFN screening is poor (46–80%) but the negative predictive value is better, up to 99.5% for delivery within 7 days
- Actim Partus test detects IGFBP-1, a protein present in amniotic fluid in large concentrations, but absent in semen, urine and blood. A swab of cervicovaginal secretions gives a positive or negative result (10–15 minutes). Positive predictive values of 40–50% and negative predictive values of 98% have been reported. The test has not been consistently associated with CL changes and the comparison data with fFN suggest fFN is superior in a high risk population

Management

It is important to look for a cause and assess maternal and fetal well-being. Fetal well-being can be assessed using a cardiotocograph (CTG) and ultrasound. Once it is clearly established that the patient is in PTL a decision must be made with regards to the use of steroids and tocolysis. Inhibition of labour beyond 34 weeks is not warranted.

Corticosteroids

Women in suspected PTL who are between 24^{+0} and 34^{+6} should be given a single course of antenatal corticosteroids to reduce the risk of adverse neonatal outcomes including death, necrotising enterocolitis, need for respiratory support, intraventricular haemorrhage, admission to neonatal intensive care unit (NICU) and systemic infection. In suspected PTL the ratio of women given a complete course of steroids to the number of women who actually deliver before 34 weeks' gestation is as high as 15:1. Antenatal corticosteroids can be considered for women in spontaneous PTL between 23^{+0} and 23^{+6} gestation. This decision should be individualised and made at senior level. The Royal College of Obstetricians and Gynaecologists (RCOG) recommend betamethasone 12 mg intramuscularly in two doses (usually 24 hours apart) or dexamethasone 6 mg intramuscularly in four doses (usually 12 hourly).

Tocolytic agents

The use of tocolytic agents remains an area of huge debate, not least because use is not associated with a clear reduction in perinatal or neonatal morbidity and there is some evidence that keeping a baby in a potentially hostile uterine environment may be harmful. Those most likely to benefit are

- Women in extreme PTL
- Those needing transfer to a hospital with NICU facilities
- Those who have not yet received a course of corticosteroids

Absolute contraindications to tocolysis include fetal death, fetal congenital anomaly incompatible with life and chorioamnionitis. Relative contraindications include mild haemorrhage because of placenta praevia, fetal growth restriction and multiple pregnancies. PPROM is not an absolute contraindication to delaying labour but care must be taken to exclude infection. Currently used tocolytics are compared in **Table 50**. Magnesium sulphate, antibiotics, ethanol, relaxin and electro-inhibition have also been tried as tocolytics in the past.

A recent systematic review and network meta-analysis concluded that the probability of delivery being delayed by 48 hours was highest with prostaglandin inhibitors (OR 5.39, credible interval 2.14–12.34) followed by magnesium sulphate, calcium channel blockers and Atosiban. No class of tocolytic was significantly superior to placebo in reducing neonatal respiratory distress syndrome (RDS). Prostaglandin synthetase inhibitors and calcium channel blockers had the best probability of being ranked

Table 50 Tocolytic agents currently in use.			
Tocolytic	Calcium channel blockers, e.g. nifedipine	Oxytocin receptor agonist (Atosiban)	Prostaglandin synthetase inhibitors, e.g. indomethacin
Mode of action	Inhibit the influx of calcium ions through channels in the cell membrane	Oxytocin receptor antagonist	PGF2α and PGE2 are thought to be involved in the final pathway in smooth muscle contraction. May act via anti-inflammatory effects
Licensed for PTL use in UK	No	Yes (24–33 weeks)	No
Maternal side effects	Flushing, palpitations, nausea and vomiting and hypotension	Nausea, vomiting, headache and dyspnoea	Nausea, dizziness headache, peptic ulcer disease
Fetal side effects	None	None	Renal dysfunction resulting in oligohydramnios and premature closure of ductus arteriosus (use therefore generally contraindicated after 28 w), intracranial haemorrhage and necrotising enterocollitis.
Contraindications	Maternal cardiac disease; use with caution in diabetes and multiple pregnancy because of the risks of pulmonary oedema	Not contraindicated in maternal cardiac disease or diabetes	Platelet dysfunction, hepatic dysfunction, gastrointestinal (GI) ulcer disease, renal dysfunction and asthma
Administration	Oral	Intravenous	Oral or rectal
Dosage	Initial oral dose of 20 mg followed by 10–20 mg three to four times a day for up to 48 hours. Doses > 60 mg are associated with a 3–4-fold increase in adverse events	Bolus intravenous injection of 6.75 mg over 1 minute followed by infusion of 18 mg/h for 3 hours then 6 mg/h for up to 45 hours. In clinical practice cessation of the infusion should be about 6–12 hours after uterine quiescence	100 mg PR every 24 hours or 25 mg po qds (continue for 48 hours)

in the top three medication classes for the outcomes of 48 hour delay in delivery, RDS, neonatal mortality and maternal side effects (all causes).

- The use of multiple tocolytic agents should be avoided as it is associated with a higher risk of adverse effects
- There is no evidence that maintenance therapy with any agent is effective at reducing the incidence of preterm delivery
- Antibiotics should not be used in an attempt to prolong gestation in women with PTL and intact membranes
- Neither bedrest nor hydration have been shown effective

Mode of delivery

In PTL the optimal mode of delivery is controversial. Claims that preterm caesarean delivery reduces the risk of fetal or neonatal death and birth trauma have been countered with claims that such a policy leads to risk of serious morbidity for both mother and baby. A recent Cochrane systematic review concluded that for singleton pregnancies there is not enough evidence to evaluate the use of a policy of planned immediate caesarean delivery for women in PTL. Therefore mode of delivery should be individualised considering fetal condition, presentation, gestation, estimated weight, progress in labour and likelihood of serious maternal morbidity.

Role of magnesium sulphate in fetal neuroprotection

The results of a large meta-analysis suggest that predelivery magnesium sulphate reduces the occurrence of cerebral palsy. Women who are < 30 weeks and at risk of delivering within the next 24 hours should have magnesium sulphate for neuroprotection of the fetus, infant and child. An initial intravenous 4 g loading dose (20–30 minutes duration) should be followed with a 1 g per hour maintenance infusion continued until birth or for 24 hours, whichever comes first. Magnesium should be used regardless of the number of babies in utero, of why PTB is anticipated, or of anticipated mode of delivery and whether or not corticosteroids have been given. Its use is contraindicated in myasthenia gravis and it must be given with care in renal impairment.

Further reading

RCOG Green-top Guideline No.1b. Tocolysis for women in preterm labour. London: RCOG, 2011.

Mahony R, McKeating A, Murphy T, et al. Appropriate antenatal corticosteroid use in women at risk for preterm birth before 34 weeks of gestation. BJOG 2010; 117:963–967.

Royal College of Obstetricians and Gynaecologists. Scientific Impact Paper No.29: Magnesium sulphate to prevent cerebral palsy following preterm birth. London: RCOG, 2011.

Kiefer D, Vintzileos M. The utility of fetal fibronectin in the prediction and prevention of spontaneous preterm birth. Reviews in Obstetrics and Gynaecology 2008; 1(3):106–112.

Haas D, Caldwell DM, Lirkpatrick P, et al. Tocolytic therapy for preterm delivery: systematic review and network meta-analysis. BMJ 2012; 345:317.

Related topics of interest

• Preterm prelabour rupture of membranes (p. 298)

Preterm prelabour rupture of membranes

Overview

Preterm prelabour rupture of membranes (PPROM) is defined as rupture of the fetal membranes before 37 completed weeks of pregnancy. It occurs in 2% of pregnancies but accounts for nearly 40% of preterm deliveries and results in significant neonatal morbidity and mortality. The leading causes of neonatal death in association with PPROM are sepsis, pulmonary hypoplasia and prematurity. Many of the conditions associated with premature labour are also associated with PPROM.

Latency is the interval between rupture of the membranes and the onset of labour. A number of factors affect the latency period including: pregnancy complications such as placental abruption or chorioamnionitis, gestational age, degree of oligohydramnios and number of fetuses. PPROM is associated with an increased risk of skeletal deformities secondary to oligohydramnios and cord prolapse.

Clinical features

A classical history is that of a sudden gush of fluid per vaginum followed by a constant trickle unrelated to micturition. This can occur from 16 weeks of gestation. There may be evidence of clinical chorioamnionitis including maternal tachycardia and pyrexia, uterine tenderness, offensive vaginal discharge and fetal tachycardia.

Aetiology

PPROM is often idiopathic and the mechanisms responsible are largely unknown. Suggested mechanisms include excessive stretching of the membranes, decreased collagen content, placental abruption or programmed cell death in the amnion. PPROM has been linked with a number of factors including a history of previous preterm delivery or PPROM, vaginal bleeding during pregnancy, uterine overdistension, black ethnicity, smoking, amniocentesis, infection and low socioeconomic status. 25–50% of cases are associated with intrauterine infection and inflammation.

Diagnosis

This can often be very difficult:

- Examination is with a sterile speculum. Visualisation of amniotic fluid coming from the cervix is obvious; pooling in the posterior fornix is helpful. Presence of meconium and/or vernix may help differentiate amniotic fluid from urine or vaginal discharge

A number of bedside tests are available to confirm whether the fluid found in the posterior fornix is amniotic fluid. Although none of these are recommended by the (RCOG), Amnisure and Actim Prom are in widespread clinical use.

- Amniotic fluid will cause a ferning on a glass slide. Nitrazine sticks turn dark blue in the higher pH of amniotic fluid, but false positives can occur in the presence of blood, semen and infection. These tests have been largely replaced in high income settings with more sensitive tests such as Amnisure and Actim Prom
- The Amnisure test detects placental α-microglobulin-1 (PAMG-1); the concentration of this protein in amniotic fluid is 1000–10,000 times higher than cervicovaginal fluid. Therefore, the presence of high concentrations of PAMG-1 in cervicovaginal fluid is considered evidence of ruptured membranes. It has a sensitivity close to 99% and specificity varying between 87.5% and 100%
- The Actim Prom test detects insulin-like growth factor-binding-1 (IGFBP-1), a protein present in amniotic fluid in large concentrations, but absent in semen, urine and blood. The Actim Prom test is done

using a swab which is applied to the fluid in the posterior fornix. The result is either positive, IGFBP-1 is present, or negative. As with the Amnisure test a result is obtained within 10–15 minutes. Sensitivity varies from 74–100% and specificity from 77% to 98.2%

Although a direct head-to-head comparison has not been performed, data suggest that the Amnisure test is more reliable.

Ultrasound scanning may be helpful in some cases to confirm the diagnosis (with a reduction in liquor volume) but this must be done in the context of the whole clinical picture.

Digital vaginal examination should be avoided to reduce the risk of infection.

Management

Management is dependent on gestation. Following a diagnosis of PPROM women should be examined or observed for signs of clinical chorioamnionitis, admitted to hospital and a full blood count and cardiotocography (CTG) performed dependent upon gestation. The evidence available to decide between home and outpatient monitoring versus ongoing hospital admission is insufficient. It is prudent to admit patients for at least 48 hours. Subsequent to this, management must be individualised. If the woman opts for home and outpatient monitoring she should aim to take her temperature on a 4–8-hourly basis and report any abnormality.

Very early PPROM (16–24 weeks)

The neonatal outcomes of pregnancies complicated by very early PPROM are extremely poor. In some studies fetuses with PPROM at ≤23 weeks have a perinatal survival rate of <20% compared with 50% with rupture of the membranes at 24–26 weeks. Recent studies have suggested that those with iatrogenic very early PPROM (PPROM following amniocentesis, chorionic villus sampling, cervical cerclage) have better outcomes than those with spontaneous, very early PPROM with higher gestational age at

birth and significantly higher survival rates (85% versus 25% survival to discharge in those managed conservatively).

- In the cohort of patients who present at <22 weeks' gestation termination of pregnancy is a consideration
- Erythromycin should be given for 10 days following the diagnosis of PPROM
- One of the major issues with this group is the development of pulmonary hypoplasia. This is extremely difficult to diagnose antenatally
- Some studies have looked at the use of fibrin glue to seal the chorioamniotic membranes and prevent pulmonary hypoplasia. However, there is no evidence to recommend this as routine treatment and larger studies are needed
- A pilot randomised controlled trial of serial amnioinfusion versus expectant management in women with PPROM between 16–24 weeks (AMIPROM) is currently in the follow up phase. However, at present there is insufficient evidence to recommend amnioinfusion to prevent pulmonary hypoplasia

For those women 24–34 weeks of gestation

- Erythromycin should be given for 10 days following the diagnosis of PPROM. This will reduce maternal and neonatal morbidity and delay delivery to allow corticosteroids to take effect
- Antenatal corticosteroids should be administered between 24–34 weeks' gestation. A meta-analysis including more than 1400 women with PPROM demonstrated that corticosteroids reduce the risk of respiratory distress syndrome, intraventricular haemorrhage and necrotising enterocolitis whilst not appearing to increase the risk of infection in either mother or baby. Corticosteroids may increase the maternal white cell count within 24 hours, but it should then fall. Persistently elevated levels should raise the suspicion of infection
- The use of tocolytics is not recommended as they do not improve perinatal outcomes
- More than a third of women with PPROM will have evidence of intrauterine infection as defined by positive amniotic fluid

cultures. Positive cultures are associated with a shorter latency and increased rates of neonatal sepsis. However, the role of amniocentesis in improving outcome remains to be determined and there is insufficient evidence to recommend the use of amniocentesis in the diagnosis of intrauterine infection

For those women > 34 weeks of gestation the RCOG recommends that consideration should be given to delivery at 34 weeks' gestation. However, a recently updated meta-analysis suggests that the risks of neonatal sepsis and caesarean section are no different for women with > 24 hours PPROM between 34–37 weeks randomised to either induction of labour (IOL) or expectant management with IOL on reaching 37 weeks (neonatal sepsis relative risk (RR) 1.06; 95% CI 0.64–1.76, caesarean section RR 1.27; 0.98–1.65).

In all situations delivery should be expedited if there are signs of maternal compromise, e.g. development of chorioamnionitis. If IOL is appropriate prostaglandins can be used safely if time permits and may improve the Bishop score prior to syntocinon, especially in nulliparous women. Whilst PPROM increases the risk of cord compression and fetal distress during labour there is no evidence to support amnioinfusion during labour.

Further reading

RCOG Green-top Guideline No 44. Preterm prelabour rupture of membranes. London: RCOG, 2010.

Di Renzo GC, Roura LC, Facchinetti F, et al. Guidelines for the management of spontaneous preterm labour: identification of spontaneous preterm labor, diagnosis of preterm premature rupture of membranes, and preventative tools for preterm birth. J Mat-Fet and Neonatal Medicine 2011; 24(5):659–667.

Van der Ham DP, et al. Induction of labour versus expectant management in women with preterm prelabour rupture of the membranes between 34–37 weeks: a randomised controlled trial. PLoS Med 2012; 9(4): e1001208.

Related topics of interest

Prolonged pregnancy

Overview

The International Federation of Gynecology and Obstetrics (FIGO) quote World Health Organization (WHO) criteria to define prolonged pregnancy as a 'pregnancy lasting 42 completed weeks (294 days) or more'. The frequency of prolonged pregnancy is approximately 10% when the estimated date of delivery (EDD) is certain and 15% when EDD is uncertain. Thus, use of dating scan in the first trimester of pregnancy has reduced the incidence of prolonged pregnancy.

Aetiology

This is unknown. Previously, aetiological factors included fetal abnormalities such as anencephaly, but this is now much rarer as affected pregnancies are now identified in the first or second trimester. In a very small proportion of prolonged pregnancies, factors have been identified which could explain the phenomenon such as placental sulphatase deficiency or low thyroid hormone levels. Prolonged pregnancy may recur; woman who have had one prolonged or two prolonged pregnancies have a 30% or 40% chance of a further prolonged pregnancy respectively. Other factors associated with prolonged pregnancy are nulliparity, maternal obesity and maternal ethnicity.

Fetal and neonatal implications

Expectant management in prolonged pregnancies carries a risk of increased perinatal morbidity and mortality due to 'unexplained' intrauterine death, intrapartum hypoxia and meconium aspiration syndrome. At 41–42 weeks of gestation the perinatal mortality rate is 1.2–1.27 per 1000 ongoing pregnancies; at 42–43 weeks it is 1.2–1.9 per 1000; beyond 43 weeks' gestation the risk of fetal demise is 1.58–6.3 per 1000.

Fetuses in a prolonged pregnancy have greater degrees of ossification and a quarter of them will weigh more than 4000 g. Macrosomic babies tend to have increased risks such as prolonged labour and shoulder dystocia with the added risk of trauma to both fetus and mother. Notwithstanding these factors, there is no documented increase in the incidence of fetal distress in labour for prolonged uncomplicated singleton pregnancies.

Meconium stained liquor may be more common, but this may be a reflection more of dominant vagal tone which increases with gestation than of true fetal distress.

Oligohydramnios can be associated with prolonged pregnancy, with potential of non-reassuring cardiotocography (CTG) both antepartum and intrapartum due to cord compression.

The long term effect of prolonged pregnancies is still unknown and is a controversial topic.

Diagnosis

The diagnosis of prolonged pregnancy is assisted by determining the exact age of the fetus by ultrasound scan in the first or early second trimester. Where this is not routinely available (e.g. low-income countries) EDD may be estimated from last menstrual period or uterine size.

Management of prolonged pregnancy

Induction of labour

Induction of labour (IOL) at 41 weeks and beyond appears to be supported by:

- The increase risk of fetal compromise and stillbirth rises after 42 weeks of gestation from a low baseline. On the basis of this the National Institute of Health and Clinical Excellence (NICE) recommend that at all pregnancies should be offered IOL between 41–42 weeks of gestation
- Randomised controlled trials suggest that elective IOL at 41 weeks of gestation and beyond may be associated with a decrease in both the risk of caesarean delivery and meconium-stained liquor and may be cost-effective

- There is no increase in the risk of caesarean section with IOL as compared to expectant management beyond 41 weeks of gestation
- Women report increased satisfaction with an offer of IOL at 41 weeks compared to expectant management

Therefore, women should be appropriately counselled in order to make an informed choice between scheduled IOL for a prolonged pregnancy or monitoring without IOL (delayed IOL).

Prior to pharmacological IOL a membrane sweep should be offered at 40–41 weeks for nulliparous women and after 41 weeks for multiparous women. A membrane sweep releases endogenous prostaglandins and increases the incidence of spontaneous labour before 42 weeks.

Conservative management

If a woman declines IOL after appropriate counselling her wishes should be respected. However, it is advisable to initiate tests of fetal well-being consisting of twice weekly CTG and ultrasound determination of the liquor volume. Studies looking at Doppler have failed to indicate any benefit of performing these in prolonged pregnancies. Oligohydramnios indicates need for IOL but is associated in these circumstances with increase risk of abnormal CTG, increased admission to neonatal intensive care unit and decreased Apgar scores.

Further reading

Bakketeig, LS, Bergsjo, P. Post-term pregnancy: magnitude of the problem. In: Enkin M, Keirse MJ, Chalmers I (Eds). Effective Care in Pregnancy and Childbirth. Oxford: Oxford University Press, 1989.

NICE Clinical Guideline No. 70. Induction of labour. London: NICE 2008.

Nakling J, Backe B. Pregnancy risk increases from 41 weeks of gestation. Acta Obstet Gynecol Scand 2006; 85(6):663.

Myers ER, Blumrick R, Christian AL, et al. Management of Prolonged Pregnancy. Rockville (MD): Agency for Healthcare Research and Quality (US), 2002.

Caughey AB, et al. Maternal and neonatal outcomes of elective induction of labor. Evide Rep Technol Assess 2009; 176:1–257.

Gulmezoglu AM, Crowther CA, Middleton P, Heatley E. Induction of labour for improving birth outcomes for women at or beyond term. Cochrane Database Systematic Reviews 2012; 13(6):CD004945.

Related topics of interest

Puerperal psychosis and postnatal depression

Overview

The first few weeks after giving birth are frequently a time of significant emotional adjustment. Most women experience a sense of elation and excitement immediately after the birth of their child. For many women between the 3rd and 5th day following delivery can be associated with feelings of inadequacy, anxiety and tearfulness. This is common (50–80%) and is self-limiting; it may be referred to as the 'baby blues'.

Approximately 10% of women will go on to develop some form of postnatal depressive illness. The nature and severity of illness that comprises this group is diverse and not all respond to the same treatment. In contrast to the 'blues', it is unlikely that women suffering from postnatal depression will improve without some form of intervention. Untreated patients may have a prolonged illness continuing into a subsequent pregnancy.

Puerperal psychosis is a distinct entity and refers to the development of a psychotic episode shortly following childbirth in a previously well woman. The terminology can be used for a women who has developed her first ever episode of psychosis or a woman who has previously suffered from a psychotic illness who was well prior to delivery. Puerperal psychosis is uncommon, with an incidence of 2 per 1000 births. Psychosis may have tragic consequences of suicide or infanticide. Early recognition and prompt action is essential to help prevent serious sequelae. The importance of adequate mental health care is recurrently highlighted by the frequency of psychiatric illness as a cause of indirect maternal deaths (13 deaths from 2006–2008).

Clinical features

The features and severity of symptoms of postnatal depression are very varied as with depression occurring at any time in a person's life. Postnatal depression develops most commonly within the first 4 months after birth, but can occur within the first 12 months. The onset of symptoms tends to be insidious but occasionally acute episodes develop. The symptoms may include:
- Sadness/despair
- Insomnia
- Poor appetite
- Anxiety (may also focus excessively on child's well-being)
- Lack of interest in daily activities
- May or may not have components of anxiety or obsessive behaviour

As with other forms of depression, the illness can be graded as mild, moderate or severe. Even mild depressive illness can have a detrimental impact on the quality of life for the entire family as often these illnesses are often under-recognised and can be protracted if not treated.

Puerperal psychosis develops acutely and may rapidly deteriorate after delivery. Although most women (50%) present within the first week following delivery, the first 3 months following delivery remain a high risk time. The clinical features displayed are very similar to any other psychotic episodes and include:
- Labile mood ranging from severe depression to elation
- Persecutory feelings, often with mistrust/suspicion of staff and family
- Grandiose ideas
- Inability to sleep
- Lack of interest in food or self-care
- Delusional ideations (occasionally concerning the infant)

Aetiology

As with all depressive illness, postnatal depression may develop due to a complex combination of inheritable, biological and social factors. The following are known risk factors for developing postnatal depression:
- Depression/anxiety during pregnancy
- Lack of social support

- Recent adverse life events (particularly if these include previous traumatic delivery experiences)
- Ambivalence towards pregnancy

Puerperal psychosis is not as strongly linked to psychosocial risk factors as postnatal depression, but there does appear to be strong biological risk factors:

- Previous personal history of puerperal psychosis or bipolar illness
- Family history of bipolar illness or puerperal psychosis

Diagnosis

Staff caring for women in pregnancy and in the postnatal period should have an understanding of the risk factors for and signs of mental health problems. Ideally attempts to predict those at risk for developing these illnesses should start at the booking visit where a series of relevant questions are asked. Depending on the perceived risk, the woman should be offered care accordingly. For women at significant risk of serious mental health problems this may mean being cared for by a perinatal psychiatrist and specialist mental health care team. For lower risk women, this may include supportive visits from a caseload midwife with escalation of service if this is needed. Staff awareness of symptoms and of the expected time frame of presentation should then allow the detection of illness.

Although there are conflicting guidelines regarding screening for mental health problems, tools such as the Edinburgh Postnatal Depression Scale (EPDS) have been extensively studied as means of detecting postnatal depression and can be used by health care professionals to aid detection of illness. It is most likely that the onset of postnatal depression will arise in the community setting.

The diagnosis of puerperal psychosis is made based on the presence of clinical symptoms. In the initial stages care must be taken not to attribute these symptoms to the 'baby blues' as both can begin to subtly develop as insomnia, agitation and tearfulness within the first few days following delivery. The symptoms of the 'blues' will alleviate with reassurance and support and will resolve within 24–48 hours, whilst in stark contrast, the symptoms of puerperal psychosis will dramatically deteriorate within the same time frame. Due to the acute nature of the latter, if psychosis is suspected on the maternity ward, an urgent psychiatric assessment should be requested. It is important to exclude physical causes (especially sepsis) for an acute confusional state by performing a careful physical examination including assessment of pulse, blood pressure and temperature.

Management

Postnatal depression is pharmacologically managed in the same way as depression occurring at any other time in life. However, this is a time where increased social and psychological support is likely to be of particular value as the woman has the additional challenge of a highly dependent newborn. Pharmacological treatments include tricyclic antidepressants (excretion in breast milk does occur but is very low) such as imipramine or amitriptyline. Doxepin should be avoided due to reports of serious neonatal sedation. Selective serotonin reuptake inhibitors (SSRIs) are widely used in depression outwith pregnancy and include fluoxetine, paroxetine and citalopram. SSRI excretion in breast milk is higher than that of tricyclic antidepressants. The breastfed infant of mothers taking SSRIs should be observed for poor feeding, jitteriness and poor sleep.

Women who develop puerperal psychosis need to be urgently assessed by a psychiatrist and ideally cared for in a specialised mother and baby unit. The pharmacological management of this illness include the use of antipsychotic medication (typical antipsychotic agents include: haloperidol and chlorpromazine or newer drugs such as olanzapine), mood stabilisers (e.g. Lithium Carbonate) and at times an antidepressant. Care must be taken when the woman continues to breastfeed her child when taking such medication.

Women suffering from both conditions will need long term follow-up and discussion about prevention and risk of recurrence in future pregnancies.

Further reading

Oates M. Postnatal Affective Disorders. Part 1: an introduction. The Obstetrician and Gynaecologist 2008; 10:145–150.

O'Hara MW, Swain AM. Rates and risk of postpartum depression – a meta-analysis. Int Rev Psychiatry 1996; 8:37–54.

NICE Guidline Number No. 45. Antenatal and postnatal mental health. London: NICE, 2007.

Related topics of interest

- Maternal death (p. 255)

Puerperium and breastfeeding

The puerperium

The puerperium is defined as the time after completion of the third stage of labour until the changes of pregnancy revert to their non-pregnant state; this period is traditionally held to be 6 weeks. However, this is an arbitrary definition with little or no underlying physiological evidence. Although the puerperium is traditionally regarded as low risk for complications compared to antenatal or intrapartum periods, many problems can occur at this stage such as sepsis or thromboembolic disease, or a pre-existing problem such as mental health disorder or cardiac disease could deteriorate potentially severely enough to endanger the woman's life.

Puerperal changes

Structural   Uterine involution occurs when uterine weight reduces from 1000 g to 50–100 g within a number of weeks. This is also return of abdominal muscular tone, fading of striae gravidarum, return of normal renal tract dimensions, tone and bladder volume, loss of vaginal distensibility and return of normal elasticity and capacity (may be delayed by breastfeeding). Cessation of the lochia, that is shedding of the superficial layer of the decidua and blood with an estimated loss of 200–500 mL occurs; this usually occurs in the first 4 weeks after delivery, but in up to 15% of women loss of lochia can take up to 6–8 weeks. The cervix takes up to 1 week to reduce to < 1 cm dilatation and the small circular cervical opening of a pre-pregnancy nulliparous woman becomes a large transverse slit.

Hormonal   Falling levels of sex steroids and prolactin (unless breastfeeding), return of ovarian function (may be delayed by breastfeeding) secondary to cyclical gonadotrophin release from the pituitary, falling thyroid hormones, a short-lived rise then a fall of urinary 17-ketosteroids, declining plasma cortisol, testosterone, androstenedione, renin, angiotensin II and aldosterone, and a loss of the relative insulin resistance. Human chorionic gonadotrophin returns to normal in 2–4 weeks after delivery but on occasion this return to normality may be prolonged. Menstruation occurs by the 12th week in 70% of women.

Weight   There is an average loss of 12.5 kg from the weight gain of pregnancy, consisting of water loss and products of conception (5 kg) and then a slower loss of 4.25 kg until by 10 weeks postnatally the woman is 2.25 kg heavier than in the non-pregnant state. However, retention of some of the weight gained leads to the increased incidence in obesity in developed countries. 14–25% of women will gain more than 4.5 kg postpartum.

Cardiovascular and haematological   After an immediate rise, a 4-day fall occurs in the haemotocrit and haemoglobin, which is followed by a steady rise again. There is also a fall in plasma volume and leucocyte count and fibrinogen levels as well as a rise in plasma proteins and osmolality and platelets. The incidence of anaemia is up to 30%, which should be treated with oral iron supplementation (e.g. ferrous sulphate).

The physiological hypercoagulable state of pregnancy lasts for about 6 weeks postpartum, which has implications for the duration of thromboembolic treatment. There is a slow fall in cardiac output and circulating blood volume. Blood pressure may remain elevated for a week.

Obstetric pelvic floor and sexual function   Up to 85% of women in the UK will have a degree of perineal trauma during vaginal delivery with approximately 1% having anal sphincter injuries. Urinary incontinence occurs in up to 30% of women postnatally. Women who have minor incontinence problems after delivery and subsequently resolve are at risk of recurrence of their incontinence after another vaginal delivery, with potential long term problems. Sexual health problems can occur with pelvic pain, dyspareunia and decreased arousal impacting upon psychological well-being.

Psychological   The health care professional must be able to differentiate between normal and abnormal. At least 10% of new mothers undergo a clinical postnatal depressive illness (over and above the so-called 'baby blues') and this needs to be appreciated by obstetricians, midwives, health visitors, general practitioners, partners and families of new mothers. Contributing factors will include a relevant past psychiatric or obstetric history (e.g. previous depression), poor socioeconomic circumstances, a difficult pregnancy, labour and delivery, preterm delivery, baby in special care, a baby with abnormalities, stillbirth or neonatal death. One in 500–1000 women will have a puerperal psychosis. 10% will develop a new depressive illness and 2% will need referral to a psychiatrist. Although severe psychiatric disease can affect all socioeconomic groups of women, women with language barrier are at particular risk.

Breastfeeding

The glandular breast tissue is derived from ectoderm and radiates out from the nipple in 15–20 ducts that lead to ductules and then to secretory alveolar cells. Each alveolus is surrounded by oxytocin-sensitive, contractile, myoepithelial cells, and each duct and ductule is lined by longitudinal contractile cells, resulting in milk release at the nipple under the stimulus of the milk let-down reflex. The milk let-down reflex is mediated by oxytocin and acts synergistically with the prolactin neuroendocrine reflex and both are required for successful lactation.

The breast shows significant hyperplasia and hypertrophy in pregnancy under the influence of oestrogen, growth hormone, glucocorticoids, progesterone, prolactin and human placental lactogen. Prolactin, the main hormone in lactation, is manufactured by lactotrophs in the anterior pituitary. Its release is augmented by a neuroendocrine reflex initiated by nipple stimulus, e.g. suckling. Such a stimulus blocks release of prolactin inhibitory factors, e.g. dopamine, from the hypothalamus and stimulates release of prolactin-releasing factors, e.g. thyroid-releasing hormone. Prolactin binds to receptors on the alveolus and acts at multiple sites to stimulate synthesis of milk constituents. The initial early milk, or colostrum, has high concentrations of proteins, including immunoglobulins. Milk contains all of the constituents necessary for at least the first 6 months of the baby's life. The average daily volume of milk released is of the order of 800–1200 mL and a lactating mother requires a calorific intake of 2000–3000 kcal/day to maintain it. Lactation is associated with amenorrhoea and suppression of ovulation. Breastfeeding is not a reliable contraceptive, with between 1–10% of women conceiving while breastfeeding.

Up to two-thirds of women will have minor problems breastfeeding. Mastitis may occur due to a blocked duct or *Staphylococcus aureus* or *Candida albicans*. If the symptoms do not respond to antibiotics or a mass is palpated, ultrasound may locate an abscess necessitating drainage and prolonged antibiotic therapy.

Further reading

Amorim AR, Linne YM, Lourenco PM. Diet or exercise, or both, for weight reduction in women after childbirth. Cochrane Database Systematic Reviews 2007; CD005627.

Lone F, Sultan A, Thakar R. Obstetric pelvic floor and anal injuries. The Obstetrician and Gynaecologist 2012; 14(4):255–266.

Related topics of interest

- Puerperal psychosis and postnatal depression (p. 303)

Reduced fetal movements

Background

Most women are aware of fetal movements by 20 weeks of gestation. The frequency of fetal movements remains constant after 32 weeks gestation; there is no reduction in fetal movements in late pregnancy. Reduced fetal movements are a common reason for presentation to the maternity service in the third trimester of pregnancy, 6–15% of women present on at least one occasion.

A confidential enquiry into 422 antepartum stillbirths described suboptimal care relating to stillbirth in 69 cases.

Clinical features

Fetal movements should be assessed by maternal perception of fetal movements. There is no evidence that using specific thresholds to define 'reduced fetal movements' (e.g. < 10 movements in 12 hours) is useful. The only threshold developed in a 'normal' obstetric population was < 10 movements in 2 hours of focussed counting, but this is rarely used in clinical practice.

Formal fetal movement counting using kick charts does not appear to increase maternal anxiety, but there is no evidence that it reduces perinatal mortality. Therefore, women should be advised to be aware of their baby's pattern of movements after 28 weeks of pregnancy and present to their maternity service provider if they notice reduced or absent fetal movements.

Clinical associations with reduced fetal movements

Reduced or absent fetal movements can be a symptom of intrauterine fetal death (IUFD).

In babies that are alive at presentation, reduced fetal movements are associated with an increased risk of subsequent stillbirth or fetal growth restriction (FGR) by placental insufficiency. This association is present in many studies from different countries over a 30-year period.

Other associations include fetomaternal haemorrhage and congenital anomalies particularly those affecting the neurological and musculoskeletal systems.

Placentas from women who present with reduced fetal movement are smaller, show more signs of infarction, greater number of syncytial knots, reduced villous vascularity and impaired placental amino-acid transport.

Approximately 70% of women who present with reduced fetal movements have a normal pregnancy outcome.

Management

The aim of management is to confirm fetal viability and then to exclude acute fetal compromise and FGR. Initially, a history should be taken from the patient which should include the presence or absence of fetal movements and the time period over which this occurred. An algorithm for the management of reduced fetal movements is shown in **Figure 27**.

Fetal viability should be confirmed by auscultation of the fetal heart with Pinard stethoscope or handheld Doppler device. If the fetal heart cannot be located, ultrasound scan should be performed (see Topic 104 – Stillbirth and late IUFD).

After 28 weeks gestation acute fetal compromise should be excluded by cardiotocography (CTG).

The risk of FGR should be assessed by maternal history (obstetric history, past medical history, cigarette/alcohol/drug misuse). A clinical examination including measurement of symphysis-fundal height plotted on a customised growth chart should be performed.

An ultrasound scan to assess fetal biometry, liquor volume and umbilical artery Doppler should be offered if the woman has risk factors for or evidence of FGR or where reduced fetal movements persist despite a normal CTG. Women with more than two presentations with reduced fetal movements have an increased risk of poor perinatal outcome.

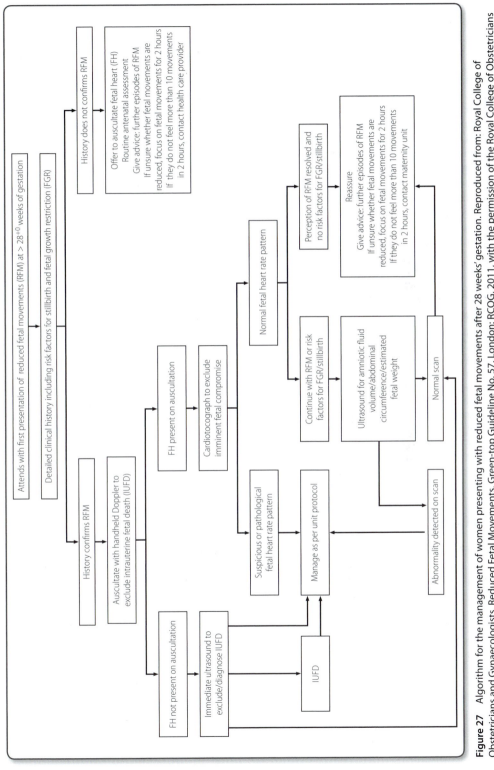

Figure 27   Algorithm for the management of women presenting with reduced fetal movements after 28 weeks' gestation. Reproduced from: Royal College of Obstetricians and Gynaecologists. Reduced Fetal Movements. Green-top Guideline No. 57. London: RCOG, 2011, with the permission of the Royal College of Obstetricians and Gynaecologists.

If fetal anatomy has not been examined by ultrasound (e.g. second-trimester anomaly scan) prior to the examination assessment of fetal morphology should be carried out.

In Norway, routinely performing an ultrasound scan for fetal growth, liquor volume and umbilical artery Doppler identified an abnormality in 11.6% of scans, and reduced perinatal mortality from 3.0 per 1000 live births to 2.0 per 1000 live births.

If a woman presents with reduced fetal movements before 28 weeks of gestation, a thorough history should be taken to assess her risk of stillbirth, then fetal viability should be confirmed with a handheld Doppler device. If there is evidence of FGR an ultrasound scan to measure fetal growth, liquor volume and umbilical artery Doppler should be performed.

Follow-up

If all investigations are normal, women with reduced fetal movements should contact their maternity unit if they have another period of reduced fetal movements. There are no data to support giving women who have presented with reduced fetal movements a kick chart to assist with formal fetal movement counting. At present there are no data to support induction of labour for reduced fetal movements at term if the investigation findings are normal.

Further reading

RCOG Green-top Guideline No. 57, Reduced fetal movements. London: RCOG, 2011.

Heazell AE, Green M, Wright C, et al. Midwives and obstetricians knowledge and management of women presenting with decreased fetal movements. Acta Obstet Gynecol Scand 2008; 87(3):331–339.

Dutton PJ, Warrander LK, Roberts SA, et al. Predictors of poor perinatal outcome following maternal perception of reduced fetal movements – a prospective cohort study. PLoS One 2012; 7(7):e39784.

Heazell AE, Frøen JF. Methods of fetal movement counting and the detection of fetal compromise. J Obstet Gynaecol 2008; 28(2):147–154.

Warrander LK, Batra G, Bernatavicius G, et al. Maternal perception of reduced fetal movements is associated with altered placental structure and function. PLoS One 2012; 7(4):e34851.

Tveit JV, Saastad E, Stray-Pedersen B, et al. Reduction of late stillbirth with the introduction of fetal movement information and guidelines – a clinical quality improvement. BMC Pregnancy Childbirth 2009; 22(9):32.

Related topics of interest

Renal disease in pregnancy

Overview

Renal disease can be divided into acute disease caused by pregnancy, chronic disease which has been revealed during pregnancy and pre-existing renal disease known prior to pregnancy.

Renal physiology in pregnancy

There is dilatation and distortion of the ureters (right more than left because of uterine dextrorotation) up to the calyces, which is the result of smooth muscle relaxation (secondary to hormones) and uterine pressure on the ureters. There is no marked increase in vesicoureteric reflux in pregnancy, but the ureteric dilatation and reduced motility may exacerbate urinary stasis and predispose to infection. The kidneys enlarge by up to 1 cm because of this dilatation and there is an increased glomerular filtration rate (GFR) which is 60% higher by 16 weeks, remaining at this level until term. Renal plasma flow is 30–50% higher than before pregnancy by 20 weeks. Consequently, average values for creatinine and urea decrease during pregnancy and proteinuria increases (with a normal upper limit of 300 mg per 24 hours collection or a protein/creatinine ratio of 30 mg/mmol creatinine). Plasma albumin declines early in pregnancy and then remains static until term.

Acute renal disease in pregnancy

Asymptomatic bacteriuria

This is when true bacteriuria exists without symptoms or signs of an acute urinary tract infection (UTI) with a midstream specimen of urine (MSU) showing > 1,000,000 colonies per mL; E. coli is the most common organism. Up to 40% of such women may have an upper renal tract infection and there is a link between UTI, low birthweight and preterm labour. Reinfection and relapse occur in about 15% of such patients. Antibiotic therapy should be administered.

Acute UTI/pyelonephritis

Lower UTI affects about 1% of pregnant women. Upper UTI, i.e. acute pyelonephritis, is the commonest renal complication of pregnancy. Once upper UTI has been diagnosed, it should be treated promptly with intravenous antibiotics and fluids, initially in a hospital setting. Thereafter, patients should have their urine cultured a minimum of monthly. If a patient has two proven UTIs during pregnancy, consideration should be given to administration of low dose antibiotics as a prophylactic measure for the remainder of the pregnancy.

Renal disease unmasked by pregnancy

Any renal disease may be unmasked by pregnancy. Abnormal renal function and/or significant proteinuria, especially prior to 24 weeks of pregnancy, should always raise the possibility of chronic renal disease. Appropriate management would include renal and liver function tests, blood pressure (BP) reading, quantification of urinary protein [by 24 hour urine collection or protein: creatinine ratio (PCR)], a renal ultrasound and an autoantibody screen. A renal physician should be involved in the plan of investigations and care for the patient.

Rarely a renal biopsy can be required in pregnancy to aid management decisions; this is rarely performed after 26 weeks' gestation. This is generally performed in the prone position which may not be technically possible in late pregnancy. Complications include perirenal haemorrhage, bleeding, ureteric colic secondary to blood clot and trauma to surrounding organs and haematoma. There are conflicting data on whether these complications are more frequent in pregnancy compared to all patients undergoing renal biopsy.

Pre-existing renal disease in pregnancy

Ideally all women with pre-existing renal disease should have preconception counselling. This can advise on the timing of pregnancy in relation to disease flares/transplant, optimise baseline disease and BP control and advise on medication – sometimes changing drugs to those more suitable for pregnancy or advising the woman what medication she needs to stop/switch in early pregnancy.

Women with pre-existing renal disease have variable pregnancy outcomes depending on the disease itself, the degree of renal impairment and the degree of proteinuria/associated hypertension. These pregnancies should be managed in a multidisciplinary team setting with an obstetrician, a renal/obstetric physician and a specialist midwife.

It is important that women are aware of the risks of pregnancy, with some groups of patients having an increased risk of fetal growth restriction (FGR), preterm birth, anaemia and long term renal deterioration. Unless there are contraindictions all patients with pre-existing renal disease should commence low dose aspirin (75 mg) in early pregnancy because of the increased risk of pre-eclampsia. BP control needs to be maintained within strict parameters in these patients, with a target BP of < 140/90 mmHg. For some women with significant renal impairment or proteinuria the target BP level may need to be lowered. Anaemia may be unresponsive to iron supplementation alone and the use of erythropoietin (EPO) may be required to maintain the haemoglobin > 100 g/L. EPO is given as an intravenous or subcuticular injection and is contraindicated with uncontrolled hypertension.

Glomerulonephritis

This is a group of inflammatory conditions of the kidney which are often asymptomatic, slowly progressive and are characterised by the presence of haematuria ± proteinuria, oedema and variable degrees of renal impairment. In the absence of significant hypertension, proteinuria or renal compromise these patients generally have a favourable pregnancy outcome. However, patients with IgA nephropathy can have rapidly progressive disease during pregnancy.

Nephrotic syndrome

The definition of nephrotic syndrome is variable, but proteinuria of > 3 g per 24 hours is often used as the discriminatory level. The most common cause in pregnancy is pre-eclampsia but nephrotic syndrome can be secondary to primary glomerular disease. Serum albumin values of < 25 g/L should also raise suspicion about the possibility of such being present. Fetal complications (e.g. FGR) are increased in such women. Nephrotic syndrome also confers an increased risk of venous thromboembolism. The use of low molecular weight heparin thromboprophylaxis in these patients should be strongly considered in the antenatal and postnatal periods.

Renal transplant

Pregnancy is estimated to occur in 12% of transplanted patients of childbearing age. It is recommended that pregnancy should be delayed until 12–24 months post-transplant and > 12 months after a rejection episode. The patient should be on maintenance immunosuppression and non-teratogenic drugs. Mycophenolate mofetil (MMF) has traditionally been considered unsafe in pregnancy. Its use has been associated with an increased risk of malformations and first-trimester pregnancy loss and ideally should be stopped 6 weeks prior to conception. Standard immunosuppression with azathioprine, tacrolimus, cyclosporin and prednisolone is compatible with pregnancy. The graft function should be stable, with minimal/no proteinuria and optimal control of hypertension (if present). The incidence of a serious rejection episode in pregnancy is the same as the background transplant population.

During pregnancy there should be frequent surveillance/management of renal function, proteinuria, BP and monitoring for pre-eclampsia and FGR. If tacrolimus and prednisolone are used as immunosuppression, screening for gestational diabetes should be performed.

In the absence of obstetric complications, delivery should be planned for 38–39 weeks of gestation. Unless contraindicated the aim should be vaginal delivery. If a caesarean section is planned, a senior obstetrician should be present and if prior surgery has been multiple or complicated the presence of a transplant surgeon is beneficial.

Dialysis

Pregnancy outcome is improved in patients who conceive off dialysis and then require it in later pregnancy compared to those women who conceive on dialysis. Conception on dialysis is infrequent due to reduced fertility.

After conception on dialysis spontaneous miscarriage is more common. Although the live birth rate can approach 80% there is significant perinatal mortality and morbidity that follows such births. The average gestation for delivery is 32 weeks. Polyhydramnios is a common feature of pregnancies on dialysis and the maternal and fetal complications of hypertension, pre-eclampsia, preterm labour, abruption and FGR are common.

Further reading

Renal Disease in Pregnancy, Consensus views arising from the 54th Study Group. Renal disease in Pregnancy. RCOG, 2008.
Kapoor N, Makanjuola D, Shehata H. Review – management of women with chronic renal disease in pregnancy. The Obstetrician & Gynaecologist 2011; 11(3):185–191.
Bramham K, Soh MC, Nelson-Piercy C. Pregnancy and renal outcomes in lupus nephritis: an update and guide to management. Lupus 2012; 21(12):1271–1283.
Bramham K, Nelson-Piercy C, Gao H, et al. Pregnancy in renal transplant recipients: a UK national cohort study. Clin J Am Soc Nephrol 2012; Oct 18.
Nevis IF, Reitsma A, Dominic A, et al. Pregnancy outcomes in women with chronic kidney disease: a systematic review. Clin J Am Soc Nephrol 2011; 6(11):2587–2598.

Related topics of interest

Rhesus disease

Overview

Red cell isoimmunisation, followed by placental transfer of antibodies (IgG), is most commonly due to sensitisation of a Rhesus negative mother by red cells positive for the Rhesus antigen, which was discovered by Landsteiner and Wiener in 1940. In the case of Rhesus negative women, Rhesus positive fetal erythrocytes are antigenically different from mother's red cell, which leads to a maternal immune response with subsequent antibody production.

The volume of fetal erythrocytes transferred to maternal circulation increases with gestation. The development of anti-D has led to a dramatic decrease in the incidence of Rhesus disease (RhD). The perinatal mortality has now dropped from 46 per 1000 to 1.9 per 1000.

Approximately 16% of Caucasians are Rhesus negative because of the deletion of the gene. To prevent future occurrence of Rhesus-associated haemolytic disease of the newborn the Royal College of Obstetricians and Gynaecologists (RCOG) recommend that all non-sensitised Rhesus negative women should be routinely offered a single dose of 1500 IU anti-D immunoglobulin between 28–30 weeks of pregnancy. Prophylaxis against isoimmunisation is also recommended by injection of anti-D when there is increased risk of fetomaternal haemorrhage, e.g. antepartum haemorrhage or at delivery.

Aetiology

The Rhesus antigen is produced from a complex area on chromosome 1; at least three genes, C, D and E, are involved. The D antigen appears to be the most clinically relevant, with over 95% of cases of Rhesus incompatibility being due to the D antigen, which is inherited by simple Mendelian principles. Maternal Anti-D antibodies account for 85% of all haemolytic disease of the newborn.

Clinical features

The clinical presentation of fetal haemolytic anaemia is late and easily missed and depends on the degree of haemolysis of the affected fetus. The pregnancy may result in miscarriage, intrauterine death or the birth of a severely hydropic infant with attendant obstetric complications (related to fetal size and fetal distress), i.e. fetal growth restriction (FGR) fetus or with ultrasound appearances of polyhydramnios associated with hydrops, pleural effusion and pericardial effusion and oedema of skin. RhD may lead to neonatal anaemia or jaundice leading to kernicterus.

Diagnosis

- A history of Rhesus isoimmunisation or features suggestive of isoimmunisation may be apparent (e.g. polyhydramnios)
- Routine maternal antibody screening at the antenatal booking visit will generally identify first time sensitised pregnancies when the maternal serum is screened for ABO blood group and Rhesus (D) antibodies
- In Rhesus negative women the presence of antibodies is followed up by serial direct assays for antibody titres. Serial measurements indicate whether the level of antibody is increasing
- The Rhesus status of baby may be investigated by establishing genotype of father as the D antigen is inherited as autosominal dominant. If father is rhesus negative (i.e. genotype d/d) it is likely that anti-D antibody in a Rhesus negative woman would have developed from exposure to some other source of incompatibility, e.g. previous blood transfusion or previous partner and if confident of parent paternity the fetus will not be affected and further action is not necessary
- If the father is homozygous for D (i.e. gentoype D/d) the baby may be Rh D +ve and hence at risk
- Where there is uncertainty fetal blood group can be determined by examining cell free fetal DNA from maternal blood sample (accuracies of 100% for RhD genotyping in Rhesus negative women).

Management

Management depends on the degree of haemolysis and the gestation.

Principles of management are similar for RhD regardless of the levels of antibody present (in anti-Kell antibodies severity does not correlate with antibody titres).

Due to the rarity of the disease referral is recommended to a tertiary fetal medicine centre for monitoring of fetal anaemia by measurement of peak systolic velocity (PSV) in the middle cerebral artery (MCA).

MCA-PSV has superseded amniocentesis, the traditional method of choice for the surveillance of the severity of fetal anaemia (**Figure 28**). Measurement of blood flow in the MCA is a non-invasive test; in MCA the hyperkinetic circulation correlates well with degree of anaemia and predicts the necessity for further treatment in terms of intrauterine transfusion.

Measurement of MCA-PSV is useful in pregnancies after those complicated by haemolytic disease of the newborn/RhD as maternal titres are no longer predictive of the risk of fetal anaemia. For more information on the management of fetal anaemia please see Topic 76 – Hydrops fetalis.

Advanced RhD may present with decreased fetal movements. On the cardiotocography there may be evidence of poor variability, decelerations or a sinusoidal trace.

In pregnancies complicated by RhD cord blood should be collected for haemoglobin,

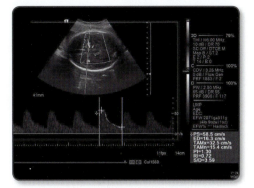

Figure 28 Middle cerebral artery Doppler trace demonstrating increased peak systolic velocity indicative of fetal anaemia in Rhesus disease.

platelets and blood group, bilirubin and direct Coombs test after delivery.

The neonate may need to be treated for anaemia or hyperbilirubinaemia. Treatment depends on the degree of anaemia and jaundice and may include red cell transfusion, exchange transfusion and phototherapy.

Summary

Although the outcome for RhD is good, associated hydrops reduces the survival rate to 11%. Neonatal recovery may be complicated by the need for repeated blood transfusions but studies have demonstrated a satisfactory long term neurological outcome in over 90% of cases.

Further reading

Kumar S, Regan F. Management of pregnancies with RhD alloimmunization. BMJ 2005; 330:1255.

Royal College of Obstetricians and Gynaecologists. The Use of Anti-D Immunoglobulin for Rhesus D Prophylaxis. London: RCOG, 2011.

National Institute for Health and Clinical Excellence. Routine antenatal anti-D prophylaxis for women who are Rhesus D negative London: NICE, 2011.

Bullock R, Martin WL, Coomarasamy A, Kilby MD. Prediction of fetal anaemia in pregnancies with red-cell alloimmunization: comparison of middle cerebral artery peak systolic velocity and amniotic fluid OD450. Ultrasound Obstet Gynaecol 2005; 25(4):331–334.

Moise, K. Management of Rhesus alloimmunization in pregnancy. Obstetrics and Gynaecology 2008; 112(1):164–176.

Related topics of interest

Risk management in obstetrics

Overview

Clinical governance is a multi-system approach to improve the quality of patient care. Risk management is one the pillars of this alongside education and training, clinical effectiveness and audit, research and development, openness and information management.

Risk management is the identification, analysis, assessment, control, and avoidance, minimisation or elimination of unacceptable risks. Risk management can be proactive using guidelines, evidence based practice, audit results, etc. to minimise risk and improve day-to-day clinical practice. In addition, risk management can also be reactive in response to incident reporting, serious untoward investigations (SUI) and complaints. The following discussion uses examples from the National Health Service (NHS) in England.

Whose responsibility is risk management?

Risk management is the responsibility of all individuals working in any aspect of patient care. At a departmental and hospital (in the UK, the NHS trust) level there are designated multidisciplinary risk management/clinical governance teams. A good risk management programme builds a culture of safety, exhibits good and consistent leadership, supports staff, integrates risk management activity, promotes incident reporting, involves and communicates well with patients and the public, learns from its mistakes, shares safety lessons and implements solutions to prevent further harm.

Individual clinicians can reduce the danger of adverse outcomes by adopting the '6 Cs' approach:

- Correct patient
- Clear communication with patient and other staff
- Counselling
- Consent
- Competence
- Case notes documentation

National Health Service Litigation Authority (NHSLA)

The NHSLA is the organisation which manages claims against the National Health Service (NHS) in England and Wales and provides indemnity cover. They:

- Set standards for safe care and assess NHS providers against them – the Clinical Negligence Scheme for Trusts (CNST)
- Share learning from claims to help improve safety in the NHS, e.g. the report *Ten Years of Maternity Claims,* an analysis of NHSLA data published in 2012
- Ensure members' contributions are fair and reflect risk, thereby encouraging them to provide safer care that reduces claims

Maternity claims represent the highest value and second highest number of clinical negligence claims reported to the NHSLA. Between 1st April 2000 and 31st March 2010 there were 5087 maternity claims with a total value of £3.1 billion. During a similar time period from 2000–2009 inclusive, there were 5.5 million births in England. Thus, < 0.1% of these births had become the subject of a claim, indicating that the vast majority of births do not result in a clinical negligence claim. The three most frequent categories of claim were those relating to management of labour (14.05%), caesarean section (13.24%) and cerebral palsy (10.65%). Two of these categories, namely cerebral palsy and management of labour, along with cardiotocography (CTG) interpretation, were also the most expensive and together accounted for 70% of the total value of all the maternity claims.

Clinical negligence scheme for trusts (CNST)

The NHSLA indemnifies English NHS bodies against claims for clinical negligence through CNST. A separate set of CNST standards was developed for maternity services in 2003, because of the disproportionate scale of maternity claims. These are now updated annually. The standards and assessment process are designed to:

- Improve the safety of women and their babies
- Provide a framework to focus risk management activities to support the delivery of quality improvements in patient care, organisational governance, and the safety of women and their babies
- Assist in the identification of risk
- Embed risk management into the maternity services' culture
- Focus maternity services on increasing incident reporting whilst decreasing the overall severity of incidents
- Encourage awareness of and learning from claims
- Reflect risk exposure and enable maternity services to determine how to manage their own risks
- Encourage and support maternity services in taking a proactive approach to improvement
- Provide information to the organisation, other inspecting bodies and stakeholders on how areas of risk covered by the standards are being managed

There are three progressive levels of assessment and for each level minimum requirements are set:
- Level 0 maternity services must be assessed annually until such time as they achieve Level 1
- Level 1 services must be assessed at least once in any 2-year period
- Level 2 and 3 must be assessed at least once in any 3-year period

An incentive scheme, in the form of a discount payment for achieving each level exists.

The five CNST standards are: organisation, clinical care, high risk conditions, communication and postnatal and newborn care. Each standard has 10 individual criteria.

Level 1 is concerned with policy documentation, i.e. existence of up to date guidelines. Level 2 is concerned with practice implementation and audit. The assessors review health records from a minimum sample size agreed in advance. Level 3 is the demonstration that action plans must be developed for any failings identified and changes made to reduce risks which have

been demonstrated through reaudit. The pass mark for each level is a minimum of 40 out of the 50 criteria, with no fewer than 7 criteria passed in any one standard.

Incident reporting systems

The maternity department will have a system to report critical incidents as they occur. A trigger list should be available in all departments to prompt the minimum that individuals should report. Triggers can be related to clinical outcomes (e.g. maternal – postpartum haemorrhage, uterine rupture, fetal – unexpected admission to the neonatal unit, staff – needlestick injury, injury at work) or infrastructure/organisational factors (e.g. lack of equipment, lack of beds, insufficient staffing issues).

Risk register

A risk register is a centrally held document which should contain all the risks identified by the maternity department. The register can be populated from incidents, complaints, national alerts and local compliance with national guidelines. All risks are given a 'rating' according to how high the impact of the risk is (financially, in terms of media exposure and patient harm) and the likelihood of occurrence. The controls for minimising the said risk should be outlined and the future action plans to further minimise or abolish the risk. This risk register should be regularly reviewed to assess progress against the proposed action plans.

Serious untoward incidents

From reviews of incident reporting, further higher level investigations or SUIs may be undertaken either because the 'incident' is unexpected or caused/had the potential to cause serious harm. Many hospitals have their own triggers for when a SUI should be commenced. These investigations make use of root cause analysis (RCA), a problem solving exercise that tries to identify the root cause(s) that caused the event(s) that led to the incident.

The report by a multidisciplinary team should include:
- Define the problem and its significance
- Outline the causal relationships that combined to cause the problem and the identified root causes – these may be identified as problems with quality of care and service delivery problems
- Explain how the action plan will prevent the recurrence of the defined problem(s)

There are many tools and methods that are employed to identify the root causes of an SUI. More than one approach may often be required for each investigation, e.g. events and causal factor charting, barrier analysis, tree diagrams, why-why chart to name a few tools used in RCA.

SUI reports enable the maternity unit to actively learn from incidents and to ensure that where required changes are identified and that they become embedded into practice.

Further reading

NHS Litigation Authority. Ten years of Maternity Claims. London: NHSLA, 2012.

Harding K. Risk management in obstetrics. Obstetrics, Gynaecology and Reproductive Medicine 2012; 22(1):1–6.

Gillham J. Pitfalls in our practice, examples from three cases of obstetric litigation. Obstetrics, Gynaecology & Reproductive Medicine 2012; 22(8):229–236.Royal College of Obstetricians and Gynaecologists. Improving Patient Safety: Risk Management for Maternity and Gynaecology, 3rd edn. London: RCOG, 2009.

Related topics of interest

- Caesarean section (p. 198)
- Monitoring in labour (p. 262)

Shoulder dystocia

Overview

Shoulder dystocia is defined as a requirement for additional obstetric manoeuvres to deliver the fetal body after gentle traction has failed following delivery of the head. Shoulder dystocia is a bony problem, caused by the anterior shoulder impacting on the maternal symphysis, or the posterior shoulder on the sacral promontory. The incidence is between 0.58% and 0.7%. Shoulder dystocia is associated with maternal complications: postpartum haemorrhage (11%) and third or fourth degree tears (3.8%). Potential fetal complications include: death, hypoxic-ischaemic encephalopathy, brachial plexus injuries (BPI) in 2.3–16% of deliveries, and fractures of the humerus and clavicle in approximately 4.2–9.5% of cases.

Clinical features

As shoulder dystocia is largely unpredictable it is important be vigilant especially if the following features are evident at delivery:
- Difficulty in delivery of the face and chin
- The 'turtle neck' sign, where the head is seen to retract
- Failure of head restitution and shoulder descent

Risk factors

The following features are associated with increased risk of shoulder dystocia: previous shoulder dystocia, macrosomia (defined as birth weight > 4.5 Kg), diabetes mellitus, raised body mass index (> 30 Kg/m^2) and induction of labour (IOL). Features to be aware of in labour include prolonged first stage and second stage of labour, secondary arrest, oxytocin augmentation and instrumental delivery. In non-diabetic women with a macrosomic fetus, IOL should not be offered routinely as it does not prevent shoulder dystocia. Diabetic women have a 2–4-fold increased risk of shoulder dystocia compared with fetuses of equal weight in non-diabetic women, thus the incidence of shoulder dystocia can be reduced if IOL occurs at term. Elective caesarean section can be offered to reduce risks in diabetic women with a macrosomic fetus. If the woman has a previous history of shoulder dystocia, she can be offered either a vaginal delivery or caesarean section, after antenatal discussion with informed consent. If risk factors are present at delivery an obstetric registrar should be available on the delivery suite.

Diagnosis

Prompt recognition of features suggestive of shoulder dystocia should alert staff to the risk of difficult delivery. Failure to deliver the fetus following routine traction in an axial direction confirms the diagnosis.

Management

Shoulder dystocia should be managed in a systematic fashion. To avoid hypoxia and acidosis, delivery should ideally be achieved in > 5 minutes if possible, and should be performed effectively and with care to try and avoid injury. The mnemonic **HELPERR** can be adopted to prompt the immediate management of this obstetric emergency.

H   Call for **HELP**, the emergency buzzer should be pulled, additional and senior staff requested, and on attendance staff should be informed that the emergency is shoulder dystocia. It is important to tell the mother to stop pushing, and to avoid any fundal pressure, to lie flat and to position the buttocks at the end of the bed.

E   **Evaluate** for **episiotomy**. This is not always required. It is performed to allow room for internal manoeuvres.

L   **Legs**. The woman should be placed in McRoberts' position. It involves laying the back of the woman's bed flat and flexing and abducting her hips. This brings her thighs up to her abdomen, with one assistant on each side supporting each leg. This opens up the pelvis, straightening the lumbosacral angle and increasing the anterior–posterior pelvic diameter. McRoberts' position is very effective (reported success rates of up to 90%) and should be performed first.

P   Suprapubic pressure. This improves the success rate of the McRoberts' manoeuvre. Pressure should be applied in a downward and lateral direction at the side of the fetal back, in a continuous pressure for 30 seconds and then a 'rocking' pressure for 30 seconds during which time efforts should be continued to deliver the baby. Suprapubic pressure reduces the bisacromial diameter, dislodging the anterior shoulder impacted behind the symphysis, bringing it into the oblique position to allow subsequent delivery with routine traction.

There is a choice to perform either of the following two manoeuvres first, depending upon the situation and the individual clinician's decision.

E   Enter the vagina, for performing 'internal manoeuvres'. In the Rubin II manoeuvre, two fingers are placed on the posterior aspect of the anterior shoulder and forward pressure is applied to adduct the shoulders, moving them into the oblique position. This causes disimpaction, allowing delivery with routine traction. If unsuccessful, the Woods' screw manoeuvre can be employed. Two fingers of the opposite hand press on the anterior aspect of the posterior shoulder; this can be combined with the Rubin II manoeuvre. If unsuccessful, the Reverse Woods' screw can be employed, by placing two fingers on the posterior aspect of the posterior shoulder to rotate it in the opposite direction.

R   Removal of the posterior arm. The fingers are introduced to the fetal axilla to bring the shoulder down, and deliver the posterior arm. If required, pressure can be applied in a posterior direction on the cubital fossa, to cause downward displacement of the arm. This allows the fetal hand to be grasped and swept over the face and chest.

R   Roll the woman onto all fours. This is called the 'Gaskin' manoeuvre, and can be attempted if appropriate.

If there is still no success with these manoeuvres, consideration must be given to the following additional manoeuvres: cleidotomy (division of the clavicle), symphysiotomy (dividing the anterior fibres of the symphyseal ligament), and the Zavanelli manoeuvre (replacement of the head and delivery by caesarean section). Careful consideration must be given before performing these latter techniques as they are associated with significant maternal morbidity.

Following delivery, clinicians must be aware of potential risks of postpartum haemorrhage and third and fourth degree tears. Cord pH should be taken and the baby should be carefully assessed by a neonatologist. It is very important to debrief the parents.

Given the relative infrequency of severe shoulder dystocia, it is imperative that clinicians are trained with regular 'skills drills' this approach has been shown to improve performance in obstetric emergencies, such as shoulder dystocia.

Further reading

RCOG Green-top Guideline No.42, Shoulder dystocia. London: RCOG, 2012.

Grady K, Howell C, Cox C. Managing Obstetric Emergencies and Trauma, 2nd edn. London: RCOG, 2007; 221–231.

Related topics of interest

Stillbirth

Overview

The definition of stillbirth varies between different countries. The definition employed by the World Health Organization (WHO) is an infant delivered without signs of life after 22 weeks of gestation or weighing ≥ 500 g when gestation is unknown. The legal definition applied in the UK is an infant born after 24 completed weeks' gestation who shows no signs of life.

The stillbirth rate in the UK is approximately 5/1000 live births; this has not reduced significantly for over 20 years.

Stillbirth has a long-lasting psychological and social impact on both parents, including increased anxiety, depression and post-traumatic stress disorder. The care provided at the time of stillbirth may reduce or contribute to this burden.

Clinical features and diagnosis

Lack of fetal movements and the absence of fetal heart sounds may be the first symptoms or signs of intrauterine fetal death (IUFD).

While useful to suspect IUFD auscultation of the fetal heart with a Pinard stethoscope or handheld Doppler devices have insufficient accuracy in diagnosing IUFD.

IUFD should be diagnosed by real-time ultrasound scan of the fetal heart; ideally with a second opinion. Other signs that may be evident on ultrasound scan include skull collapse/overlapping of skull bones (Spalding's sign). It may be helpful to show the women the findings. Women should be warned that they may perceive passive fetal movements.

The diagnosis of IUFD should be made in a clear, but sensitive manner. If the patient is alone, an offer to contact partner, family or friends should be made.

Aetiology

The aetiology of stillbirth differs depending on the situation, with differences between low-income countries and high-income countries. In high-income countries with good access to midwifery and obstetric services intrapartum stillbirth is rare.

Attributing causality of stillbirth to a specific cause can be difficult. There are many different classification systems to describe the causes/associations with stillbirth. More modern classification systems such as ReCoDe, TULIP and CODAC have much lower rates of unexplained stillbirth (15.2%–16.2%) than older systems such as Wigglesworth or Aberdeen classifications (47.4–66%).

In the UK, important causes of stillbirth include fetal growth restriction, infection, congenital anomaly, placental abruption and multiple pregnancies (particularly those with a monochorionic placenta).

Investigations should be offered to parents to identify the cause of stillbirth (see below).

Management of birth

In most cases induction of labour is offered, unless specific contraindications to vaginal delivery are present (> 2 previous caesarean sections, placenta praevia, immediate threat to maternal life). Maternal preferences regarding the mode of delivery should be discussed. Expectant management is associated with deterioration in the baby's appearance, a reduced value of postmortem examination and an increased risk of coagulopathy (although this is small).

In women with an unscarred uterus, mifepristone (an antiprostagen) in combination with a prostaglandin preparation is recommended. 200 mg mifepristone reduces the length of time to induce labour but requires 24–48 hours to work. Women should be warned they may go into spontaneous labour and should be given the contact details of the maternity unit if they go home. Misoprostol or PGE2 can be used to induce labour, they are equally safe, but misoprostol appears slightly more effective (NB: misoprostol use is 'off-label' in the UK). Misoprostol should be administered vaginally (less side effects) and should be adjusted according to gestational age (100 µg 6-hourly before 26 weeks; 25–50 µg 4-hourly at 27 weeks or more).

In women who have a scarred uterus, the decision for mode of delivery/induction of labour should be made by a consultant obstetrician and the patient. Mifepristone alone increases the chance of labour within 72 hours. Misoprostol can be safely used in women with one previous caesarean section at lower doses (e.g. 25–50 µg). Women should be closely monitored for signs of scan rupture.

While membranes remain intact the chances of infection are negligible; there is no need for routine antibiotics for women with IUFD.

Patients can have the same range of analgesia routinely used for labour. Full blood count and clotting should be checked prior to epidural analgesia to exclude coagulopathy.

Management after delivery

After delivery, women (and their birth partner/families) should be allowed to spend time and hold their baby if they wish. In general, parents value mementoes of their child which include photographs, palm and footprints and/or locks of hair; these should be offered. If parents decline, they should have the option for these to be held in the medical notes. Parents may wish to name their child; if they do, this name should be used by all health professionals.

Parents should have access to spiritual and emotional support, e.g. chaplain/faith representative or bereavement support worker. Bereavement support and contact numbers for support groups, e.g. Sands (Stillbirth and Neonatal Death Charity) should be offered.

Women should be offered cabergoline 1 mg for lactation suppression.

A medical certificate of stillbirth should be completed by the obstetrician caring for the patient. If no obstetrician has cared for the patient then a midwife can complete the medical certificate of stillbirth. Parents have 42 days (21 in Scotland) to register the stillbirth. In many places the registrar of births, marriages and deaths will attend the hospital. A stillbirth certificate is then issued which allows cremation or burial.

Investigations to determine the cause of stillbirth

There are many investigations that may be carried out to determine the cause of stillbirth. The clinical context should be used to direct investigation. Parents should be counselled by a senior member of staff and ideally this should be supplemented with written information.

The investigations that are most likely to provide useful information regarding the cause of death are: postmortem, histopathological examination of the placenta, chromosomal analysis and Kleihauer (to check for fetomaternal haemorrhage). The rationale for these tests and likelihood that they will demonstrate useful information is shown in **Table 51**.

Consent for postmortem should be documented on a consent form approved by the Human Tissue Authority.

Other tests should be dictated by the clinical presentation and are shown in **Table 52**. Evidence of fetal growth restriction or placental infarction should prompt thrombophilia screen, serology for toxoplasmosis, rubella, cytomegalovirus and herpes (TORCH). Relevant blood tests should be performed for pre-eclampsia, maternal diabetes or obstetric cholestasis if maternal history or observations suggest these complications may have been present.

Rarely, investigations may be required by the coroner to determine the cause of death, usually to differentiate between a stillbirth and neonatal death (as coroners have no jurisdiction in stillbirth).

Parents should be counselled that despite full investigation a cause for the stillbirth may not be found. This can be reassuring, as these parents have little increased risk of a stillbirth in a subsequent pregnancy.

Table 51 Recommended investigations for most stillbirths/late intrauterine fetal death with rationale for their use and likelihood of obtaining positive information.			
Test	Rationale	Likelihood of obtaining useful information	Likelihood of obtaining unique information
Postmortem	Highest diagnostic yield of any investigation after stillbirth. Will identify structural anomalies, infection, evidence of fetal growth restriction, fetomaternal haemorrhage. Usually performed with histological examination of the placenta	57–89%	9–34%
Placental pathology	Histological examination of the placenta and cord can identify transplacental infection, evidence of maternal disease (diabetes, hypertension), placental infarction / vascular disorders, inflammatory disorders of the placenta (e.g. villitis). Examination of the placenta reduces the proportion of unexplained stillbirth	52–84%	16–19%
Chromosomal analysis	Aneuploidy is related to stillbirth (increased risk in Trisomy 21, Trisomy 18, Trisomy 13). Also increased risk of stillbirth in confined placental mosaicism	5–29%	Uncertain
Kleihaur	Identify occult fetomaternal haemorrhage, a recognised cause of stillbirth	12%	Uncertain

The results of the investigations should be given to the patient in a timely manner by an obstetrician, ideally one already known to the patient, and a plan made for subsequent pregnancies.

Care in a subsequent pregnancy

Women who experience a stillbirth are at a 2–10-fold increased risk of stillbirth in a subsequent pregnancy. This is particularly evident in women who have a placental cause of their stillbirth, e.g. abruption/fetal growth restriction. Women who have had a previous stillbirth should receive obstetric-led care in subsequent pregnancies.

The case notes of the stillbirth should be reviewed or information obtained from other units.

If there is a recurrent cause, then additional assessment of fetal growth and well-being should be performed.

Additional psychological support may be required as a subsequent pregnancy may reawaken negative feelings from the stillbirth. Women who have had a stillbirth are at increased risk of postnatal depression following a successful subsequent pregnancy.

Table 52 Investigations which may be indicated dependent upon clinical presentation.			
Test	Rationale	Examples of Relevant Clinical Presentations	Additional Information
Maternal blood tests			
Urea and electrolytes, liver function tests, uric acid	Stillbirth associated with pre-eclampsia and HELLP syndrome	Maternal hypertension and proteinuria	
C-reactive protein	Stillbirth can be associated with infection	Prolonged rupture of membranes, maternal sepsis	

Contd...

Contd...

Bile acids	Obstetric cholestasis (OC) is associated with stillbirth	Term stillbirth, evidence of maternal liver disease including symptoms of OC	
Random serum glucose and glycosylated haemoglobin	Diabetes (particularly if poorly controlled) associated with stillbirth	Macrosomic or severely growth restricted fetus. Rarely, a patient may present with diabetic ketoacidosis in pregnancy	
Thyroid function tests	Undiagnosed thyroid disease associated with stillbirth	Fetal growth restriction with no other cause. Maternal symptoms of thyroid disease	
Full blood count	Stillbirth associated with pre-eclampsia and HELLP syndrome, placental abruption	Maternal hypertension and proteinuria, symptoms of abruption	
Thrombophilia screen (Congenital and acquired)	Epidemiological link between stillbirth and maternal thrombophilia	Fetal growth restriction or small baby at delivery. Past medical history of stillbirth or pregnancy loss (antiphospholipid syndrome)	Some components of thrombophilia screen e.g. Protein S are reduced by pregnancy. If anti-phospholipid antibodies or lupus anticoagulant positive need repeating after 6 weeks to confirm diagnosis
Blood cultures	Stillbirth can be associated with infection	Prolonged rupture of membranes, maternal sepsis	
Placental swab / Genital tract swabs	Stillbirth can be associated with infection	Prolonged rupture of membranes, maternal sepsis	
Urine for toxicology	Cocaine and amphetamine associated with placental abruption	Placental abruption History suggestive of substance misuse	
Serology including: toxoplasma, rubella, cytomegalovirus, herpes simplex, syphilis, parvovirus B19.	Occult maternal-fetal infection is associated with stillbirth	Fetal hydrops, fetal growth restriction, history suggestive of maternal infection	Can be compared with booking sample to see if new or reactivated infection
Anti-red cell antibodies (e.g. Anti-D)	Severe hydrops associated with stillbirth	Fetal hydrops in Rhesus negative patient	
Anti-Ro and Anti-La antibodies	Congenital heart block can result from maternal autoimmune disease	Fetal hydrops or calcification of AV node on postmortem.	
Anti-platelet antibodies	Fetal haemorrhage can result from maternal antiplatelet antibodies	Evidence of fetal haemorrhage on postmortem.	

Further reading

RCOG Green-top Guideline No. 55. Late intrauterine fetal death and stillbirth London: RCOG, 2010.

Lawn JE, Blencowe H, Pattinson R, et al. Lancet's Stillbirths Series steering committee. Stillbirths: Where? When? Why? How to make the data count? Lancet 2011; 377(9775):1448–1463.

Cousens S, Blencowe H, Stanton C, et al. National, regional, and worldwide estimates of stillbirth rates in 2009 with trends since 1995: a systematic analysis. Lancet 2011; 377(9774):1319–1330.

Flenady V, Koopmans L, Middleton P, et al. Major risk factors for stillbirth in high-income countries: a systematic review and meta-analysis. Lancet 2011; 377(9774):1331–1340.

Flenady V, Middleton P, Smith GC, et al. Lancet's Stillbirths Series steering committee. Stillbirths: the way forward in high-income countries Lancet 2011; 377(9778):1703–1717.

Heazell AE, Leisher S, Cregan M, et al. Sharing experiences to improve bereavement support and clinical care after stillbirth. Acta Obstet Gynecol Scand 2012; 92(3):352–361.

Related topics of interest

Teratogenic agents

Overview

Teratology is derived from the Greek 'to study monsters or marvels'; in modern times it means study of abnormalities of physiological development. Therefore, a teratogenic agent is one which causes a congenital malformation of an embryo or fetus or disrupts development. Teratogenic effects can either be identified in utero, at birth or in infancy. Teratogenic effects in pregnancy may result from a number of agents including: chemicals, prescription drugs, substance misuse (including alcohol), environmental factors, infections and maternal disease. Teratogenicity depends upon the ability of the agent to cross the placenta.

Due to obvious ethical considerations, trials to establish teratogenicity are not conducted in humans. Therefore much of the information obtained on effects in pregnancy has been as a result of cohort or case-control studies. Many manufacturers of drugs advise to avoid in pregnancy because of a lack of data. However, there are actually very few drugs (< 30) proven to be teratogenic. Results from animal studies may provide information on teratogenicity in humans, especially when similar anomalies are seen in different species; caution must be taken as no experimental animal is identical both physiologically and metabolically to humans. The effects of thalidomide provide an example of this; although widely tested on rats with no adverse effects or outcome, the same was not true for humans who had limb, ear and cardiac defects. As a result of this tragedy, more rigorous systems are in place to provide information on drug effects in pregnancy – in the UK, the National Teratology Information Service (NTIS) and in the United States the Food and Drug Administration (FDA).

Clinical features

Clinical features are dependent on the teratogenic agent involved and timing of embryonic or fetal exposure. Not all embryos exposed to a known potential teratogen will result in teratogenic effects. Examples of known teratogens and their effects are listed in **Table 53**.

Aetiology

Susceptibility to teratogens depends on the stage of development of the embryo and fetus, the most crucial time being that of rapid cell division. The 'all or none' period describes the time from conception to implantation. If the embryo is exposed to a teratogen during this period, the result may either be death of the embryo or survival of a normal embryo. This is because the embryo is still undifferentiated and repair of cells is still possible. The embryonic period from 18 to 54–60 days after conception is the period of rapid cell division when organogenesis occurs. Effects of teratogens at this stage are dependent on which embryonic systems are differentiating at the time of teratogenic exposure and usually results in structural abnormalities. The fetal phase describes the time from the embryonic phase to term. During this phase most growth and maturation of organs occurs, therefore exposure of the fetus to teratogens may result in fetal growth restriction (FGR), rather than structural abnormalities. If targeted to a specific system the drug can induce specific fetotoxic effects (e.g. angiotensin converting enzyme inhibitors act on the kidney – oligohydramnios). The fetal brain develops and matures during both the embryonic and fetal phases, as a result exposure to teratogens at either of these phases may result in developmental delay. There are six teratogenic mechanisms associated with medication use: folate antagonism, neural crest cell disruption, endocrine disruption, oxidative stress, vascular disruption and specific receptor- or enzyme-mediated teratogenesis.

Diagnosis

Structural or anatomical abnormalities resulting from teratogenic agents may be

Table 53 Important human teratogens

Teratogenic agent		Teratogenic effect
Chemical		
Warfarin	First trimester	Abnormal cartilage and bone formation
	Second and third trimesters	Fetal cerebral haemorrhage and microcephaly
Tetracycline		Dentition staining
Angiotensin-converting enzyme (ACE) inhibitors		Fetal renal dysgenesis, oligohydramnios
Retinoic acid		Craniofacial abnormalities, cleft palate, thymic aplasia and neural tube defects
Anticonvulsants most notably phenytoin and sodium valproate		Neural tube defects, oral clefts and cardiac defects
Benzodiazepines		Facial cleft and skeletal abnormalities
Cocaine		Microcephaly, neurodevelopmental abnormalities
Heroin		Developmental delay
Amphetamines		Heart defects, gastroschisis and small intestinal atresias and cleft lip and palate
Alcohol		Fetal alcohol spectrum disorder
Disease		
Maternal diabetes		Congenital heart disease, renal, gastrointestinal and central nervous system malformations such as neural tube defects
Infection		
Cytomegalovirus	Late gestation	Fetal growth restriction, micromelia, chorioretinitis, blindness, microcephaly, cerebral calcifications, mental retardation and hepatosplenomegaly
Rubella	Early gestation	Cataracts, cardiac malformation and deafness
	Late gestation	Deafness and developmental delay
Varicella zoster	8–20 weeks of gestation	Congenital varicella syndrome (CVS) is characterised by dermatomal scarring, ocular abnormalities, low birth weight, cortical atrophy and mental impairment
Toxoplasmosis	Early gestation	Increased risk of miscarriage
	Late gestation	60% babies affected Congenital toxoplasmosis can include: hydrocephalus, epilepsy, deafness, eye infections and blindness
Syphilis	Pregnancy complications	Miscarriage, stillbirth, hydrops, polyhydramnios and preterm labour.
	Early congenital syphilis	Occurs before the age of 2 years, signs and symptoms include: hepatosplenomegaly, pneumonia, bullous skin rashes, failure to thrive
	Late congenital syphilis	Occurs after the age of 2 years. Signs and symptoms include: hepatosplenomegaly, lymphadenopathy, skeletal abnormalities, skin rashes, blunted teeth, deafness and blindness. In 63% of cases symptoms of Hutchinson's triad occurs – Hutchinson's teeth (notched incisors), keratitis and deafness

diagnosed during the antenatal period, at birth or later in life.

A clear and concise drug and exposure history should be elicited from every pregnant woman at booking. Those known to be at risk should be counselled regarding risks and offered detailed ultrasound scanning to assess for structural abnormalities.

At birth, structural abnormalities may be present on the surface of the body or internal to the viscera. Those babies known to be at risk should be examined and assessed during the neonatal period.

Some teratogenic effects are not diagnosed until later in life. For example, alcohol use in pregnancy affecting the central nervous system may cause disturbances of behaviour and intellect.

Management

Many women will have been exposed to potential teratogens before realising they were pregnant. In this situation, accurate dating of the gestation is required along with information regarding the potential teratogen. In the case of both prescribed and illicit drug use – the timing of exposure, dose, route of administration and disease treated is important to obtain.

In some cases reassurance may be given if exposure has been prior to conception or after the organogenesis period. If exposure has been during this period, counselling should include explanation of the background risk of abnormalities in the general population and if the fetus is at increased risk, which abnormalities are associated with the teratogen and if it can be diagnosed antenatally. For certain teratogens such as isotretinoin, women can be counselled that there is a definite risk of abnormalities with use of this drug during organogenesis; in such cases therapeutic options would involve termination of pregnancy (TOP).

Ideally, women taking essential medication for chronic diseases such as thrombotic disease, diabetes, hypertension or epilepsy should be counselled prenatally to discuss the effect of both the disease process and medication on the pregnancy. In some circumstances an alternative drug can be used, e.g. low molecular weight heparin in place of warfarin. In other conditions the risk of untreated maternal disease outweighs the risk of teratogenicity to the fetus. If medication is required to treat a condition diagnosed in pregnancy, consideration should again be given to the risk–benefit ratio.

Further reading

Koren G (Ed.) Maternal-Fetal Toxicology: A Clinician's Guide, 3rd edn. New York: Marcel Dekker, 2001.

van Gelder MM, van Rooij IA, Miller RK, et al. Teratogenic mechanisms of medical drugs. Hum Reprod Update 2010; 16(4):378–394.

Wattendorf DJ, Muenke M. Fetal alcohol spectrum disorders. Am Fam Physician 2005; 72:279–785.

Henderson J, Gray R, Brocklehurst P. Systematic review of effects of low-moderate prenatal alcohol exposure on pregnancy outcome. BJOG 2007; 114:243–252.

Related topics of interest

Thyroid and pregnancy

Overview

- Thyroid disease is the second most common endocrine disorder in pregnancy
- The thyroid is a bilobed gland composed of follicles lined by cuboidal epithelium; the main function of these cells is the synthesis of thyroxine (T4) and triiodothyronine (T3). Secretion of these is under the control of thyroid-stimulating hormone (TSH) secreted from the anterior pituitary. T3 and T4 provide negative feedback to TSH
- In pregnancy, the thyroid gland increases in size by 10–20% as a result of the increase in thyroid blood flow and follicular hyperplasia arising from the increased metabolic demands of pregnancy
- Iodine is required for the formation of T3 and T4. Pregnancy is associated with relative iodine deficiency as a result of iodine transfer to the fetus and increased renal clearance; as a result the thyroid gland increases its uptake of iodine from the blood
- In normal pregnancy circulating levels of thyroid-binding globulin (TBG) rise as a result of increased hepatic synthesis and increased oestrogens. This results in a small increase in total T3 and T4 concentrations. Although TSH levels usually remain within normal limits, the increase of human chorionic gonadotrophin (hCG) in early pregnancy stimulates the TSH receptor, which can result in decreased TSH levels and increased T4 concentration
- Total T3 and T4 measurements are not reliable when assessing thyroid function in pregnancy, and free hormone levels should be measured. Levels usually plateau at around 20 weeks of gestation. The thyroid returns to normal 3–6 months after delivery

The fetus

The fetal thyroid forms at 5 weeks of gestation, but thyroid hormone synthesis does not occur until 10–12 weeks of gestation. Maternal T3 and T4 cross the placenta and are very important for early fetal growth until the fetal thyroid becomes autonomous. TSH, T3 and T4 levels continue to rise until 35–37 weeks when they reach mature levels. The fetal levels of TSH are high in comparison to the amount of T4 produced, and the fetal thyroid concentrates iodine at a higher rate than the adult thyroid, hence the reason to avoid radioactive iodine therapy in pregnancy.

Clinical features

The clinical features of hypothyroidism and hyperthyroidism are listed in **Table 54**.

Aetiology

Pregnancy may mimic both hypothyroidism and hyperthyroidism, e.g. thyroid enlargement, tachycardia, bounding pulses, warm extremities, profound lassitude and excess weight gain.

Hyperthyroidism

The incidence of hyperthyroidism in the pregnant population is 1 in 500. Causes include:

- Graves disease (90%)
- Toxic nodule
- Toxic multinodular goitre
- Subacute thyroiditis

Maternal complications in uncontrolled hyperthyroidism include: miscarriage, maternal thyrotoxic crisis, cardiac failure, gestational hypertension and pre-eclampsia.

Well controlled maternal hyperthyroidism rarely causes problems for the fetus. However, poorly controlled disease or thyrotoxicosis is associated with adverse outcomes for the fetus. Complications include: miscarriage, fetal growth restriction (FGR), premature delivery, stillbirth and increased perinatal mortality. There is a 1% risk of neonatal thyrotoxicosis in women affected by Graves' disease due to transplacental transfer of anti-TSH receptor antibodies. Antithyroid drugs will cross over into the fetal circulation but rarely cause neonatal hypothyroidism. After delivery the neonate should be closely

	Hypothyroidism	Hyperthyroidism
Symptoms	Low mood, lethargy, depression	Emotional lability, irritability, frenetic activity
	Weight gain	Weight loss (despite increased appetite)
	Constipation	Frequent stools
	Menorrhagia	Oligomenorrhoea
	Dislike of cold	Dislike of hot weather
Signs	Bradycardia	Tachycardia
	Dry skin and hair	Warm peripheries
	Slow relaxing reflexes	Fine tremor
	Non-pitting oedema	Thyroid enlargement, thyroid bruit

Table 54 Clinical features of hypothyroidism and hyperthyroidism

examined for stigmata of hyperthyroidism or hypothyroidism.

Hypothyroidism

The incidence of hypothyroidism in the pregnant population is 1%. Causes include:
- Autoimmune – Hashimoto's thyroiditis
- Iatrogenic – thyroid surgery, treatment with antithyroid medication, lithium or amiodarone
- Postpartum thyroiditis

Maternal complications in well controlled hypothyroidism are rare. In untreated hypothyroidism complications include: infertility, miscarriage, gestational hypertension and pre-eclampsia.

Overt maternal hypothyroidism has been linked to FGR and a slight reduction in IQ in the fetus.

Diagnosis

The majority of women with thyroid disease in pregnancy will have been diagnosed prenatally.

Diagnosis of hyperthyroidism in early pregnancy can be difficult, and hyperemesis and trophoblastic disease must be excluded. If symptoms persist beyond 12 weeks an elevated T3 or T4 with suppressed TSH levels are diagnostic. TSH levels are elevated in hypothyroidism, with normal T4 levels in subclinical hypothyroidism and low T4 levels in overt hypothyroidism.

Management
Hyperthyroidism

The two main drugs used to treat hyperthyroidism are carbimazole and propylthiouracil which inhibit thyroid hormone synthesis. There are conflicting opinions on which drug is best for use in pregnancy. Although both side effects are rare carbimazole has been linked with a risk of fetal aplasia cutis and propylthiouracil has been linked to liver failure. Therefore, the general consensus is to leave women with well controlled disease on their current medication.

Surgical treatment is rarely called for in pregnancy and block and replace regimens should not be used. Radioiodine must not be used in pregnancy.

Thyroid function tests should be undertaken every 4–6 weeks with an aim to keep free T4 levels in the upper limit of normal.

Hypothyroidism

Thyroxine replacement is given to women with hypothyroidism. Doses of thyroxine often need increasing in pregnancy and should be increased in increments of 25–50 µg. Therapeutic ranges of TSH vary between the literature; however, general consensus appears to be that of < 2–2.5 milliunits/L.

Further reading

Girling JC. Thyroid disease in pregnancy. The Obstetrician and Gynaecologist 2008; 10(4):237–243.

Turnbull Sir AC, Chamberlain GC. Indexed Thyroid References. Obstetrics. Edinburgh: Churchill Livingstone, 1989.

Related topics of interest

Vaginal birth after caesarean

Overview

In 2008 approximately 148,000 pregnant women in the UK had caesarean deliveries, i.e. approximately 24%. This number seems likely to increase. The increase in caesarean sections (CS) has led to an increase in women with a previous CS. Women are more likely to have a repeat CS if they have had one previously, with a vaginal delivery rate of 72–76%. Vaginal birth after caesarean section (VBAC) is a reasonable and safe choice for the majority of women with prior caesarean.

Antenatal counselling

Women should be given information to make an informed choice as to the mode of delivery after a previous lower segment caesarian section (LSCS).

Where possible the case notes of the women should be reviewed to determine the indication for CS, any complications during or after the procedure. Where notes are not available efforts should be made to contact the clinician who was responsible for the care in pregnancy ending in CS.

Women with a classical CS or inverted T incision are not suitable for VBAC in view of increased risk of uterine rupture during labour.

The Royal College of Obstetricians and Gynaecologists (RCOG) recommends that in any woman with one previous transverse LSCS, VBAC is a reasonable option, with the alternative option of elective repeat caesarean section should (ERCS).

The counselling involves shared decision making between the health care professional and the woman. The main risks of an ERCS are bladder, ureteric or bowel injury, hysterectomy, venous thromboembolism (VTE), haemorrhage, transfusion requirement, wound infection, endometritis and rarely maternal death.

The main complications of undergoing a vaginal birth after a previous CS are uterine rupture or dehiscence or necessity for an emergency CS during labour with all of the complications above at an increased rate. A low anaesthetic risk is quoted independent of mode of delivery. There are also risks of ERCS to the fetus including laceration of presenting part and respiratory distress particularly if performed before 39 weeks' gestation. All discussions should be clearly documented in the antenatal notes and an information leaflet should be given to the woman.

A cautious approach to counselling should be undertaken in the presence of additional antenatal risk factors such as twins, fetal macrosomia or a short interdelivery interval. Both maternal and fetal harm and benefits are essential in the antenatal counselling of mode of delivery.

If after thorough discussion the woman does not wish to labour she may be offered an ERCS after 39 weeks of gestation; however, some women may prefer to labour, if they go into spontaneous labour prior to the planned CS date (up to 10%). This decision should be clearly documented in the notes.

Success rates

The overall success rate for a successful VBAC is in the region of 72–76% for women who have one previous CS. This rate increases up to 90% with a previous successful vaginal delivery, particularly a previous successful VBAC. Success rate is decreased in women with no previous vaginal deliveries, increased body mass index (BMI), induction of labour, increased maternal age and < 24 months since previous CS.

Benefits of vaginal birth

The benefits of vaginal delivery are that it removes the risk of complications of repeat CS such as visceral injury and wound infection. More women are likely to suffer from a VTE or urine infection after a CS. In one meta-analysis the rates of maternal hysterectomy, haemorrhage, and transfusions did not differ significantly between VBAC and ERCS. Women should be informed that attempting VBAC probably reduces the risk that their baby will have respiratory problems after delivery from 2–3% with a planned VBAC as opposed to 3–4% with ERCS. Apart from the above physical benefits there are improved recovery period and potential psychological benefits.

The risks of placenta praevia and placenta accreta increase after every CS from 0.13% after two CS, to 2.13% after four CS and to 6.74% after six or more CS. Maternal mortality is rare irrespective of the mode of delivery; however, it is increased after an ERCS (13.4 per 100,000) as opposed to trial of labour (3.8 per 100,000).

Risks of VBAC

The main risk of VBAC is uterine rupture which has significant implications for mother and infant. Uterine rupture is defined as: the disruption of the uterine muscle extending to and involving the uterine serosa or disruption of the uterine muscle with extension to the bladder or broad ligament. Previous CS is the main risk factor, especially in the presence of a classical or T or J shaped previous incision or short pregnancy interval after CS.

Women considering planned VBAC should be informed that this decision carries a 2–3 per 10,000 additional risk of intrapartum-related perinatal death and an 8 per 10,000 risk of hypoxic-ischaemic encephalopathy when compared with ERCS; this is due to uterine rupture and consequent fetal asphyxia.

The rate of uterine rupture for all women with prior caesarean is approximately 2.2–7.4 per 1000 and the risk is significantly increased with VBAC.

Signs and symptoms of uterine rupture include abnormal fetal heart rate trace on cardiotocography (CTG), severe abdominal pain, scar tenderness, haematuria, and cessation of uterine activity, disappearance of presenting part and maternal tachycardia or shock. Although the overall rate of uterine rupture is low women should be aware that the overall rate increases up to 2–3-fold with induction of labour (particularly with prostaglandins). Thus, induction or augmentation labour after a previous CS should be approached with due consideration; the decision should be made by a consultant obstetrician. Clear information should be given to the woman and documented accordingly in the birth notes.

Due to the risks of uterine rupture it is essential that VBAC should be undertaken where there is immediate recourse to emergency delivery, e.g. consultant-led unit. Monitoring of the fetus in terms of continuous CTG after onset of regular contractions and maternal progress in labour are essential. Many uterine ruptures are preceded by abnormalities of the fetal heart rate.

Vaginal birth after multiple CS

Those women considering a vaginal birth after two or more previous CS must have appropriate counselling of success and complications with regards to maternal and fetal outcomes. The evidence suggests that there are similar success rates in those undergoing a vaginal birth after two CS as opposed to trial of labour after one CS, with a uterine rupture of 1 in 70 and a comparative morbidity as compared to the ERCS option. The woman should be supported in her decision as long as she has been fully counselling by a consultant obstetrician with an individualised management plan. This should be fully documented in the antenatal notes with the appropriate information leaflet given.

Further reading

Guise JM, Eden K, Emeis C, et al. Vaginal birth after caesarean: new insights. Evid Rep Technol Assess 2010; 191:1–397.

Tahseen S, Griffiths M. Vaginal birth after two CSs (VBAC-2) – a systematic review with meta-analysis of success rate and adverse outcomes of VBAC-2 versus VBAC-1 and repeat (third) caesarean sections. BJOG 2010; 117(1):5–19.

Al-Zirqi I, Stray-Pedersen B, Forsén L, Vangen S. Uterine rupture after previous caesarean section. BJOG 2010; 117(7):809–820.

RCOG Green-top Guideline No. 45. Birth after Previous Caesarean Birth. London: RCOG, 2007.

Thomas J, Paranjothy S. National Sentinel CS Audit Report. London: RCOG, 2001.

Related topics of interest

• Induction of labour (p. 240)

• Placenta praevia and morbidly adherent placenta (p. 283)

Venous thromboembolism

Overview

Venous thromboembolism (VTE) remains a leading cause of preventable maternal death in the UK. The incidence in pregnancy is 1:1000, with the postnatal period being highest risk. In pregnancy, VTE is 10 times more common than in non-pregnant women of similar age. Women should be assessed for thromboprophylaxis antenatally, on hospital admission and postnatally. Thromboprophylaxis includes mobility and hydration advice, graduated compression stockings and low molecular weight heparins (LMWH). Royal College of Obstetricians and Gynaecologists (RCOG) guidelines suggest:

- Women with three or more of the risk factors in **Table 55** should be considered for LMWH antenatally. Assessment should occur early in pregnancy (i.e. at booking)
- Women with two or more of the risk factors postnatally in **Table 55** should be considered for 1 week LMWH

- All women with a body mass index (BMI) > 40 kg/m², those delivered by emergency caesarean section (CS) and or elective CS and one other risk factor should receive 7 days postnatal LMWH. Six weeks treatment should be considered in women with additional significant risk factors or until the risk factors have ceased
- Women receiving antenatal LMWH should usually receive it for 6 weeks postnatally

Clinical features

Symptoms can be similar to those of normal pregnancy but should be taken seriously, especially in women with risk factors.
Symptoms of deep vein thrombosis (DVT):
- Leg pain and swelling (usually unilateral)
- Increased redness and swelling of the affected limb
- Lower abdominal pain
- Dilation of superficial leg veins

Symptoms of pulmonary embolism (PE):
- Dyspnoea

Table 55.1 VTE risk factors in pregnant women		
Underlying risk factors	**Antenatal/Pregnancy Factors**	**Transient risk factors**
Previous VTE	Multiple pregnancy	Surgical procedure
Inherited or acquired thrombophilias	Assisted reproductive treatment	Hyperemesis or dehydration for other reasons
Medical disorders such as cancer, active systemic lupus erythematosus, inflammatory conditions, nephrotic syndrome, sickle cell disease, intravenous drug use, cardiac disease	Pre-eclampsia	Ovarian hyperstimulation
Over 35 years	Caesarean section	Hospital admission > 3 days or other significant restriction on mobility
BMI > 30 kg/m²	Prolonged labour or mid-cavity rotational instrumental delivery in theatre	Systemic infection needing antibiotic therapy
Parity ≥ 3	Postpartum haemorrhage or need for transfusion	Long distance travel > 4 hours
Smoking		
Gross varicose veins (symptomatic, above the knee or with skin changes/phlebitis)		
Paraplegia		

Adapted from the RCOG Green-top Guideline No. 37a. Reducing the risk of thrombosis and embolism during pregnancy and puerperium. London: RCOG, 2009.

- Chest pain, typically pleuritic
- Haemoptysis
- Abdominal pain
- Low grade pyrexia
- Collapse

Aetiology

Physiology of pregnancy increases the risk of thrombosis (covered in Topic 64). DVT usually precedes PE, as the latter is usually the result of a clot detaching and travelling through the venous system, and lodging within the smaller vessels of the lung.

Diagnosis

- Baseline tests of full blood count, coagulation, liver function and urea and electrolytes should be conducted. Thrombophilia screens are not usually recommended in pregnancy, and if taken should be interpreted by specialist haematologists. D-dimers are unhelpful as they are usually 2–3-fold higher in pregnancy
- Compression Duplex ultrasound scan should be used to exclude DVT. If the scan is negative but a high degree of clinical suspicion persists, the scan should be repeated in a week and anticoagulation continued in the interim. Magnetic resonance imaging (MRI) or contrast venography may be useful if iliac vein thrombosis is suspected
- Chest X-ray is the first investigation for suspected PE (**Figure 29**). This is usually normal in PE, but it is used to exclude other diagnoses, and to guide subsequent investigations
- If the chest X-ray is normal, bilateral leg Doppler should be performed. If these show a DVT, no further investigation is needed, thus limiting exposure to radiation
- If the leg Doppler and chest X-ray are normal, further investigation is with ventilation-perfusion (VQ) scan or computed tomography pulmonary angiogram (CTPA)

- If the chest X-ray is abnormal, the alternative diagnosis indicated should be treated. If there remains a high clinical suspicion of PE, CTPA should be performed, as VQ scans are unhelpful in the presence of an abnormal chest X-ray
- CTPA and VQ scanning involve risks of radiation, thus the women should be involved in the decision making process. VQ scanning carries a 1 per 280,000 risk of fatal childhood cancer compared to 1 per 1,000,000 from CTPA (fetal radiation exposure 10% of VQ). CTPA is associated with an increased lifetime risk of breast cancer of 13.6% (background 1 per 200). Breast tissue is particularly sensitive in pregnancy and previous chest computed tomography (CT) scanning and family history should be considered. Neonatal hypothyroidism has also been reported, but is very rare.
- To reduce radiation exposure from VQ scanning, half-dose perfusion scanning may be used, only proceeding to the ventilation part if the perfusion scan shows a defect
- CTPA has higher specificity and sensitivity (99% negative predictive value), and can diagnose alternative pathology but may miss small peripheral thrombi
- VQ scans lack discrimination in pregnancy in that 20% of women will have an indeterminate probability scan and up to 20% of women with a high probability result do not have a PE. Although PE can be excluded with a low probability scan (likely in 75% of women), if there remains a high degree of clinical suspicion, further CTPA may be needed

Management

- Women with suspected VTE should be commenced on a therapeutic dose of LMWH whilst the diagnosis is being confirmed or refuted. The therapeutic dose of LMWH is weight related, and is given twice daily for Dalteparin and Enoxaparin and once daily for Tinzaparin
- If VTE is confirmed, LMWH should be continued for the rest of the pregnancy

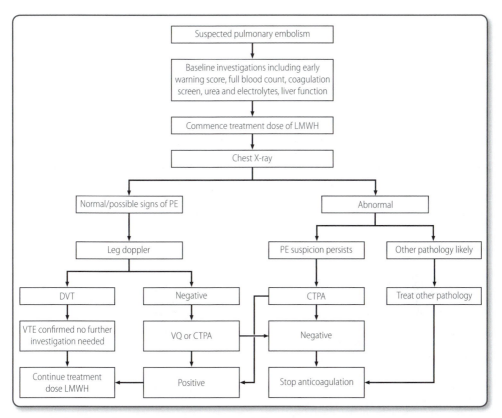

Figure 29 Flow chart of the diagnosis of pulmonary embolism (PE) in pregnancy. CTPA, computed tomography pulmonary angiogram; DVT, deep vein thrombosis; LMWH, low molecular weight heparins; PE, pulmonary embolism; VQ, ventilation-perfusion; VTE, venous thromboembolism.

and for 6 weeks into the postnatal period. If this is less than 3–6 months, further anticoagulation for this period after the clot is needed. Duration of anticoagulation should be discussed with haematologists

- Although monitoring of anti-Xa levels is not routinely recommended, this should be conducted if body weight is > 90 kg or < 50 kg and in renal impairment.
- Although unfractionated heparin may cause low platelets, this has not been reported in pregnant women on LMWH who have never received unfractionated heparin. Therefore, regular platelet counts are not needed
- Side effects of LMWH include rashes, bruising/haematomas at injection sites, and there may be a long term risk of osteopenia/ osteoporosis (less than with unfractionated

heparin). If an allergic reaction occurs, use of an alternative preparation can be considered, or the use of danaparoid sodium or fondaparinux under the advice of a specialist haematologist

- Heparin does not cross the placenta
- Warfarin should not be used in pregnancy as it crosses the placenta and is associated with miscarriage, congenital abnormality and fetal intracerebral bleeding. Warfarin embryopathy is a risk with exposure between 6–9 weeks' gestation and comprises: saddle nose, nasal and mid-face hypoplasia, frontal bossing and short stature, calcification of thyroid cartilage, cardiac lesions, low-set ears, mental retardation and blindness
- Women taking LMWH should be advised to stop heparin once labour commences.

Regional analgesia should not be used until 24 hours after the last therapeutic dose. There is a 2% risk of wound haematoma at CS. Therefore the wound should be closed with interrupted sutures, and surgical drains considered
- Treatment doses of LMWH should be recommenced once any risk of bleeding has ceased a minimum of 4 hours after spinal analgesia or removal of an epidural catheter. RCOG guidelines suggest an initial prophylactic dose 4 hours post elective CS, then treatment dose in the evening

- Warfarin can be commenced when the risk of bleeding has passed or on postnatal day 3
- Breastfeeding on warfarin or heparin is safe
- Breastfeeding women undergoing VQ scanning should be advised to express and discard breast milk for 12–24 hours
- Acute massive PE associated with maternal collapse should be managed with multidisciplinary resuscitation. Thrombolysis can be considered

Further reading

RCOG Green-top Guideline No 37a. Reducing the risk of thrombosis and embolism during pregnancy and puerperium. London: RCOG, 2009.

RCOG Green-top Guideline No 37b. The acute management of thrombosis and embolism during pregnancy and the puerperium. London: RCOG, 2010.

Matthews S. Imaging pulmonary embolism in pregnancy: what is the most appropriate imaging protocol? British Journal of Radiology 2006; 79:441–444.

Related topics of interest

Index

Note: Page numbers in **bold** or *italic* refer to tables or figures, respectively.